THE OFFICIAL PARENT'S SOURCEBOOK

on

SUDDEN INFANT DEATH SYNDROME

JAMES N. PARKER, M.D.
AND PHILIP M. PARKER, PH.D., EDITORS

ii

3 9082 11430 6072

ICON Health Publications
ICON Group International, Inc.
4370 La Jolla Village Drive, 4th Floor
San Diego, CA 92122 USA

Printed in the United States of America.

Last digit indicates print number: 10 9 8 7 6 4 5 3 2 1

Publisher, Health Care: Philip Parker, Ph.D.
Editor(s): James Parker, M.D., Philip Parker, Ph.D.

Publisher's note: The ideas, procedures, and suggestions contained in this book are not intended as a substitute for consultation with your child's physician. All matters regarding your child's health require medical supervision. As new medical or scientific information becomes available from academic and clinical research, recommended treatments and drug therapies may undergo changes. The authors, editors, and publisher have attempted to make the information in this book up to date and accurate in accord with accepted standards at the time of publication. The authors, editors, and publisher are not responsible for errors or omissions or for consequences from application of the book, and make no warranty, expressed or implied, in regard to the contents of this book. Any practice described in this book should be applied by the reader in accordance with professional standards of care used in regard to the unique circumstances that may apply in each situation, in close consultation with a qualified physician. The reader is advised to always check product information (package inserts) for changes and new information regarding dose and contraindications before administering any drug or pharmacological product. Caution is especially urged when using new or infrequently ordered drugs, herbal remedies, vitamins and supplements, alternative therapies, complementary therapies and medicines, and integrative medical treatments.

Cataloging-in-Publication Data

Parker, James N., 1961-
Parker, Philip M., 1960-

    The Official Parent's Sourcebook on Sudden Infant Death Syndrome: A Revised and Updated Directory for the Internet Age/James N. Parker and Philip M. Parker, editors
         p.   cm.
    Includes bibliographical references, glossary and index.
    ISBN: 0-497-11060-1
    1. Sudden Infant Death Syndrome-Popular works.   I. Title.

Disclaimer

This publication is not intended to be used for the diagnosis or treatment of a health problem or as a substitute for consultation with licensed medical professionals. It is sold with the understanding that the publisher, editors, and authors are not engaging in the rendering of medical, psychological, financial, legal, or other professional services.

References to any entity, product, service, or source of information that may be contained in this publication should not be considered an endorsement, either direct or implied, by the publisher, editors, or authors. ICON Group International, Inc., the editors, or the authors are not responsible for the content of any Web pages nor publications referenced in this publication.

Copyright Notice

Dedication

To the healthcare professionals dedicating their time and efforts to the study of sudden infant death syndrome.

Acknowledgements

The collective knowledge generated from academic and applied research summarized in various references has been critical in the creation of this sourcebook which is best viewed as a comprehensive compilation and collection of information prepared by various official agencies which directly or indirectly are dedicated to sudden infant death syndrome. All of the *Official Parent's Sourcebooks* draw from various agencies and institutions associated with the United States Department of Health and Human Services, and in particular, the Office of the Secretary of Health and Human Services (OS), the Administration for Children and Families (ACF), the Administration on Aging (AOA), the Agency for Healthcare Research and Quality (AHRQ), the Agency for Toxic Substances and Disease Registry (ATSDR), the Centers for Disease Control and Prevention (CDC), the Food and Drug Administration (FDA), the Healthcare Financing Administration (HCFA), the Health Resources and Services Administration (HRSA), the Indian Health Service (IHS), the institutions of the National Institutes of Health (NIH), the Program Support Center (PSC), and the Substance Abuse and Mental Health Services Administration (SAMHSA). In addition to these sources, information gathered from the National Library of Medicine, the United States Patent Office, the European Union, and their related organizations has been invaluable in the creation of this sourcebook. Some of the work represented was financially supported by the Research and Development Committee at INSEAD. This support is gratefully acknowledged. Finally, special thanks are owed to Tiffany Freeman for her excellent editorial support.

About the Editors

James N. Parker, M.D.

Dr. James N. Parker received his Bachelor of Science degree in Psychobiology from the University of California, Riverside and his M.D. from the University of California, San Diego. In addition to authoring numerous research publications, he has lectured at various academic institutions. Dr. Parker is the medical editor for the *Official Parent's Sourcebook* series published by ICON Health Publications.

Philip M. Parker, Ph.D.

Philip M. Parker is the Eli Lilly Chair Professor of Innovation, Business and Society at INSEAD (Fontainebleau, France and Singapore). Dr. Parker has also been Professor at the University of California, San Diego and has taught courses at Harvard University, the Hong Kong University of Science and Technology, the Massachusetts Institute of Technology, Stanford University, and UCLA. Dr. Parker is the associate editor for the *Official Parent's Sourcebook* series published by ICON Health Publications.

About ICON Health Publications

In addition to sudden infant death syndrome, *Official Parent's Sourcebooks* are available for the following related topics:

- The Official Patient's Sourcebook on Down Syndrome
- The Official Patient's Sourcebook on Fragile X Syndrome
- The Official Patient's Sourcebook on Infantile Apnea
- The Official Patient's Sourcebook on Klinefelter Syndrome
- The Official Patient's Sourcebook on Mccune Albright Syndrome
- The Official Patient's Sourcebook on Phenylketonuria
- The Official Patient's Sourcebook on Pituitary Tumors
- The Official Patient's Sourcebook on Primary Immunodeficiency

To discover more about ICON Health Publications, simply check with your preferred online booksellers, including Barnes&Noble.com and Amazon.com which currently carry all of our titles. Or, feel free to contact us directly for bulk purchases or institutional discounts:

ICON Group International, Inc.
4370 La Jolla Village Drive, Fourth Floor
San Diego, CA 92122 USA
Fax: 858-546-4341
Web site: **www.icongrouponline.com/health**

Table of Contents

INTRODUCTION

Overview

Dr. C. Everett Koop, former U.S. Surgeon General, once said, "The best prescription is knowledge."[1] The Agency for Healthcare Research and Quality (AHRQ) of the National Institutes of Health (NIH) echoes this view and recommends that all parents incorporate education into the treatment process. According to the AHRQ:

> Finding out more about your [child's] condition is a good place to start. By contacting groups that support your [child's] condition, visiting your local library, and searching on the Internet, you can find good information to help guide your decisions for your [child's] treatment. Some information may be hard to find—especially if you don't know where to look.[2]

As the AHRQ mentions, finding the right information is not an obvious task. Though many physicians and public officials had thought that the emergence of the Internet would do much to assist parents in obtaining reliable information, in March 2001 the National Institutes of Health issued the following warning:

> The number of Web sites offering health-related resources grows every day. Many sites provide valuable information, while others may have information that is unreliable or misleading.[3]

---

[1] Quotation from **http://www.drkoop.com**.
[2] The Agency for Healthcare Research and Quality (AHRQ):
http://www.ahcpr.gov/consumer/diaginfo.htm.
[3] From the NIH, National Cancer Institute (NCI):
http://cancertrials.nci.nih.gov/beyond/evaluating.html.

Since the late 1990s, physicians have seen a general increase in parent Internet usage rates. Parents frequently enter their children's doctor's offices with printed Web pages of home remedies in the guise of latest medical research. This scenario is so common that doctors often spend more time dispelling misleading information than guiding children through sound therapies. *The Official Parent's Sourcebook on Sudden Infant Death Syndrome* has been created for parents who have decided to make education and research an integral part of the treatment process. The pages that follow will tell you where and how to look for information covering virtually all topics related to sudden infant death syndrome, from the essentials to the most advanced areas of research.

The title of this book includes the word "official." This reflects the fact that the sourcebook draws from public, academic, government, and peer-reviewed research. Selected readings from various agencies are reproduced to give you some of the latest official information available to date on sudden infant death syndrome.

Given parents' increasing sophistication in using the Internet, abundant references to reliable Internet-based resources are provided throughout this sourcebook. Where possible, guidance is provided on how to obtain free-of-charge, primary research results as well as more detailed information via the Internet. E-book and electronic versions of this sourcebook are fully interactive with each of the Internet sites mentioned (clicking on a hyperlink automatically opens your browser to the site indicated). Hard copy users of this sourcebook can type cited Web addresses directly into their browsers to obtain access to the corresponding sites. Since we are working with ICON Health Publications, hard copy *Sourcebooks* are frequently updated and printed on demand to ensure that the information provided is current.

In addition to extensive references accessible via the Internet, every chapter presents a "Vocabulary Builder." Many health guides offer glossaries of technical or uncommon terms in an appendix. In editing this sourcebook, we have decided to place a smaller glossary within each chapter that covers terms used in that chapter. Given the technical nature of some chapters, you may need to revisit many sections. Building one's vocabulary of medical terms in such a gradual manner has been shown to improve the learning process.

We must emphasize that no sourcebook on sudden infant death syndrome should affirm that a specific diagnostic procedure or treatment discussed in a research study, patent, or doctoral dissertation is "correct" or your child's best option. This sourcebook is no exception. Each child is unique. Deciding on appropriate options is always up to parents in consultation with their children's physicians and healthcare providers.

Organization

This sourcebook is organized into three parts. Part I explores basic techniques to researching sudden infant death syndrome (e.g. finding guidelines on diagnosis, treatments, and prognosis), followed by a number of topics, including information on how to get in touch with organizations, associations, or other parent networks dedicated to sudden infant death syndrome. It also gives you sources of information that can help you find a doctor in your local area specializing in treating sudden infant death syndrome. Collectively, the material presented in Part I is a complete primer on basic research topics for sudden infant death syndrome.

Part II moves on to advanced research dedicated to sudden infant death syndrome. Part II is intended for those willing to invest many hours of hard work and study. It is here that we direct you to the latest scientific and applied research on sudden infant death syndrome. When possible, contact names, links via the Internet, and summaries are provided. It is in Part II where the vocabulary process becomes important as authors publishing advanced research frequently use highly specialized language. In general, every attempt is made to recommend "free-to-use" options.

Part III provides appendices of useful background reading covering sudden infant death syndrome or related disorders. The appendices are dedicated to more pragmatic issues facing parents. Accessing materials via medical libraries may be the only option for some parents, so a guide is provided for finding local medical libraries which are open to the public. Part III, therefore, focuses on advice that goes beyond the biological and scientific issues facing children with sudden infant death syndrome and their families.

Scope

While this sourcebook covers sudden infant death syndrome, doctors, research publications, and specialists may refer to your child's condition using a variety of terms. Therefore, you should understand that sudden infant death syndrome is often considered a synonym or a condition closely related to the following:

- Cot Death
- Crib Death

In addition to synonyms and related conditions, physicians may refer to sudden infant death syndrome using certain coding systems. The International Classification of Diseases, 9th Revision, Clinical Modification (ICD-9-CM) is the most commonly used system of classification for the world's illnesses. Your physician may use this coding system as an administrative or tracking tool. The following classification is commonly used for sudden infant death syndrome:[4]

- 798.0 sudden infant death syndrome

For the purposes of this sourcebook, we have attempted to be as inclusive as possible, looking for official information for all of the synonyms relevant to sudden infant death syndrome. You may find it useful to refer to synonyms when accessing databases or interacting with healthcare professionals and medical librarians.

Moving Forward

Since the 1980s, the world has seen a proliferation of healthcare guides covering most illnesses. Some are written by parents, patients, or their family members. These generally take a layperson's approach to understanding and coping with an illness or disorder. They can be uplifting, encouraging, and highly supportive. Other guides are authored by physicians or other healthcare providers who have a more clinical outlook. Each of these two styles of guide has its purpose and can be quite useful.

---

[4] This list is based on the official version of the World Health Organization's 9th Revision, International Classification of Diseases (ICD-9). According to the National Technical Information Service, "ICD-9CM extensions, interpretations, modifications, addenda, or errata other than those approved by the U.S. Public Health Service and the Health Care Financing Administration are not to be considered official and should not be utilized. Continuous maintenance of the ICD-9-CM is the responsibility of the federal government."

As editors, we have chosen a third route. We have chosen to expose you to as many sources of official and peer-reviewed information as practical, for the purpose of educating you about basic and advanced knowledge as recognized by medical science today. You can think of this sourcebook as your personal Internet age reference librarian.

Why "Internet age"? When their child has been diagnosed with sudden infant death syndrome, parents will often log on to the Internet, type words into a search engine, and receive several Web site listings which are mostly irrelevant or redundant. Parents are left to wonder where the relevant information is, and how to obtain it. Since only the smallest fraction of information dealing with sudden infant death syndrome is even indexed in search engines, a non-systematic approach often leads to frustration and disappointment. With this sourcebook, we hope to direct you to the information you need that you would not likely find using popular Web directories. Beyond Web listings, in many cases we will reproduce brief summaries or abstracts of available reference materials. These abstracts often contain distilled information on topics of discussion.

While we focus on the more scientific aspects of sudden infant death syndrome, there is, of course, the emotional side to consider. Later in the sourcebook, we provide a chapter dedicated to helping you find parent groups and associations that can provide additional support beyond research produced by medical science. We hope that the choices we have made give you and your child the most options in moving forward. In this way, we wish you the best in your efforts to incorporate this educational approach into your child's treatment plan.

The Editors

PART I: THE ESSENTIALS

ABOUT PART I

Part I has been edited to give you access to what we feel are "the essentials" on sudden infant death syndrome. The essentials typically include a definition or description of the condition, a discussion of who it affects, the signs or symptoms, tests or diagnostic procedures, and treatments for disease. Your child's doctor or healthcare provider may have already explained the essentials of sudden infant death syndrome to you or even given you a pamphlet or brochure describing the condition. Now you are searching for more in-depth information. As editors, we have decided, nevertheless, to include a discussion on where to find essential information that can complement what the doctor has already told you. In this section we recommend a process, not a particular Web site or reference book. The process ensures that, as you search the Web, you gain background information in such a way as to maximize your understanding.

Chapter 1. The Essentials on Sudden Infant Death Syndrome: Guidelines

Overview

Official agencies, as well as federally funded institutions supported by national grants, frequently publish a variety of guidelines on sudden infant death syndrome. These are typically called "Fact Sheets" or "Guidelines." They can take the form of a brochure, information kit, pamphlet, or flyer. Often they are only a few pages in length. The great advantage of guidelines over other sources is that they are often written with the parent in mind. Since new guidelines on sudden infant death syndrome can appear at any moment and be published by a number of sources, the best approach to finding guidelines is to systematically scan the Internet-based services that post them.

The National Institutes of Health (NIH)[5]

The National Institutes of Health (NIH) is the first place to search for relatively current guidelines and fact sheets on sudden infant death syndrome. Originally founded in 1887, the NIH is one of the world's foremost medical research centers and the federal focal point for medical research in the United States. At any given time, the NIH supports some 35,000 research grants at universities, medical schools, and other research and training institutions, both nationally and internationally. The rosters of those who have conducted research or who have received NIH support over the years include the world's most illustrious scientists and physicians.

---

[5] Adapted from the NIH: http://www.nih.gov/about/NIHoverview.html.

Among them are 97 scientists who have won the Nobel Prize for achievement in medicine.

There is no guarantee that any one Institute will have a guideline on a specific medical condition, though the National Institutes of Health collectively publish over 600 guidelines for both common and rare disorders. The best way to access NIH guidelines is via the Internet. Although the NIH is organized into many different Institutes and Offices, the following is a list of key Web sites where you are most likely to find NIH clinical guidelines and publications dealing with sudden infant death syndrome and associated conditions:

- Office of the Director (OD); guidelines consolidated across agencies available at **http://www.nih.gov/health/consumer/conkey.htm**

- National Library of Medicine (NLM); extensive encyclopedia (A.D.A.M., Inc.) with guidelines available at **http://www.nlm.nih.gov/medlineplus/healthtopics.html**

- National Institute of Child Health and Human Development (NICHD); guidelines available at **http://www.nichd.nih.gov/publications/pubskey.cfm**

Among those listed above, the National Institute of Child Health and Human Development (NICHD) is especially noteworthy. The mission of the NICHD, a part of the National Institutes of Health (NIH), is to support and conduct research on topics related to the health of children, adults, families, and populations. NICHD research focuses on the idea that events that happen prior to and throughout pregnancy as well as during childhood have a great impact on the health and well-being of adults. The following guideline is one the NICHD provides concerning sudden infant death syndrome.[6]

What Is Sudden Infant Death Syndrome?[7]

Sudden Infant Death Syndrome (SIDS) is the diagnosis given for the sudden death of an infant under one year of age that remains unexplained after a complete investigation, which includes an autopsy, examination of the death scene, and review of the symptoms or illnesses the infant had prior to dying and any other pertinent medical history. Because most cases of SIDS occur

---

[6] This and other passages have been adapted from the NIH and NICHD: http://www.nichd.nih.gov/default.htm. "Adapted" signifies that the text has been reproduced with attribution, with some or no editorial adjustments.

[7] Adapted from The National Institute of Child Health and Human Development (NICHD): http://www.nichd.nih.gov/publications/pubs/sidsfact.htm.

when a baby is sleeping in a crib, SIDS is also commonly known as crib death.

SIDS is the leading cause of death in infants between 1 month and 1 year of age. Most SIDS deaths occur when a baby is between 1 and 4 months of age. African American children are two to three times more likely than white babies to die of SIDS, and Native American babies are about three times more susceptible. Also, more boys are SIDS victims than girls.

What Are the Risk Factors for SIDS?

A number of factors seem to put a baby at higher risk of dying from SIDS. Babies who sleep on their stomachs are more likely to die of SIDS than those who sleep on their backs. Mothers who smoke during pregnancy are three times more likely to have a SIDS baby, and exposure to passive smoke from smoking by mothers, fathers, and others in the household doubles a baby's risk of SIDS. Other risk factors include mothers who are less than 20 years old at the time of their first pregnancy, babies born to mothers who had no or late prenatal care, and premature or low birth weight babies.

What Causes SIDS?

Mounting evidence suggests that some SIDS babies are born with brain abnormalities that make them vulnerable to sudden death during infancy. Studies of SIDS victims reveal that many SIDS infants have abnormalities in the "arcuate nucleus," a portion of the brain that is likely to be involved in controlling breathing and waking during sleep. Babies born with defects in other portions of the brain or body may also be more prone to a sudden death. These abnormalities may stem from prenatal exposure to a toxic substance, or lack of a vital compound in the prenatal environment, such as sufficient oxygen. Cigarette smoking during pregnancy, for example, can reduce the amount of oxygen the fetus receives.

Scientists believe that the abnormalities that are present at birth may not be sufficient to cause death. Other possibly important events occur after birth such as lack of oxygen, excessive carbon dioxide intake, overheating or an infection. For example, many babies experience a lack of oxygen and excessive carbon dioxide levels when they have respiratory infections that hamper breathing, or they rebreathe exhaled air trapped in underlying bedding when they sleep on their stomachs. Normally, infants sense such inadequate air intake, and the brain triggers the babies to wake from sleep and cry, and changes their heartbeat or breathing patterns to compensate for the insufficient oxygen and excess carbon dioxide. A baby with a flawed arcuate nucleus, however, might lack this protective mechanism and succumb to SIDS. Such a scenario might explain why babies who sleep on their stomachs are more susceptible to SIDS, and why a disproportionately large number of SIDS babies have been reported to have respiratory infections prior to their deaths. Infections as a trigger for sudden infant death may explain why more SIDS cases occur during the colder months of the year, when respiratory and intestinal infections are more common.

The numbers of cells and proteins generated by the immune system of some SIDS babies have been reported to be higher than normal. Some of these proteins can interact with the brain to alter heart rate and breathing during sleep, or can put the baby into a deep sleep. Such effects might be strong enough to cause the baby's death, particularly if the baby has an underlying brain defect.

Some babies who die suddenly may be born with a metabolic disorder. One such disorder is medium chain acylCoA dehydrogenase deficiency, which prevents the infant from properly processing fatty acids. A build-up of these acid metabolites could eventually lead to a rapid and fatal disruption in breathing and heart functioning. If there is a family history of this disorder or childhood death of unknown cause, genetic screening of the parents by a blood test can determine if they are carriers of this disorder. If one or both parents is found to be a carrier, the baby can be tested soon after birth.

What Might Help Lower the Risk of SIDS?

There currently is no way of predicting which newborns will succumb to SIDS; however, there are a few measures parents can take to lower the risk of their child dying from SIDS.

Good prenatal care, which includes proper nutrition, no smoking or drug or alcohol use by the mother, and frequent medical check-ups beginning early in pregnancy, might help prevent a baby from developing an abnormality that could put him or her at risk for sudden death. These measures may also reduce the chance of having a premature or low birthweight baby, which also increases the risk for SIDS. Once the baby is born, parents should keep the baby in a smoke-free environment.

Parents and other caregivers should put babies to sleep on their backs as opposed to on their stomachs. Studies have shown that placing babies on their backs to sleep has reduced the number of SIDS cases by as much as a half in countries where infants had traditionally slept on their stomachs. Although babies placed on their sides to sleep have a lower risk of SIDS than those placed on their stomachs, the back sleep position is the best position for infants from 1 month to 1 year. Babies positioned on their sides to sleep should be placed with their lower arm forward to help prevent them from rolling onto their stomachs.

Many parents place babies on their stomachs to sleep because they think it prevents them from choking on spit-up or vomit during sleep. But studies in countries where there has been a switch from babies sleeping predominantly on their stomachs to sleeping mainly on their backs have not found any evidence of increased risk of choking or other problems.

In some instances, doctors may recommend that babies be placed on their stomachs to sleep if they have disorders such as gastroesophageal reflux or certain upper airway disorders which predispose them to choking or breathing problems while lying on their backs. If a parent is unsure about the best sleep position for their baby, it is always a good idea to talk to the baby's doctor or other health care provider.

A certain amount of tummy time while the infant is awake and being observed is recommended for motor development of the shoulder. In addition, awake time on the stomach may help prevent flat spots from developing on the back of the baby's head. Such physical signs are almost always temporary and will disappear soon after the baby begins to sit up.

Parents should make sure their baby sleeps on a firm mattress or other firm surface. They should avoid using fluffy blankets or covering as well as pillows, sheepskins, blankets, or comforters under the baby. Infants should not be placed to sleep on a waterbed or with soft stuffed toys.

Recently, scientific studies have demonstrated that bedsharing, between mother and baby, can alter sleep patterns of the mother and baby. These studies have led to speculation that bedsharing, sometimes referred to as co-sleeping, may also reduce the risk of SIDS. While bedsharing may have certain benefits (such as encouraging breast feeding), there are not scientific studies demonstrating that bedsharing reduces SIDS. Some studies actually suggest that bedsharing, under certain conditions, may increase the risk of SIDS. If mothers choose to sleep in the same beds with their babies, care should be taken to avoid using soft sleep surfaces. Quilts, blankets, pillows, comforters, or other similar soft materials should not be placed under the baby. The bedsharer should not smoke or use substances such as alcohol or drugs which may impair arousal. It is also important to be aware that unlike cribs, which are designed to meet safety standards for infants, adult beds are not so designed and may carry a risk of accidental entrapment and suffocation.

Babies should be kept warm, but they should not be allowed to get too warm because an overheated baby is more likely to go into a deep sleep from which it is difficult to arouse. The temperature in the baby's room should feel comfortable to an adult and overdressing the baby should be avoided.

There is some evidence to suggest that breast feeding might reduce the risk of SIDS. A few studies have found SIDS to be less common in infants who have been breast fed. This may be because breast milk can provide protection from some infections that can trigger sudden death in infants.

Parents should take their babies to their health care provider for regular well baby check-ups and routine immunizations. Claims that immunizations increase the risk of SIDS are not supported by data, and babies who receive their scheduled immunizations are less likely to die of SIDS. If an infant ever has an incident where he or she stops breathing and turns blue or limp, the baby should be medically evaluated for the cause of such an incident.

Although some electronic home monitors can detect and sound an alarm when a baby stops breathing, there is no evidence that such monitors can prevent SIDS. A panel of experts convened by the National Institutes of Health in 1986 recommended that home monitors not be used for babies who do not have an increased risk of sudden unexpected death. The monitors are recommended, however, for infants who have experienced one or more severe episodes during which they stopped breathing and required resuscitation or stimulation, premature infants with apnea, and siblings of two or more SIDS infants. If an incident has occurred or if an infant is on a monitor, parents need to know how to properly use and maintain the device, as well as how to resuscitate their baby if the alarm sounds.

How Does a SIDS Baby Affect the Family?

A SIDS death is a tragedy that can prompt intense emotional reactions among surviving family members. After the initial disbelief, denial, or numbness begins to wear off, parents often fall into a prolonged depression. This depression can affect their sleeping, eating, ability to concentrate, and general energy level. Crying, weeping, incessant talking, and strong feelings of guilt or anger are all normal reactions. Many parents experience unreasonable fears that they, or someone in their family, may be in danger. Over-protection of surviving children and fears for future children is a common reaction.

As the finality of the child's death becomes a reality for the parents, recovery occurs. Parents begin to take a more active part in their own lives, which begin to have meaning once again. The pain of their child's death becomes less intense but not forgotten. Birthdays, holidays, and the anniversary of the child's death can trigger periods of intense pain and suffering.

Children will also be affected by the baby's death. They may fear that other members of the family, including themselves, will also suddenly die. Children often also feel guilty about the death of a sibling and may feel that they had something to do with the death. Children may not show their feelings in obvious ways. Although they may deny being upset and seem unconcerned, signs that they are disturbed include intensified clinging to parents, misbehaving, bed wetting, difficulties in school, and nightmares. It is important to talk to children about the death and explain to them that the baby died because of a medical problem that occurs only in infants in rare instances and cannot occur in them. The National Institute of Child Health and Human Development (NICHD) continues to support research aimed at uncovering what causes SIDS, who is at risk for the disorder, and ways to lower the risk of sudden infant death. Inquiries regarding research programs should be directed to Dr. Marian Willinger, 301-496-5575.

Families with a baby who has died from SIDS may be aided by counseling and support groups. Examples of these groups include the following:

Association of SIDS and Infant Mortality Programs
c/o Minnesota SIDS Center
2525 Chicago Ave. South
Minneapolis, MN 55404
1-612-813-6285

National SIDS Resource Center
2070 Chain Bridge Road
Suite 450
Vienna, VA 22181
1-703-821-8955

SIDS Alliance (a national network of SIDS support groups)
1314 Bedford Avenue
Suite 210
Baltimore, MD 21208
1-800-221-7437 or
1-410-653-8226

More Guideline Sources

The guideline above on sudden infant death syndrome is only one example of the kind of material that you can find online and free of charge. The remainder of this chapter will direct you to other sources which either publish or can help you find additional guidelines on topics related to sudden infant death syndrome. Many of the guidelines listed below address topics that may be of particular relevance to your child's specific situation, while certain guidelines will apply to only some children with sudden infant death syndrome. Due to space limitations these sources are listed in a concise manner. Do not hesitate to consult the following sources by either using the Internet hyperlink provided, or, in cases where the contact information is provided, contacting the publisher or author directly.

Topic Pages: MEDLINEplus

For parents wishing to go beyond guidelines published by specific Institutes of the NIH, the National Library of Medicine has created a vast and parent-oriented healthcare information portal called MEDLINEplus. Within this Internet-based system are "health topic pages." You can think of a health topic page as a guide to patient guides. To access this system, log on to **http://www.nlm.nih.gov/medlineplus/healthtopics.html**. From there you can either search using the alphabetical index or browse by broad topic areas. Recently, MEDLINEplus listed the following as being relevant to sudden infant death syndrome:

African-American Health
http://www.nlm.nih.gov/medlineplus/africanamericanhealth.html

Arrhythmia
http://www.nlm.nih.gov/medlineplus/arrhythmia.html

Child Safety
http://www.nlm.nih.gov/medlineplus/childsafety.html

Infant and Newborn Care
http://www.nlm.nih.gov/medlineplus/infantandnewborncare.html

Infant and Toddler Health
http://www.nlm.nih.gov/medlineplus/infantandtoddlerhealth.html

Sudden Infant Death Syndrome
http://www.nlm.nih.gov/medlineplus/suddeninfantdeathsyndrome
.html

Within the health topic page dedicated to sudden infant death syndrome, the following was recently recommended to parents:

- General/Overviews

    JAMA Patient Page: Sudden Infant Death Syndrome
    Source: American Medical Association
    http://www.medem.com/medlb/article_detaillb.cfm?article_ID=ZZ
    Z1I7HB09D&sub_cat=2001

    Questions & Answers on Sudden Infant Death Syndrome (SIDS)
    Source: Sudden Infant Death Syndrome Alliance
    http://www.sidsalliance.org/documents/Q_and_A.asp

    Rock-a-bye Baby... on Their Backs
    Source: American Medical Association
    http://www.medem.com/medlb/article_detaillb.cfm?article_ID=ZZ
    ZZNDKTIAC&sub_cat=14

    SIDS: Sudden and Silent
    Source: Nemours Foundation
    http://kidshealth.org/parent/general/sleep/sids.html

    What is SIDS?
    Source: National Sudden Infant Death Syndrome Resource Center
    http://www.sidscenter.org/SIDSFACT.HTM

- Coping

    After Sudden Infant Death Syndrome: Facing Anniversaries, Holidays, and Special Events
    Source: National Sudden Infant Death Syndrome Resource Center
    http://www.sidscenter.org/FACING.HTM

    Friends and Relatives: Some Suggestions on How to Help
    Source: Sudden Infant Death Syndrome Alliance
    http://www.sidsalliance.org/Documents/Support/Friends_Relative
    s.asp

If Your Baby Has Died of SIDS...
Source: Sudden Infant Death Syndrome Alliance
http://www.sidsalliance.org/Documents/Support/Baby_has_Died_f
rom_SIDS.asp

- Specific Conditions/Aspects

    Protecting America's Infants - Safe Sleep Practices and the Hazards of the Adult Bed
    Source: Sudden Infant Death Syndrome Alliance
    http://www.sidsalliance.org/index/protectamerica.html

    Safe Sleep for My Grandbaby
    Source: Maternal and Child Health Bureau, National SIDS & Infant Death Program Support Center, Sudden Infant Death Syndrome Alliance
    http://sids-id-psc.org/_documents/pdf/grandparents.pdf

    Sudden Infant Death Syndrome (SIDS) and Vaccination
    Source: National Immunization Program
    http://www.cdc.gov/nip/vacsafe/concerns/SIDS/default.htm

    Sudden Infant Death Syndrome and the Child Care Provider
    Source: Maternal and Child Health Bureau, National SIDS & Infant Death Program Support Center, Sudden Infant Death Syndrome Alliance
    http://sids-id-psc.org/_documents/pdf/childcare_provider.pdf

- From the National Institutes of Health

    L.A. Summit Seeks to Reduce SIDS in Western U.S. African American Communities
    Source: National Institute of Child Health and Human Development
    http://www.nih.gov/news/pr/mar2003/nichd-13.htm

    Sudden Infant Death Syndrome
    Source: National Institute of Child Health and Human Development
    http://www.nichd.nih.gov/publications/pubs/sidsfact.htm

- Latest News

    SIDS Risk Factors Identified in Large Study
    Source: 04/23/2004, Reuters Health
    http://www.nlm.nih.gov//www.nlm.nih.gov/medlineplus/news/f
    ullstory_17322.html

- Organizations

  American Academy of Pediatrics
  http://www.aap.org/

  National Institute of Child Health and Human Development
  http://www.nichd.nih.gov/

  National SIDS & Infant Death Program Support Center
  http://sids-id-psc.org/

  National Sudden Infant Death Syndrome Resource Center
  Source: Dept. of Health and Human Services, Maternal and Child Health Bureau
  http://www.sidscenter.org/

  Sudden Infant Death Syndrome (SIDS) Alliance
  Source: Sudden Infant Death Syndrome Alliance
  http://www.sidsalliance.org/index/default.asp

- Prevention/Screening

  Campaign's Resource Kit Seeks to Reduce Incidence of SIDS in African American Communities
  Source: National Institute of Child Health and Human Development
  http://www.nichd.nih.gov/new/releases/sids.cfm

  SIDS Facts: Reducing the Risk of SIDS
  Source: Sudden Infant Death Syndrome Alliance
  http://www.sidsalliance.org/documents/Reducing_the_Risk_of_SIDS.asp

- Research

  Bed Sharing with Siblings, Soft Bedding, Increase SIDS Risk
  Source: Centers for Disease Control and Prevention, National Institute of Child Health and Human Development
  http://www.nih.gov/news/pr/may2003/nichd-05.htm

  Higher SIDS Risk Found in Infants Placed in Unaccustomed Sleeping Position
  Source: National Institute of Child Health and Human Development, National Institute on Deafness and Other Communication Disorders
  http://www.nih.gov/news/pr/feb2003/nichd-28.htm

Most Definitive Study of Its Kind Shows That Sleeping on the Stomach Increases Infant SIDS Risk
Source: Centers for Disease Control and Prevention, National Institute of Child Health and Human Development, National Institute on Deafness and Other Communication Disorders
http://www.nih.gov/news/pr/oct2002/nichd-07.htm

NICHD-Funded Researchers Uncover Abnormal Brain Pathways in SIDS Victims
Source: National Institute of Child Health and Human Development
http://www.nichd.nih.gov/new/releases/sidsbrainstem.cfm

Research on Sudden Infant Death Syndrome (SIDS)
Source: National Institute of Child Health and Human Development
http://www.nichd.nih.gov/womenshealth/sids_research.cfm

Study Estimates 20 Percent of SIDS Deaths Occur in Child Care Settings
Source: American Academy of Pediatrics
http://www.aap.org/advocacy/archives/augsidz.htm

Study Raises Questions about Relationship between SIDS and Events Detected by Home Monitors
Source: National Institute of Child Health and Human Development
http://www.nih.gov/news/pr/may2001/nichd-01.htm

Summits Seek to Reduce SIDS Risk in African American Community
Source: National Institute of Child Health and Human Development
http://www.nih.gov/news/pr/jan2003/nichd-30.htm

- Statistics

   Infant Mortality
   Source: National Center for Health Statistics
   http://www.cdc.gov/nchs/fastats/infmort.htm

   SIDS Statistics
   Source: Sudden Infant Death Syndrome Alliance
   http://www.sidsalliance.org/documents/Back_to_Sleep/Statistics.asp

You may also choose to use the search utility provided by MEDLINEplus at the following Web address: **http://www.nlm.nih.gov/medlineplus/**. Simply type a keyword into the search box and click "Search." This utility is similar to the NIH search utility, with the exception that it only includes materials that are linked within the MEDLINEplus system (mostly patient-oriented information). It also has the disadvantage of generating unstructured results. We recommend, therefore, that you use this method only if you have a very targeted search.

The Combined Health Information Database (CHID)

CHID Online is a reference tool that maintains a database directory of thousands of journal articles and educational guidelines on sudden infant death syndrome and related conditions. One of the advantages of CHID over other sources is that it offers summaries that describe the guidelines available, including contact information and pricing. CHID's general Web site is **http://chid.nih.gov/**. To search this database, go to **http://chid.nih.gov/detail/detail.html**. In particular, you can use the advanced search options to look up pamphlets, reports, brochures, and information kits. The following was recently posted in this archive:

- **Volunteering and Raising Funds to Fight Sudden Infant Death Syndrome**

  Source: Atlanta, GA: American Sudden Infant Death Syndrome Institute. 1996. 4 p.

  Contact: Available from American Sudden Infant Death Syndrome Institute, 6065 Roswell Road, Suite 876, Atlanta, GA 30328. (404) 843-1030, (800) 232-7437 (Nationwide), (800) 847-7437 (in GA), (404) 843-0577 (Fax), prevent@sids.org (Email), http://www.sids.org (Website). Free of charge.

  Summary: The American **Sudden Infant Death Syndrome** (SIDS) Institute in Atlanta, Georgia, is dedicated to the prevention of sudden infant death and the promotion of infant health through research, clinical services, family support, and professional education. The institute depends heavily on the financial support of individuals and organizations to achieve its goals. This brochure provides interested persons with a wide variety of ideas for raising funds for SIDS. The ideas include a beautiful baby contest, a canister drive, a car wash, a fun run, a garage sale, money from mall fountains, a walk-a-thon or other marathon event, and requests for memorials. The brochure lists items that the institute can offer fund raisers to assist them in their activities, such as a public service announcement tape, stationery, donation forms, their nonprofit tax ID number, solicitation letters, and brochures. The brochure also includes an event planning checklist and 11 basic facts about SIDS.

- **Raising Funds to Fight Sudden Infant Death Syndrome**

  Source: Atlanta, GA: American Sudden Infant Death Syndrome Institute. 1995. 4 p.

  Contact: Available from American Sudden Infant Death Syndrome Institute, 6065 Roswell Road, Suite 876, Atlanta, GA 30328. (404) 843-1030, (800) 232-7437 (Nationwide), (800) 847-7437 (in GA), (404) 843-0577 (Fax), prevent@sids.org (Email), http://www.sids.org (Website). Free of charge.

  Summary: The American SIDS Institute in Atlanta, Georgia, is dedicated to the prevention of sudden infant death and the promotion of infant health through research, clinical services, family support, and professional education. The institute depends heavily on the financial support of individuals and organizations to achieve its goals. This brochure provides interested persons with a wide variety of ideas for raising funds for SIDS. The ideas include a beautiful baby contest, a canister drive, a car wash, a fun run, a garage sale, money from mall fountains, a walk-a-thon or other marathon event, and requests for memorials. The brochure lists items that the institute can offer fundraisers to assist them in their activities, such as a public service announcement tape, stationery, donation forms, their nonprofit tax ID number, solicitation letters, and brochures. The brochure also includes an event planning checklist and 11 basic facts about SIDS.

- **Reduce the Risk of Sudden Infant Death Syndrome. Reduciendo el Riesgo del Sindrome de Muerte Infantil Repentina**

  Source: Rancho Cordova, CA: California SIDS Program. 2000. 8 p.

  Contact: Available from California SIDS Program, 3164 Gold Camp, Suite 220, Rancho Cordova, CA 95670. (916) 463-0146, (800) 369-7437 (in CA), (916) 536-0167 (Fax), info@californiasids.com (E-mail), http://www.californiasids.com (Web Site). Free to CA residents; $0.50 each plus shipping and handling for residents of other states.

  Summary: This bilingual Spanish-English brochure provides parents and other child care providers with information on reducing the risk of **sudden infant death syndrome** (SIDS). The brochure states that most SIDS deaths occur by 6 months of age, more boys are victims than girls, and most deaths occur during the fall, winter, and early spring months. SIDS cannot be predicted or prevented, but parents and caregivers are urged to follow certain infant care practices to significantly reduce the risk of SIDS: place your baby to sleep on his or her back; keep the area around your baby smoke-free; make sure your baby sleeps on a firm mattress in a safety-approved crib and not on a waterbed, sheepskin, pillow, or other soft surface; keep fluffy blankets, comforters, stuffed toys, bumper pads, and pillows out of the crib; keep your baby warm, but not hot; receive early and regular prenatal care and do not smoke or use alcohol or drugs while pregnant; and breast feed your baby, if possible. The brochure states that babies who roll over onto their stomachs on their own should not be forced to stay on their back. Parents are urged to talk to their doctor or nurse if they have any questions about their baby's sleep position or health.

- **Sudden Infant Death Syndrome: Information for Coroners and Coroner's Investigators in California**

  Source: Berkeley, CA: California Sudden Infant Death Syndrome Program. June 1992. 8 p.

  Contact: Available from California Sudden Infant Death Syndrome Program, 5330 Primrose Drive, Suite 231, Fair Oaks, CA 95628-3542. (916) 536-0146, (800) 369-7437 (in CA), (916) 536-0167 (Fax). Free to CA residents; $0.71 per copy for residents of other States.

  Summary: This booklet provides coroners and their investigators with basic information about **sudden infant death syndrome** (SIDS) and guidelines for conducting a death scene investigation of a possible SIDS death in California. The first part of the booklet outlines the coroner's responsibilities in a presumptive SIDS death investigation according to California State codes; describes the three types of information the pathologist needs to arrive at a diagnosis of SIDS, and which information is the responsibility of the coroner; and describes a typical SIDS history and typical death scene and autopsy findings. The second part of the booklet provides coroners with six guidelines to follow in dealing with parents or caregivers: explain the purpose of the investigation; treat the baby with kindness and respect; ask open-ended, nonjudgmental questions; explain what will happen next; be reassuring; and make sure that both you and the parents know how to contact each other later. Specific information is provided for each guideline.

- **Eastern Connecticut Sudden Infant Death Syndrome Network**

  Source: Ledyard, CT: Eastern Connecticut Sudden Infant Death Syndrome Network. December 1993. 2 pp.

  Contact: Available from Sudden Infant Death Syndrome Network, P.O. Box 520, Ledyard, CT 06339. (860) 892-7042, ext. 551 (Voicemail), (860) 887-7309 (Fax), sidsnet@sids-network.org (E-mail), http://sids-network.org (Web site).

  Summary: This brochure describes the mission and services of the **Sudden Infant Death Syndrome** Network in Ledyard, CT. The Network is a nonprofit, voluntary agency whose mission is threefold: to eliminate **sudden infant death syndrome** (SIDS) through the support of SIDS research projects, to provide support for persons who have been touched by the tragedy of SIDS, and to raise public awareness of SIDS through education. The network offers the following services: a website that is accessible worldwide, peer counseling and crisis intervention counseling, monthly support group meetings, referrals to other agencies and professional services, educational programs for health professionals and community service professionals, resource materials on SIDS, public service announcements, and a newsletter. The brochure also includes basic information about SIDS.

- **Sudden Infant Death Syndrome Resources, Inc**

  Source: St. Louis, MO: Sudden Infant Death Syndrome Resources, Inc. 0000. 2 p.

  Contact: Available from Sudden Infant Death Syndrome Resources, Inc., 143 Grand Avenue, St. Louis, MO 63122. (314) 822-2323, (800) 421-3511 (in MO), (314) 822-2098 (Fax).

  Summary: This brochure describes the services of **Sudden Infant Death Syndrome** Resources (SIDS), Inc., a nonprofit organization dedicated to helping people who are affected by **Sudden Infant Death Syndrome** (SIDS) in Missouri. The organization began as a federally funded project in 1974, and in 1982 the project was awarded a contract by the State to provide SIDS services. Today, the organization offers the following services: family support services, including family counseling, home visits, support groups, peer contact, research update meetings, and a quarterly newsletter; training for health professionals, police, and other emergency workers who are first responders in SIDS cases; community awareness activities; and research support. The brochure includes a list of facts about SIDS.

- **Babies sleep safest on their backs: Reduce the risk of Sudden Infant Death Syndrome (SIDS)**

  Source: Bethesda, MD: National Institute of Child Health and Human Development. 2000. 8 pp.

  Contact: Available from National Institute of Child Health and Human Development Clearinghouse, P.O. Box 3006, Rockville, MD 20847. Telephone: (800) 370-2943 TTY: (888) 320-6942 / fax: (301) 984-1473 / e-mail: NICHDClearinghouse@mail.nih.gov / Web site: http://www.nichd.nih.gov/publications/info.htm. Available at no charge.

Summary: This brochure discusses **Sudden Infant Death Syndrome** (SIDS) and ways for parents to prevent harm to their infant. Topics include facts about SIDS, why babies should sleep on their backs, ways to lower the risk of SIDS, and other ways parents can keep their baby healthy. Information is provided for contacting the Back to Sleep Campaign for more information. The brochure is available in English and Spanish.

- **Sudden infant death syndrome**

  Source: Bethesda, MD: Public Information and Communications Branch, National Institute of Child Health and Human Development, U.S. Department of Health and Human Services. 1997. 4 pp.

  Contact: Available from National Maternal and Child Health Clearinghouse, 2070 Chain Bridge Road, Suite 450, Vienna, VA 22182-2536. Telephone: (703) 356-1964 or (888) 434-4MCH / fax: (703) 821-2098 / e-mail: nmchc@circsol.com / Web site: http://www.nmchc.org. Available at no charge.

  Summary: This brochure explains what **sudden infant death syndrome** (SIDS) is, what the risk factors for it are, what causes it, what might help lower the risk, and how a SIDS baby affects the family. Examples of SIDS counseling and support groups are provided.

- **Sudden Infant Death Syndrome: What Every Young Adult Should Know. Revised Edition**

  Source: Seattle, WA: SIDS Foundation of Washington. January 1996. 2 p.

  Contact: Available from SIDS Foundation of Washington, 4649 Sunnyside Avenue N., Room 328, Seattle, WA 98103. (206) 548-9290 (Seattle), (509) 456-0505 (Spokane), (800) 533-0376 (WA, ID, OR only), (206) 548-9445 (Fax), sids- wa@zipcon.net (Email), http://www.zipcon.net/sids-wa (Website). $0.15 each plus shipping and handling.

  Summary: This brochure introduces adolescents and young adults to **sudden infant death syndrome** (SIDS). The brochure is intended to prepare them for the possibility of SIDS occurring in their life, whether they experience it as a family member, babysitter, close friend, or parent. The brochure answers the following questions: What is SIDS?; Why should young adults know about SIDS?; What are the known facts about SIDS?; How can you prepare to face SIDS or another emergency as a babysitter?; What should you know as a new parent to help reduce the risk of SIDS occurring?; When SIDS occurs, what is its impact?; and What can you do to help a parent, sibling, or friend who has experienced a SIDS death?.

- **About Sudden Infant Death Syndrome (SIDS)**

  Source: Camberwell, Australia: National SIDS Council of Australia Ltd. October 1991. 4 p.

  Contact: Available from National SIDS Council of Australia Ltd., 357 Burwood Road, Hawthorn, VIC 3122 Australia. 011-61-03-9819-9277.

  Summary: This brochure presents basic information about **sudden infant death syndrome** (SIDS). The brochure covers the following topics: the definition of SIDS, possible causes, whether the baby smothered or choked on vomit or food, whether the baby suffered, whether SIDS is contagious, whether the death was anyone's fault, why the police are called in SIDS deaths, normal grief reactions, the reactions of other children, having another baby, current research objectives, and sources of information and help. Contact information is provided for nine organizations that are located throughout Australia.

- **Prevent Sudden Infant Death Syndrome**

  Source: New Brunswick, NJ: New Jersey Sudden Infant Death Syndrome Resource Center. 1996. 2 p.

  Contact: Available from SIDS Center of New Jersey, 254 Easton Avenue, New Brunswick, NJ 08903. (908) 249-2160, (800) 545-7437 (NJ Hotline), (908) 249-6306 (Fax), esposili@umdnj.edu (Email), http://www2.umdnj.edu/sids/home.htm (Website).

  Summary: This brochure presents guidelines to parents, relatives, and caregivers of infants for reducing the risk for **sudden infant death syndrome** (SIDS). The guidelines are as follows: don't smoke and avoid exposure to smoky atmospheres (infants who are exposed to smoke have five times the risk for SIDS as infants who are not exposed to smoke); place infants on their backs to sleep, near the foot of the bed, with blankets or sheets covering no further than the shoulders; make sure the infant sleeps on a firm mattress, never a pillow or a soft surface; do not overheat the infant by bundling him or her with excess bedding and bed clothes; remove the infant's outdoor clothing, including any head covering, upon going indoors into a building, car, train, or bus so the infant can vent excess heat; learn to recognize the signs of a serious illness in the infant (e.g., a high-pitched or weak cry, unresponsiveness and limpness, paleness, grunting while breathing, a lowered intake of fluids, vomiting green fluid, passing blood during bowel movements, or fever); learn to recognize when an infant needs urgent medical attention (i.e., when the infant stops breathing or turns blue, is unresponsive or shows no awareness of what is going on around him or her, has glazed eyes and does not focus on anything, or cannot be awakened); and breastfeed the infant, if possible. The brochure is printed in color. A companion risk-reduction poster also is available.

- **Reduce the Risks of Sudden Infant Death Syndrome**

  Source: Hackensack, NJ: CJ Foundation for SIDS. 1996.

  Contact: Available from CJ Foundation for SIDS, Don Imus-WFAN Pediatric Center, Hackensack University Medical Center, 30 Prospect Avenue, Hackensack, NJ 07601. (201) 996-5111, (201) 996-5326 (Fax), SUSANCJ@aol.com (Email). Free of charge.

  Summary: This brochure presents parents and child care providers with six steps for reducing the risk for **sudden infant death syndrome** (SIDS). These steps are as follows: put a healthy infant on his or her back to sleep; do not smoke near the infant; do not let the infant get too hot; put the infant to sleep on a firm mattress; take good care of yourself and the infant; and breast feed the infant, if possible. The brochure stresses that infants should be put to sleep on their backs whether they are being put down for a nap or to bed for the night. If an infant has problems breathing or spits up a lot after feeding, parents should ask their pediatrician about the appropriate sleep position for their child. Basic facts about SIDS are included in the brochure.

- **American Sudden Infant Death Syndrome Institute**

  Source: Atlanta, GA: American Sudden Infant Death Syndrome Institute. 1994. 4 p.

  Contact: Available from American Sudden Infant Death Syndrome Institute, 6065 Roswell Road, Suite 876, Atlanta, GA 30328. (404) 843-1030, (800) 232-7437 (Nationwide), (800) 847-7437 (in GA), (404) 843-0577 (Fax), prevent@sids.org (Email), http://www.sids.org (Website). Free of charge.

  Summary: This brochure provides a description of the American **Sudden Infant Death Syndrome** (SIDS) Institute in Atlanta, Georgia, and its activities. The nonprofit organization dedicates itself to a comprehensive national program of research, education, and health care. The Institute encourages collaborative research efforts between members of its staff and investigators from other institutions throughout the country. In terms of health care, the Institute's clinic in Atlanta provides medical services for infants at risk for SIDS, regardless of the family's financial situation. The clinic also provides diagnostic evaluation and a comprehensive program of home monitoring. In the event of a SIDS death, the Institute provides bereavement services to families and friends that include crisis phone counseling, bereavement counseling, and grief literature. The Institute also organizes conferences, workshops, and teaching programs to provide rapid dissemination of the latest research to professional groups, including health care providers, first responders, and researchers. In 1992, the Institute began the SIDS Prevention Campaign to inform both physicians and the general public about research findings that have implications for reducing the incidence of SIDS.

- **Facts About Sudden Infant Death Syndrome and Reducing the Risks for SIDS. Revised Edition**

Source: Baltimore, MD: Sudden Infant Death Syndrome Alliance. 1997. 4 p.

Contact: Available from Sudden Infant Death Syndrome Alliance, 1314 Bedford Avenue, Suite 210, Baltimore, MD 21208. (410) 653-8226, (800) 221-7437, (410) 653-8709 (Fax), sidshq@charm.net (Email). $0.10 each; $10.00 per packet of 100.

Summary: This brochure provides parents and child care providers with basic information on **sudden infant death syndrome** (SIDS) and recommendations for reducing the risk for SIDS that are based on the latest medical evidence. These recommendations are supported by the **Sudden Infant Death Syndrome** Alliance, a national not-for-profit voluntary health organization dedicated to the support of SIDS families, education, and research. The brochure recommends that parents and caregivers place their baby on his or her back to sleep but allow the baby supervised awake time on its tummy to promote infant development and prevent head- flattening. Back sleep is preferable to side sleep and wedges are not recommended to keep a baby propped on the side. Research findings show that women who smoke cigarettes during or after pregnancy put their infants at increased risk for SIDS. Parents are advised not to smoke during pregnancy and the first year of the baby's life, and not to allow anyone else to smoke around the baby either. Other recommendations are to use firm, flat bedding; avoid overheating the baby; and take good care of oneself and the baby during pregnancy and infancy. Breastfeeding is good for the baby and is recommended, and parents should follow the recommended schedule for their baby's immunizations. Bedsharing has not been shown to protect against SIDS and may be hazardous under some conditions. The same recommendations for safest sleep conditions apply whether one's baby sleeps alone in a crib or shares a bed with a parent. Though bedsharing may boost breastfeeding and promote the bond between mother and infant, bedsharing with family members other than the parents is not recommended. Parents are encouraged to turn to the SIDS Alliance for help, and to consider becoming a SIDS volunteer, educator, fundraiser, or activist for the Alliance affiliate in their area.

- **Back to Sleep. Reduce the Risk of Sudden Infant Death Syndrome (SIDS). Revised Edition**

  Source: Bethesda, MD: National Institute of Child Health and Human Development (NIH). 1997. 2 p.

  Contact: Available from Back to Sleep, P.O. Box 29111, Washington, DC 20040. (800) 505-CRIB. Free of charge.

  Summary: This brochure, a product of the national 'Back to Sleep' campaign in the United States, presents parents and child care providers with information on reducing the risk for **sudden infant death syndrome** (SIDS). The 'Back to Sleep' campaign was initiated in June 1994 to alert new parents and health professionals to sleep position as a possible risk factor for SIDS. Research has shown that the greatest risk for SIDS occurs in the prone sleep position. The safest sleep position for healthy babies is the supine position, so pediatricians now recommend that healthy infants be put down to sleep on their backs for nap time and bedtime. The side sleep position does not provide as much protection against SIDS as the back position, but it is still much safer than placing an infant to sleep on his or her stomach. Parents of infants who were born with a birth defect or who have gastrointestinal, respiratory, or heart problems should ask their doctor about which sleep position to use during naps and at night. Other things that parents can do to help reduce the risk for SIDS are as follows: make sure that the baby sleeps on a firm mattress without fluffy blankets or comforters underneath; do not let the baby sleep on a waterbed, sheepskin, pillow, or other soft material; do not place stuffed toys or pillows in the crib; keep the temperature in the baby's room where it feels comfortable to you; do not let anyone smoke around the baby; if the baby seems sick, call your doctor or clinic right away; make sure the baby receives all of his or her shots on time; get early and regular prenatal care; do not smoke or use alcohol or drugs during pregnancy; and breastfeed your baby, if possible. The brochure also is available in Spanish (MCS000501).

- **Sudden Infant Death Syndrome. Revised Edition**

  Source: Seattle, WA: SIDS Foundation of Washington. 1996. 1 p.

  Contact: Available from SIDS Foundation of Washington, 4649 Sunnyside Avenue, N., Room 438, Seattle, WA 98103. (206) 548-9290 (Seattle), (509) 456-0505 (Spokane), (800) 533-0376 (WA, ID, OR only), (206) 548- 9445

(Fax), sids-wa@zipcon.net (Email), http://www.zipcon.net/sids-wa (Website). $0.03 each plus shipping and handling.

Summary: This half-page fact sheet presents basic information about **sudden infant death syndrome** (SIDS). The fact sheet presents the definition of SIDS; its incidence in the United States; the peak age for SIDS and other demographic characteristics; and the fact that SIDS cannot be predicted or prevented, even by a physician. The fact sheet also lists causes of death that are often erroneously thought to be causes of SIDS (e.g., suffocation, child abuse, vomiting, choking), and states that SIDS is not contagious nor does it cause pain or suffering to the infant.

- **California Sudden Infant Death Syndrome Program: Mission Statement; Program Goals and Activities**

  Source: Fair Oaks, CA: California SIDS Program. June 1996. 1 p.

  Contact: Available from California Sudden Infant Death Syndrome Program, 5330 Primrose Drive, Suite 231, Fair Oaks, CA 95628-3542. (916) 536-0146, (800) 369-7437 (in CA), (916) 536-0167 (Fax).

  Summary: This information sheet describes the mission, goals, and activities of the California **Sudden Infant Death Syndrome** Program. Following a brief mission statement, specific activities are listed under each of the following program goals: to reduce the emotional suffering that accompanies a SIDS death; to provide SIDS education and training for professionals, paraprofessionals, and parents; to increase public awareness and knowledge of SIDS; and to encourage SIDS research.

- **Selected Books on Sudden Infant Death Syndrome**

  Source: McLean, VA: National Sudden Infant Death Syndrome Resource Center. May 1993. 2 p.

  Contact: Available from National SIDS Resource Center, Suite 450, 2070 Chain Bridge Road, Vienna, VA 22182-2536. (703) 821-8955, (703) 821-2098 (Fax), sids@circsol.com (Email), http://www.circsol.com/sids (Website). Free of charge; distribution limited to one per customer. Order No. S102.

  Summary: This information sheet lists 13 selected books on **sudden infant death syndrome** (SIDS) published from 1980 to the present that cover research, the impact of a SIDS death on parents and families, and the role of professionals and others in helping families deal with the loss. Publisher and/or distributor information is listed whenever possible. Three books that are no longer in print are included, as copies may still be available at a medical, university, or public library, or through interlibrary loan arrangements at these institutions.

- **Reduce the Risks of Cot Death**

  Source: London, England: The Foundation for the Study of Infant Deaths. 1992. 4 p.

  Contact: Foundation for the Study of Infant Deaths, 14 Halkin Street, London SW1X 7DP, England. 011-44-171-235-0965, 011-44-171- 235-1721 (Helpline), 011-44-171-823-1986 (Fax).

  Summary: This pamphlet identifies factors that may reduce the risk for **sudden infant death syndrome** (SIDS), including placing a baby on his or her back or side to sleep, avoiding smoking before and after a baby is born, and taking care not to make a baby either too hot or too cold. Suggestions for helping parents maintain the proper thermal environment include the following: indoors, babies over 1 month old do not need more clothes than their parents; warm outdoor clothes should be removed when the baby is brought indoors; 65 degrees F. is the ideal room temperature for a baby; a baby's room should be kept at an even temperature throughout the night; and in terms of clothing, a baby does not need more than a nappy, vest, and babygro to sleep in. A table shows the amount of bedding an infant needs at different room temperatures. The brochure also includes guidelines for caring for a baby that is unwell. In addition, lists are presented of physical symptoms that require urgent medical attention and those that indicate that a serious illness may be present.

- **Sudden Infant Death Syndrome: The Facts**

  Source: Milwaukee, WI: Wisconsin Sudden Infant Death Center. 1993. 2 p.

  Contact: Available from Wisconsin Sudden Infant Death Center, Children's Hospital of Wisconsin, P.O. Box 1997, Milwaukee, WI 53201-0997. (414) 266- 2743, (414) 266-2653 (Fax). Order No. 10k TJ93.

  Summary: This pamphlet, intended for the general public, provides the following information about **sudden infant death syndrome** (SIDS): a definition, facts about SIDS that are based on research, the characteristics of SIDS victims and the circumstances typically surrounding SIDS deaths, common misconceptions about its cause and prevention, the importance of an autopsy to a SIDS diagnosis, and the chances of recurrence within the same family.

- **When Your Baby Has Died of Sudden Infant Death Syndrome**

  Source: Toronto, Ontario: The Canadian Foundation for the Study of Infant Deaths. 1991. 5 p.

Contact: Canadian Foundation for the Study of Infant Deaths, 586 Eglinton Avenue East, Suite 308, Toronto, ON M4P 1P2 Canada. (416) 488-3260, (800) 363-7437, (416) 488-3864 (Fax), sidscanada@inforamp.net (Email), http://www.sidscanada.org/sids.html (Website).

Summary: This pamphlet, written for the parents of infants who have died from **sudden infant death syndrome** (SIDS), provides facts about SIDS; identifies common parental reactions to the death of a baby (i.e., guilt, shock, anger, fear); describes the physical symptoms of grief; and discusses the issue of subsequent children. The pamphlet also discusses the unique grief reactions of mothers and fathers, single parents, siblings, and grandparents, and advises parents on talking to their other children about the death. The pamphlet also is available in French (MCS000477).

- **Reducing the Risk of Sudden Infant Death Syndrome in Canada**

    Source: Toronto, Ontario: The Canadian Foundation for the Study of Infant Deaths. August 1993. 2 pp.

    Contact: Canadian Foundation for the Study of Infant Deaths, 586 Eglinton Avenue East, Suite 308, Toronto, ON M4P 1P2 Canada. (416) 488-3260, (800) 363-7437, (416) 488-3864 (Fax), sidscanada@inforamp.net (E-mail), http://www.sidscanada.org/sids.html (Web site).

    Summary: This position statement on reducing the risks for **sudden infant death syndrome** is supported by the Canadian Foundation for the Study of Infant Deaths, the Canadian Institute of Child Health, the Canadian Paediatric Society, and Health Canada. The recommendations include placing healthy infants in the supine or lateral position for sleep, caring for infants in a smoke-free environment, dressing and covering infants in a manner that avoids overheating, and breastfeeding infants whenever possible.

The National Guideline Clearinghouse™

The National Guideline Clearinghouse™ offers hundreds of evidence-based clinical practice guidelines published in the United States and other countries. You can search their site located at **http://www.guideline.gov** by using the keyword "sudden infant death syndrome" or synonyms. The following was recently posted:

- **(1) Distinguishing sudden infant death syndrome from child abuse fatalities; (2) Distinguishing sudden infant death syndrome from child abuse fatalities (Addendum)**

  Source: American Academy of Pediatrics - Medical Specialty Society; 2001 February (addendum published 2001 Sep); 5 pages

  http://www.guideline.gov/summary/summary.aspx?doc_id=2763&nbr=1989&string=sudden+AND+infant+AND+death+AND+syndrome

- **Apnea, sudden infant death syndrome, and home monitoring**

  Source: American Academy of Pediatrics - Medical Specialty Society; 2003 April; 4 pages

  http://www.guideline.gov/summary/summary.aspx?doc_id=3732&nbr=2958&string=sudden+AND+infant+AND+death+AND+syndrome

- **Changing concepts of sudden infant death syndrome: implications for infant sleeping environment and sleep position**

  Source: American Academy of Pediatrics - Medical Specialty Society; 2000 March; 7 pages

  http://www.guideline.gov/summary/summary.aspx?doc_id=2768&nbr=1994&string=sudden+AND+infant+AND+death+AND+syndrome

Healthfinder™

Healthfinder™ is an additional source sponsored by the U.S. Department of Health and Human Services which offers links to hundreds of other sites that contain healthcare information. This Web site is located at **http://www.healthfinder.gov**. Again, keyword searches can be used to find guidelines. The following was recently found in this database:

- **Babies Sleep Safest on Their Backs: Reduce the Risk of Sudden Infant Death Syndrome**

  Source: National Institute of Child Health and Human Development, National Institutes of Health

  http://www.healthfinder.gov/scripts/recordpass.asp?RecordType=0&RecordID=3179

- **Back to Sleep Campaign**

  Summary: This website offers information for parents and health professionals on sudden infant death syndrome. Some materials are available in Spanish.

  Source: National Institute of Child Health and Human Development, National Institutes of Health

  http://www.healthfinder.gov/scripts/recordpass.asp?RecordType=0&RecordID=409

- **Frequently Asked Questions and SIDS Research Information**

  Summary: These links focus on a number of issues related to Sudden Infant Death Syndrome: smoking, sleep, sleep apnea, and vaccinations.

  Source: Sudden Infant Death Syndrome Network, Inc.

  http://www.healthfinder.gov/scripts/recordpass.asp?RecordType=0&RecordID=7705

- **healthfinder® just for you: Infants**

  Summary: healthfinder®'s just for you: Infants section features topics such as birth defects, child care, and sudden infant death syndrome (SIDS).

  Source: U.S. Department of Health and Human Services

  http://www.healthfinder.gov/scripts/recordpass.asp?RecordType=0&RecordID=7015

- **SIDS Information for New Parents**

  Summary: Here are some important tips for new parents, grandparents and infant caregivers to help reduce the risk of Sudden Infant Death Syndrome and accidental infant deaths.

  Source: Sudden Infant Death Syndrome Alliance

  http://www.healthfinder.gov/scripts/recordpass.asp?RecordType=0&RecordID=7706

- **Study Identifies SIDS Risk Factors Among American Indian Infants**

  Summary: A study of Northern Plains Indians found that infants were less likely to die of Sudden Infant Death Syndrome (SIDS) if their mothers received visits from public health nurses before and after giving

  Source: Indian Health Service

  http://www.healthfinder.gov/scripts/recordpass.asp?RecordType=0&RecordID=7136

The NIH Search Utility

After browsing the references listed at the beginning of this chapter, you may want to explore the NIH search utility. This allows you to search for documents on over 100 selected Web sites that comprise the NIH-WEB-SPACE. Each of these servers is "crawled" and indexed on an ongoing basis. Your search will produce a list of various documents, all of which will relate in some way to sudden infant death syndrome. The drawbacks of this approach are that the information is not organized by theme and that the references are often a mix of information for professionals and parents. Nevertheless, a large number of the listed Web sites provide useful background information. We can only recommend this route, therefore, for relatively rare or specific disorders, or when using highly targeted searches. To use the NIH search utility, visit the following Web page: **http://search.nih.gov/index.html**.

Additional Web Sources

A number of Web sites that often link to government sites are available to the public. These can also point you in the direction of essential information. The following is a representative sample:

- AOL: **http://search.aol.com/cat.adp?id=168&layer=&from=subcats**
- Family Village: **http://www.familyvillage.wisc.edu/specific.htm**
- Google: **http://directory.google.com/Top/Health/Conditions_and_Diseases/**
- Med Help International: **http://www.medhelp.org/HealthTopics/A.html**
- Open Directory Project: **http://dmoz.org/Health/Conditions_and_Diseases/**
- Yahoo.com: **http://dir.yahoo.com/Health/Diseases_and_Conditions/**
- WebMD®Health: **http://my.webmd.com/health_topics**

Vocabulary Builder

The material in this chapter may have contained a number of unfamiliar words. The following Vocabulary Builder introduces you to terms used in this chapter that have not been covered in the previous chapter:

Airway: A device for securing unobstructed passage of air into and out of the lungs during general anesthesia. [NIH]

Apnea: Cessation of breathing. [NIH]

Branch: Most commonly used for branches of nerves, but applied also to other structures. [NIH]

Bridge: A form of dental prosthesis which replaces one or more lost or missing teeth, being supported and held in position by attachments to adjacent teeth. [NIH]

Infancy: The period of complete dependency prior to the acquisition of competence in walking, talking, and self-feeding. [NIH]

Infections: The illnesses caused by an organism that usually does not cause disease in a person with a normal immune system. [NIH]

Monitor: An apparatus which automatically records such physiological signs as respiration, pulse, and blood pressure in an anesthetized patient or one undergoing surgical or other procedures. [NIH]

Need: A state of tension or dissatisfaction felt by an individual that impels him to action toward a goal he believes will satisfy the impulse. [NIH]

Nucleus: A body of specialized protoplasm found in nearly all cells and containing the chromosomes. [NIH]

Presumptive: A treatment based on an assumed diagnosis, prior to receiving confirmatory laboratory test results. [NIH]

Prone: Having the front portion of the body downwards. [NIH]

Supine: Having the front portion of the body upwards. [NIH]

CHAPTER 2. SEEKING GUIDANCE

Overview

Some parents are comforted by the knowledge that a number of organizations dedicate their resources to helping people with sudden infant death syndrome. These associations can become invaluable sources of information and advice. Many associations offer parent support, financial assistance, and other important services. Furthermore, healthcare research has shown that support groups often help people to better cope with their conditions.[8] In addition to support groups, your child's physician can be a valuable source of guidance and support.

In this chapter, we direct you to resources that can help you find parent organizations and medical specialists. We begin by describing how to find associations and parent groups that can help you better understand and cope with your child's condition. The chapter ends with a discussion on how to find a doctor that is right for your child.

Associations and Sudden Infant Death Syndrome

In addition to associations or groups that your child's doctor might recommend, we suggest that you consider the following list (if there is a fee for an association, you may want to check with your child's insurance provider to find out if the cost will be covered):

- **American Sudden Infant Death Syndrome Institute**
  Telephone: (770) 621-1030 Toll-free: (800) 232-7437

---

[8] Churches, synagogues, and other houses of worship might also have groups that can offer you the social support you need.

Fax: (770) 612-8277

Email: prevent@sids.org

Web Site: http://www.sids.org

Background: The American **Sudden Infant Death Syndrome** Institute is a not-for-profit organization dedicated to preventing **Sudden Infant Death Syndrome** (SIDS) and to ensuring that the medical and corporate communities, government agencies, and general public share the sense of urgency in preventing SIDS. **Sudden Infant Death Syndrome** is characterized by the sudden death of any infant or young child that is unexpected by history and for which no adequate cause of death can be found. The Institution was founded to develop a comprehensive national program of research, clinical care, and education and to focus national attention and resources on the problem of SIDS. Most importantly, the Institute searches aggressively and with a strong sense of urgency for the means to eliminate this disorder. Established in 1983, the organization provides support groups, promotes research, engages in patient and professional education, and offers clinical services. Educational materials include a newsletter entitled 'The Promise,' brochures, and pamphlets.

Relevant area(s) of interest: Cot Death, Crib Death, Sudden Infant Death Syndrome

- **National Sudden Infant Death Syndrome Resource Center**

Telephone: (703) 821-8955

Fax: (703) 821-2098

Email: sids@circlesolutions.com

Web Site: http://www.circsol.com/sids

Background: The National **Sudden Infant Death Syndrome** (SIDS) Resource Center is a professional for profit health organization that provides information services and technical assistance concerning SIDS and related topics in order to promote understanding of SIDS and to comfort those affected by a SIDS loss. Established in 1981, the Resource Center assists the National Center of Education's Maternal and Child Health Bureau (MCHB) by providing its services to State MCHB-supported projects and State SIDS programs funded through the Maternal and Child Health Block Grant. The Resource Center also offers its services to parents, family members, care providers, counselors, medical and legal professionals, researchers, program planners, policymakers, and the general public. The Resource Center maintains automated databases of SIDS technical literature, public awareness materials, MCHB materials, and organizations concerned with SIDS. The

Center also develops and distributes bibliographies of materials on SIDS, fact sheets, and other educational materials, including its 'Information Exchange' newsletter; tracks information and resources on current developments related to SIDS; conducts customized database searches; and refers those making inquiries to State SIDS programs and other regional and national organizations, as appropriate.

Relevant area(s) of interest: Sudden Infant Death Syndrome

- **Sudden Infant Death Syndrome Alliance, Inc**

  Telephone: (410) 653-8226 Toll-free: (800) 221-7437

  Fax: (410) 653-8709

  Email: info@sidsalliance.org

  Web Site: http://www.sidsalliance.org

  Background: The **Sudden Infant Death Syndrome** Alliance exists to ensure the elimination of **sudden infant death syndrome** through medical research and education, while providing support to those affected by an infant death. It is a national, non-profit voluntary health organization that unites families, caregivers, health professionals and scientists with government, business and community service groups. As a sponsor of the national Back to Sleep Campaign, the SIDS Alliance supplies information on SIDS to nwe and expectant parents and the general public via a nationwide 24-hour, tollfree hotline and its website. It works closely with the National Institute of Child Health and Human Development to advocate for a coordinated research agenda for the nation.

  Relevant area(s) of interest: Crib Death, Sudden Infant Death Syndrome

Finding Associations

There are a several Internet directories that provide lists of medical associations with information on or resources relating to sudden infant death syndrome. By consulting all of associations listed in this chapter, you will have nearly exhausted all sources for parent associations concerned with sudden infant death syndrome.

The National Health Information Center (NHIC)

The National Health Information Center (NHIC) offers a free referral service to help people find organizations that provide information about sudden infant death syndrome. For more information, see the NHIC's Web site at **http://www.health.gov/NHIC/** or contact an information specialist by calling 1-800-336-4797.

DIRLINE

A comprehensive source of information on associations is the DIRLINE database maintained by the National Library of Medicine. The database comprises some 10,000 records of organizations, research centers, and government institutes and associations which primarily focus on health and biomedicine. DIRLINE is available via the Internet at the following Web site: **http://dirline.nlm.nih.gov**. Simply type in "sudden infant death syndrome" (or a synonym) or the name of a topic, and the site will list information contained in the database on all relevant organizations.

The Combined Health Information Database

Another comprehensive source of information on healthcare associations is the Combined Health Information Database. Using the "Detailed Search" option, you will need to limit your search to "Organizations" and "sudden infant death syndrome". Type the following hyperlink into your Web browser: **http://chid.nih.gov/detail/detail.html**. To find associations, use the drop boxes at the bottom of the search page where "You may refine your search by." For publication date, select "All Years." Then, select your preferred language and the format option "Organization Resource Sheet." By making these selections and typing in "sudden infant death syndrome" (or synonyms) into the "For these words:" box, you will only receive results on organizations dealing with sudden infant death syndrome. You should check back periodically with this database since it is updated every 3 months.

The National Organization for Rare Disorders, Inc.

The National Organization for Rare Disorders, Inc. has prepared a Web site that provides, at no charge, lists of associations organized by specific medical conditions. You can access this database at the following Web site: **http://www.rarediseases.org/search/orgsearch.html**. Type "sudden infant death syndrome" (or a synonym) in the search box, and click "Submit Query."

Online Support Groups

In addition to support groups, commercial Internet service providers offer forums and chat rooms to discuss different illnesses and conditions. WebMD®, for example, offers such a service at its Web site: **http://boards.webmd.com/roundtable**. These online communities can help you connect with a network of people whose concerns are similar to yours. Online support groups are places where people can talk informally. If you read about a novel approach, consult with your child's doctor or other healthcare providers, as the treatments or discoveries you hear about may not be scientifically proven to be safe and effective.

Finding Doctors

All parents must go through the process of selecting a physician for their children with sudden infant death syndrome. While this process will vary, the Agency for Healthcare Research and Quality makes a number of suggestions, including the following:[9]

- If your child is in a managed care plan, check the plan's list of doctors first.

- Ask doctors or other health professionals who work with doctors, such as hospital nurses, for referrals.

- Call a hospital's doctor referral service, but keep in mind that these services usually refer you to doctors on staff at that particular hospital. The services do not have information on the quality of care that these doctors provide.

- Some local medical societies offer lists of member doctors. Again, these lists do not have information on the quality of care that these doctors provide.

---

[9] This section has been adapted from the AHRQ:
www.ahrq.gov/consumer/qntascii/qntdr.htm.

Additional steps you can take to locate doctors include the following:

- Check with the associations listed earlier in this chapter.

- Information on doctors in some states is available on the Internet at **http://www.docboard.org**. This Web site is run by "Administrators in Medicine," a group of state medical board directors.

- The American Board of Medical Specialties can tell you if your child's doctor is board certified. "Certified" means that the doctor has completed a training program in a specialty and has passed an exam, or "board," to assess his or her knowledge, skills, and experience to provide quality patient care in that specialty. Primary care doctors may also be certified as specialists. The AMBS Web site is located at **http://www.abms.org/newsearch.asp**.[10] You can also contact the ABMS by phone at 1-866-ASK-ABMS.

- You can call the American Medical Association (AMA) at 800-665-2882 for information on training, specialties, and board certification for many licensed doctors in the United States. This information also can be found in "Physician Select" at the AMA's Web site: **http://www.ama-assn.org/aps/amahg.htm**.

Finding a Pediatrician

The American Academy of Pediatrics (AAP) mission is "to attain optimal physical, mental, and social health and well-being for all infants, children, adolescents, and young adults."[11] The AAP maintains an online pediatrician referral service which is available to the public and free of charge. This service allows you to search the AAP's database of its 55,000 members which include pediatricians, pediatric medical subspecialists, and pediatric surgical specialists practicing in the U.S., Canada, and internationally.

To access the pediatrician referral service, log on to **http://www.aap.org/referral/** and read the terms and conditions of use. Once you accept the terms, you can search for pediatricians by name, city, state, or country. All AAP members listed in the referral service database are board-certified pediatricians.

If the previous sources did not meet your needs, you may want to log on to the Web site of the National Organization for Rare Disorders (NORD) at

---

[10] While board certification is a good measure of a doctor's knowledge, it is possible to receive quality care from doctors who are not board certified.

[11] The American Academy of Pediatrics: **http://www.aap.org/**.

http://www.rarediseases.org/. NORD maintains a database of doctors with expertise in various rare medical conditions. The Metabolic Information Network (MIN), 800-945-2188, also maintains a database of physicians with expertise in various metabolic diseases.

Selecting Your Child's Doctor[12]

When you have compiled a list of prospective doctors, call each of their offices. First, ask if the doctor accepts your child's health insurance plan and if he or she is taking new patients. If the doctor is not covered by your child's plan, ask yourself if you are prepared to pay the extra costs. The next step is to schedule a visit with your first choice. During the first visit you will have the opportunity to evaluate your child's doctor and to find out if your child feels comfortable with him or her.

Working with Your Child's Doctor[13]

Research has shown that parents who have good relationships with their children's doctors tend to be more satisfied with their children's care. Here are some tips to help you and your child's doctor become partners:

- You know important things about your child's symptoms and health history. Tell the doctor what you think he or she needs to know.

- Always bring any medications your child is currently taking with you to the appointment, or you can bring a list of your child's medications including dosage and frequency information. Talk about any allergies or reactions your child has had to medications.

- Tell your doctor about any natural or alternative medicines your child is taking.

- Bring other medical information, such as x-ray films, test results, and medical records.

- Ask questions. If you don't, the doctor will assume that you understood everything that was said.

- Write down your questions before the doctor's visit. List the most important ones first to make sure that they are addressed.

_____

[12] This section has been adapted from the AHRQ:
www.ahrq.gov/consumer/qntascii/qntdr.htm.
[13] This section has been adapted from the AHRQ:
www.ahrq.gov/consumer/qntascii/qntdr.htm.

- Ask the doctor to draw pictures if you think that this will help you and your child understand.

- Take notes. Some doctors do not mind if you bring a tape recorder to help you remember things, but always ask first.

- Take information home. Ask for written instructions. Your child's doctor may also have brochures and audio and videotapes on sudden infant death syndrome.

By following these steps, you will enhance the relationship you and your child have with the physician.

Broader Health-Related Resources

In addition to the references above, the NIH has set up guidance Web sites that can help parents find healthcare professionals. These include:[14]

- Caregivers:
  http://www.nlm.nih.gov/medlineplus/caregivers.html

- Choosing a Doctor or Healthcare Service:
  http://www.nlm.nih.gov/medlineplus/choosingadoctororhealthcareserv
  ice.html

- Hospitals and Health Facilities:
  http://www.nlm.nih.gov/medlineplus/healthfacilities.html

Vocabulary Builder

The following vocabulary builder provides definitions of words used in this chapter that have not been defined in previous chapters:

Consultation: A deliberation between two or more physicians concerning the diagnosis and the proper method of treatment in a case. [NIH]

Specialist: In medicine, one who concentrates on 1 special branch of medical science. [NIH]

---

[14] You can access this information at
http://www.nlm.nih.gov/medlineplus/healthsystem.html.

PART II: ADDITIONAL RESOURCES AND ADVANCED MATERIAL

ABOUT PART II

In Part II, we introduce you to additional resources and advanced research on sudden infant death syndrome. All too often, parents who conduct their own research are overwhelmed by the difficulty in finding and organizing information. The purpose of the following chapters is to provide you an organized and structured format to help you find additional information resources on sudden infant death syndrome. In Part II, as in Part I, our objective is not to interpret the latest advances on sudden infant death syndrome or render an opinion. Rather, our goal is to give you access to original research and to increase your awareness of sources you may not have already considered. In this way, you will come across the advanced materials often referred to in pamphlets, books, or other general works. Once again, some of this material is technical in nature, so consultation with a professional familiar with sudden infant death syndrome is suggested.

CHAPTER 3. STUDIES ON SUDDEN INFANT DEATH SYNDROME

Overview

Every year, academic studies are published on sudden infant death syndrome or related conditions. Broadly speaking, there are two types of studies. The first are peer reviewed. Generally, the content of these studies has been reviewed by scientists or physicians. Peer-reviewed studies are typically published in scientific journals and are usually available at medical libraries. The second type of studies is non-peer reviewed. These works include summary articles that do not use or report scientific results. These often appear in the popular press, newsletters, or similar periodicals.

In this chapter, we will show you how to locate peer-reviewed references and studies on sudden infant death syndrome. We will begin by discussing research that has been summarized and is free to view by the public via the Internet. We then show you how to generate a bibliography on sudden infant death syndrome and teach you how to keep current on new studies as they are published or undertaken by the scientific community.

The Combined Health Information Database

The Combined Health Information Database summarizes studies across numerous federal agencies. To limit your investigation to research studies and sudden infant death syndrome, you will need to use the advanced search options. First, go to **http://chid.nih.gov/index.html**. From there, select the "Detailed Search" option (or go directly to that page with the following hyperlink: **http://chid.nih.gov/detail/detail.html**). The trick in extracting studies is found in the drop boxes at the bottom of the search page where

"You may refine your search by." Select the dates and language you prefer, and the format option "Journal Article." At the top of the search form, select the number of records you would like to see (we recommend 100) and check the box to display "whole records." We recommend that you type in "sudden infant death syndrome" (or synonyms) into the "For these words:" box. Consider using the option "anywhere in record" to make your search as broad as possible. If you want to limit the search to only a particular field, such as the title of the journal, then select this option in the "Search in these fields" drop box. The following is a sample of what you can expect from this type of search:

- **Sudden infant death syndrome..And The SIDS Building Blocks Program**

  Source: Thanatos. 19(3): 24-28. Fall 1994.

  Contact: Available from Thanatos, Florida Funeral Directors Association, P.O. Box 6009, Tallahassee, FL 32314-6009. (904) 224-1969, (800) 226-3332, (904) 224-7965 (Fax), http://www.ffda.org (Website). 4 issues per year for $16.00; $21.00 per year for subscribers outside the U.S.

  Summary: This article describes the SIDS Building Blocks Program, which is designed to attend to the bereavement needs of children who have experienced the loss of a sibling or an infant close to them as a result of a sudden, unexpected death. The article also provides an overview of **sudden infant death syndrome** (SIDS), focusing on its epidemiology; a discussion of the need to provide support for individuals affected by a SIDS death; and a description of SIDS Resources, Inc., the developers of the SIDS Building Blocks Program. The primary goal of the program is to foster an exchange between grieving children and significant adults in their lives, such as parents, relatives, school counselors, health professionals, child care providers, and funeral directors. The adults are provided with information about the role they can play in helping children cope with grief. The following services are available free of charge through the program: counseling through home visits, telephone support, peer support, a quarterly newsletter, services of a lending library, educational programs for professionals and community organizations, and support and resources for professionals. The SIDS Building Blocks Task Force was established in 1993 to develop documents to serve individuals who had contact with the children in the program. The Task Force consisted of volunteers from the community and staff members from SIDS Recources, Inc. The documents developed by the Task Force are as follows: a program description, guides for adults who want to help children cope with a SIDS death, a book of suggestions for relatives and friends of SIDS families, a guide for helping children through the funeral process, two books intended for child care providers, and a bibliography. A description is provided for each of the eight documents. 4 references.

- **Sudden Infant Death Syndrome: Police Can Make a Difference.FBI Law Enforcement Bulletin**

Source: FBI Law Enforcement Bulletin. 67(9) : 1-5. September 1998.

Contact: Available from Federal Bureau of Investigation, J. Edgar Hoover Building, 935 Pennsylvania Avenue, NW, Washington, DC 20535-0001. (202) 324-3000, http://www.fbi.gov (Web Site). You can download this publication free of charge from <http://www.fbi.gov/publications/leb/1998/sept98.pdf>.

Summary: This journal article introduces law enforcement personnel to **sudden infant death syndrome** (SIDS) and sets forth some basic guidelines for officers to follow when responding to and investigating a possible SIDS case. One of the authors is a policeman who responded to an emergency call of an infant not breathing in February 1982. The victim was diagnosed as dying of SIDS. The officer recalls that he attended the infant's funeral, but on the night of the death, he did not document any of his observations of the death scene or additional information given by the family, actions that today are mandatory in states that have child death investigation laws. Following some basic information on the incidence and risk factors for SIDS, the article discusses the differential diagnosis of SIDS and child abuse. Although only qualified medical officials can diagnose SIDS, it can aid the investigation if the on-scene officers become familiar with the facts regarding SIDS and how SIDS cases compare to child abuse. Physically, most SIDS infants show no external signs of injury, whereas abused infants may exhibit bruises, bumps, cuts, welts, scars, signs of head trauma, or broken bones. Most SIDS infants will appear well-developed and well-nourished, while abused infants often show signs of malnourishment and neglect. Still, certain bodily appearances typically occur in SIDS cases due to the death process. Officers may notice discoloration of the skin, settling of the blood, frothy drainage from the nose or mouth that may be blood-tinged, and cooling rigor mortis. Parents of SIDS victims typically relate stories of placing their infants to sleep in the crib only to find them lifeless later. In child abuse cases, the parents' stories may sound suspicious or may not account for all the injuries to the child. Officers at the scene can help the investigation by carefully recording their observations, including the position of the infant when found, the presence of any bedding or other objects in the crib, any dangerous items in the room, any medications the child was taking, as well as room temperature and air quality. All first responders need to be good listeners. If they need more information, they can ask open-ended, nonjudgmental questions. By being sympathetic interviewers, officers will obtain the information they need while being respectful of the family's feelings. Each member of the family may react differently to the death, and in contrast to the way to officer would act. Officers need to maintain objectivity and avoid making hasty conclusions based on the family's reactions. Officers should support the family in any way they can, and keep them informed of the procedures that need to take place. They should make sure the parents get to the hospital, and that other children are taken care of at home. It is imperative that police officers and other first responders are trained to respond appropriately to possible SIDS deaths. Their observations and attention to detail could provide valuable information to researchers who are trying to find the cause of SIDS and other sudden infant and child deaths.

Federally Funded Research on Sudden Infant Death Syndrome

The U.S. Government supports a variety of research studies relating to sudden infant death syndrome and associated conditions. These studies are tracked by the Office of Extramural Research at the National Institutes of Health.[15] CRISP (Computerized Retrieval of Information on Scientific Projects) is a searchable database of federally funded biomedical research projects conducted at universities, hospitals, and other institutions. Visit CRISP at **http://crisp.cit.nih.gov/crisp/crisp_query.generate_screen**. You can perform targeted searches by various criteria including geography, date, as well as topics related to sudden infant death syndrome and related conditions.

For most of the studies, the agencies reporting into CRISP provide summaries or abstracts. As opposed to clinical trial research using patients, many federally funded studies use animals or simulated models to explore sudden infant death syndrome and related conditions. In some cases, therefore, it may be difficult to understand how some basic or fundamental research could eventually translate into medical practice. The following sample is typical of the type of information found when searching the CRISP database for sudden infant death syndrome:

---

[15] Healthcare projects are funded by the National Institutes of Health (NIH), Substance Abuse and Mental Health Services (SAMHSA), Health Resources and Services Administration (HRSA), Food and Drug Administration (FDA), Centers for Disease Control and Prevention (CDCP), Agency for Healthcare Research and Quality (AHRQ), and Office of Assistant Secretary of Health (OASH).

- **Project Title: AAV VECTOR DELIVERY TO SKELETAL MUSCLE, PLATFORM FOR THERAPEUTIC PROTEIN DELIVERY**

Principal Investigator & Institution: Flotte, Terence R.; Professor; University of Florida Gainesville, Fl 32611

Timing: Fiscal Year 2002; Project Start 30-SEP-2002; Project End 31-AUG-2003

Summary: Syndrome (SIDS) or with a combined cardiac and skeletal myopathy. Treatment of these disorders has consisted primarily of dietary manipulation and has been far less than optimal to this point. The recent development of recombinant adeno-associated virus (rAAV) vectors for highly efficient transduction of hepatocytes and myofibers present new tools for the study of FAO disorders. Specifically, our laboratory has produced rAAV vectors expressing FAO enzymes whose deficiency results in myopathy, such as short-chain acyl CoA dehydrogenase (SCAD) and long-chain acyl CoA dehydrogenase (LCAD). Human cell lines from patients deficient in these enzymes are available, and mutant mouse models exist for both of these disorders. We propose to utilize rAAV vectors expressing FAO enzymes in an attempt to unravel the pathobiology of FAO disorders and to better define endpoints for molecular or cell-based therapies of these disorders. This will be accomplished in three specific aims: (1) To assess the extent to which genetic correction of a limited percentage of SCAD deficient or LCAD deficient cells within a cell population or organ can affect biochemical correction of fatty acid oxidation. (2) To determine whether receptor binding and entry are limiting steps for stable transduction by rAAV in a intact mammalian liver or muscle bundle. (3) To test the hypothesis that the liver pathology observed in LCAD and VLCAD deficiencies are secondary to the accumulation of toxic metabolites as opposed to primary energy failure within hepatocytes. (4) To determine whether global phenotypic correction of FAO deficiency in mice is more effective after widespread vector delivery after intrauterine or neonatal IV injection. The information gained from these studies could also be used to guide the feasibility of other organ-directed therapies, potentially including stem cell transplantation.

Website: http://crisp.cit.nih.gov/crisp/Crisp_Query.Generate_Screen

- **Project Title: CALCIUM SIGNALING IN DEVELOPING CAROTID CHEMORECEPTORS**

Principal Investigator & Institution: Sterni, Laura M.; Pediatrics; Johns Hopkins University 3400 N Charles St Baltimore, Md 21218

Timing: Fiscal Year 2002; Project Start 01-JAN-1998; Project End 31-DEC-2002

Summary: (Adapted from applicants' abstract) Dr. Laura Sterni, the PI, is an assistant professor who completed her pediatric pulmonary fellowship in 1996. In this application she outlines a program to study proposed mechanisms by which the carotid chemoreceptors increase their sensitivity in early postnatal life. The carotid chemoreceptors are oxygen sensors which are almost entirely responsible for driving the ventilatory response to hypoxia. Their sensitivity is weak at birth and requires the first few days to weeks of life to reset, increase their sensitivity to hypoxia, and assume the role of defending the infant from hypoxic stress. An understanding of the mechanisms involved in this postnatal resetting is likely to be important in understanding the pathogenesis of many disorders of neonatal respiratory control, including the **Sudden Infant Death Syndrome** (SIDS), the number one killer of infants over one month of age in the United States. The PI's fellowship project demonstrated that maturation of carotid chemoreceptor sensitivity to oxygen is due, at least in part, to changes within the chemosensory type I cell. These cells respond to stimuli with an increase in cytoplasmic calcium ($[Ca2+]c$) which then triggers neurotransmitter release. Type I cells isolated from mature animals had a significantly greater $[Ca2+]c$ response to hypoxia and anoxia than cells isolated from newborns. These studies will investigate the role of intracellular Ca2+ stores in maturation of the $[Ca2+]c$ response of type I cells to hypoxia. The hypotheses that will be tested are: (1) in the mature carotid chemoreceptor cell, intracellular Ca2+ stores modulate the rise in $[Ca2+]c$ produced by voltage gated calcium entry; (2) the effect of the intracellular Ca2+ stores on the type I cell's hypoxia response changes during postnatal maturation; and (3) carotid chemoreceptor resetting is mediated partly by withdrawal of dopaminergic stimulation on Ca2+ influx and Ca2+ stores. The PI will take advantage of the strong mentoring, significant protected research time and the outstanding academic resources of the Johns Hopkins Medical Institutions to reach her goal of becoming an independent investigator in this important field.

Website: http://crisp.cit.nih.gov/crisp/Crisp_Query.Generate_Screen

- **Project Title: CARDIAC CHANNEL MUTATIONS IN SIDS**

Principal Investigator & Institution: Ackerman, Michael J.; Assistant Professor; Mayo Clinic Coll of Medicine, Rochester 200 1St St Sw Rochester, Mn 55905

Timing: Fiscal Year 2002; Project Start 07-JUN-2002; Project End 31-MAY-2006

Summary: (provided by applicant): Michael J. Ackerman, M.D., Ph.D. is a board eligible pediatric cardiologist and an Assistant Professor of

Medicine, Pediatrics, and Molecular Pharmacology & Experimental Therapeutics at Mayo Medical School. Dr. Ackerman is a physician-scientist directing a sudden death genomics laboratory and the Long QT Syndrome Clinic. His long-term objectives are to identify the underlying causes of sudden cardiac death in infants, children, adolescents, and young adults. In this proposal entitled Cardiac Channel Mutations in **Sudden Infant Death Syndrome,** the applicant sets forth to answer the fundamental question: what percentage of infants suffering a SIDS death possessed putative disease-causing mutations in the genes encoding their cardiac ion channels? Presently, SIDS continues to claim nearly 3000 apparently healthy infants each year in the United States. The fundamental causes underlying SIDS remain poorly understood. In specific aim 1, Dr. Ackerman will perform a mutational analysis of the 5 cardiac channel genes already implicated in a human arrhythmia syndrome, namely congenital long QT syndrome using temperature modulated heteroduplex analysis and denaturing high performance liquid chromatography. In specific aim 2, two non-LQTS arrhythmia syndrome ion channel genes will be investigated by mutational analysis as novel candidate SIDS genes. Finally, in specific aim 3, the possible mutations in the channel genes identified in aims 1 and 2 will be characterized functionally. These mutations will be engineered by site-directed mutagenesis into the wild type channel, expressed in transient and stable transfection cell lines, and characterized using single electrode patch clamp technologies. If the applicant's hypothesis is correct that 10% of infants with SIDS possess cardiac channel mutations, then cardiac channel genes would account for the "underlying vulnerability" for the largest identifiable subset of infants to date. Such a discovery could have significant implications on attempts to further reduce the incidence of SIDS in our country and throughout the world.

Website: http://crisp.cit.nih.gov/crisp/Crisp_Query.Generate_Screen

- **Project Title: CAROTID BODY EXCITATION--NEW CONCEPT**

Principal Investigator & Institution: Shirahata, Machiko; Associate Scientist; Environmental Health Sciences; Johns Hopkins University 3400 N Charles St Baltimore, Md 21218

Timing: Fiscal Year 2002; Project Start 05-JUL-1999; Project End 30-JUN-2004

Summary: (Applicant's abstract): The carotid body is a major chemoreceptor organ whose excitation causes reflex responses in cardiopulmonary, renal and endocrine systems. Although the mechanisms of carotid body excitation are not yet clear, essential steps include the depolarization of chemosensitive glomus cells, the increase in glomus cell intracellular calcium and the release of neurotransmitters. Many studies point to the involvement of oxygen-sensitive potassium channels, but a causal relationship between the inhibition of these channels and the depolarization of glomus cells during hypoxia has not yet been established. Since cat glomus cells release acetylcholine even under normoxic/normocapnic conditions, we hypothesize that hypoxia augments the activity of neuronal nicotinic acetylcholine receptors and/or enhances the sensitivity of acetylcholine receptors for acetylcholine. This initiates the depolarization of glomus cells and the increase in intracellular calcium. Oxygen-sensitive potassium channels and voltage-gated calcium channels participate in the later phase of the changes. Preliminary data have shown that: 1) cat glomus cells expressed alpha-4 subunit containing nicotinic acetylcholine receptors, 2) acetylcholine-induced inward current and carotid body neural output were enhanced by a mild decrease in oxygen tension from normoxic levels, 3) acetylcholine increased calcium of carotid body cells, 4) oxygen-sensitive potassium current was linearly inhibited by decreasing oxygen, and 5) increased carotid body neural output in hypoxia was inhibited by L-type voltage gated calcium channels. Specific aims are to investigate: 1) the role of acetylcholine and nicotinic acetylcholine receptors for initiating the depolarization of glomus cells and the increase in calcium, 2) the contribution of oxygen sensitive potassium channels in the late phase of glomus cell depolarization during hypoxia, 3) the contribution of voltage gated calcium channels to the late phase of the calcium increase in glomus cells during hypoxia. Patch clamp, microfluorometric, and immunocytochemical techniques are to be used. This innovative proposal will advance the understanding of the excitation mechanisms of glomus cells. Once the chemotransductive mechanisms are understood, pharmacological or genetic tools can be developed to alter the carotid body function to levels desirable for treating carotid body related pathological conditions such as **sudden infant death syndrome** and hemodynamic changes in sleep apnea patients.

Website: http://crisp.cit.nih.gov/crisp/Crisp_Query.Generate_Screen

- **Project Title: CELLULAR & CLINICAL PHENOTYPES OF NOVEL SCN5A MUTATIONS**

Principal Investigator & Institution: Makielski, Jonathan C.; Professor of Medicine and Physiology; Medicine; University of Wisconsin Madison 750 University Ave Madison, Wi 53706

Timing: Fiscal Year 2003; Project Start 15-SEP-2003; Project End 31-AUG-2007

Summary: (provided by applicant): SCN5A encodes the alpha subunit of the human voltage-dependent Na channel (hNaV1.5) found in heart. We have made the novel observation that up to four very common variants of NaV1.5 exist in human heart and at least some have functional implications. Mutations in this channel also cause sudden cardiac death in the congenitally acquired long QT syndrome (LQT3) and the Brugada Syndrome (BS). We have recently characterized four novel SCN5A mutations and found: 1) Two in **Sudden Infant Death Syndrome** (A997S, R1826H) are LQT3.2) LQT3 (M1766L) and BS (G1743) mutations have expression defects "rescued" by antiarrhythmic drugs. 3) M1766L has normal or absent current depending on the variant NaV1.5 background used to test it. We propose to investigate further the extent and mechanisms of expression defects and their "rescue" and the importance of "background". Through collaboration with Dr. Ackerman at Mayo Clinic we also have >20 additional novel SCN5A mutations to investigate for novel functional defects and arrhythrnia mechanism. We will make and express these channels in cell culture, define function by voltage clamp and immunocytochemistry, and correlate molecular function with clinical phenotype through arrhythmia mechanism. In Aim 1 we will investigate the expression and function of wild type variants, and also how mutant channel expression and function depends upon the background clone. In Aim 2 we will study novel mutants. In Aim 3 we will investigate mutants with "gain of function" and test the hypothesis that late current decay in LQT3 correlates with enhanced rate dependent QT interval adaptation, later onset, and better prognosis than mutations without late current decay. In Aim 4 we will investigate mutations with "loss of function", the mechanism for loss of function including novel trafficking defects, and test the hypothesis that this loss can be "rescued" by drugs. In Aim 5 we will co-express mutations with the beta1 and beta3 subunit, and assess effects of PKA stimulation, to test the hypothesis that these areas are critical to the mechanism of action. These studies on the novel findings will have implications for arrhythmia mechanism and genotype-phenotype correlation in both mutation arrhythmia syndromes and more generally for the variants in "normal' hearts that may generate insight into genetic predisposition to acquired arrhythmia. At a more basic level these "natural" experiments will contribute to understanding the structure-function relationship of this important channel.

Website: http://crisp.cit.nih.gov/crisp/Crisp_Query.Generate_Screen

- **Project Title: CELLULAR MECHANISMS OF MEDULLARY SEROTONERGIC NEURONS DURING DEVELOPMENT**

Principal Investigator & Institution: Richerson, George B.; Associate Professor; Children's Hospital (Boston) Boston, Ma 021155737

Timing: Fiscal Year 2003; Project Start 07-JUL-2003; Project End 31-MAR-2008

Summary: The overall goal of this program is to define the cause of SIDS. With the recent discovery of abnormal LSD binding in the medulla of SIDS infants, we have focused our efforts on the medullary serotonergic system, to define what specifically happens to serotonergic neurons to cause them to malfunction. The goal of Project 5 is to define the cellular properties of serotonergic neurons, as a means of providing a neurobiological explanation for the link between serotonin and SIDS. We have previously demonstrated that serotenergic neurons closely apposed to large arteries in the rat ventral medulla increase their firing rate in response to acidosis, and we have proposed that they are chemoreceptors that stimulete breathing, arousal and other CNS changes to restore pH homeostasis: We now plan to use a rat model to determine whether the cellular properties of serotonergic neurons can explain the three risk factors in the Triple Risk Model for SIDS. We wiil use a combination of multielectrode arrays and patch clamp recordings from serotonergic neurons in culture and in brain slices. We will: 1) Study how different subsets of serotonergic neuron respond to acidosis, hypoxia, temperature and glucose. 2) Examine how muscarinic receptor activation leads to enhancement of chemoreception. 3) Define the changes in chemosensitity of serotonergic neurons as they undergo development. 4) Determine the effects of acute and chronic (during pregnancy) nicotine exposure on the function of serotonergic neurons. 5) Compare the cellular properties of serotonergic neurons from rats with those of piglets and mice, and determine whether serotonergic neurons from these species, as well as human infants, are closely associated with large arteries of the ventral medulla. These experiments will provide information critical to a full understanding of the role of serotonergic neurons in brain function, and will lead to specific testable hypotheses about how their malfunction or maldevelopment could lead to death during sleep. URimately, the results of these experiments may provide important insights that could lead to diagnostic and therapeutic tests for those infants at highest risk of SIDS.

Website: http://crisp.cit.nih.gov/crisp/Crisp_Query.Generate_Screen

- **Project Title: COCAINE EXPOSED INFANTS--CARDIAC PROBLEMS AND OUTCOME**

  Principal Investigator & Institution: Mehta, Sudhir K.;; Case Western Reserve University 10900 Euclid Ave Cleveland, Oh 44106

  Timing: Fiscal Year 2002; Project Start 01-DEC-2001; Project End 30-NOV-2002

Summary: Infants born to mother who use cocaine during pregnancy have greater morbidity and a higher rate of sudden death. The etiology of sudden death is unclear. Preliminary observations suggest the presence of multiple cardiovascular abnormalities such as greater left ventricular mass, persistent hypertension, greater prevalence of ST segment elevations and higher vagal tone. To study the cardiovascular effects on in-utero cocaine exposure the study has the following aims: to detect the cardiovasculaar abnormalities in the newborn period; to evaluate the relationship of cord blood plasma cholinesterase activity and the above abnormalities; and to study the natural history of these abnormalities during the first 2 months of life.

Website: http://crisp.cit.nih.gov/crisp/Crisp_Query.Generate_Screen

- **Project Title: COLLABORATIVE HOME INFANT MONITORING EVALUATION (CHIME)**

  Principal Investigator & Institution: Martin, Richard J.; Professor; Case Western Reserve University 10900 Euclid Ave Cleveland, Oh 44106

  Timing: Fiscal Year 2002; Project Start 01-DEC-2001; Project End 30-NOV-2002

  Summary: This protocol is a multicenter collaborative trial of Home Infant Apnea Monitors. These devices are used to monitor breathing and heart rate in infants thought to be at risk for SIDS as well as normal controls. This study will yield extensive descriptive information regarding the efficacy of apnea monitors, their accuracy, and the ability of these devices to detect clinically important events. The follow-up of the infants continues until approximately age 1.5 yrs. The GCRC Psychometrists assist with the developmental assessments.

  Website: http://crisp.cit.nih.gov/crisp/Crisp_Query.Generate_Screen

- **Project Title: COLLABORATIVE HOME INFANT MONITORING EVALUATION (CHIME)**

  Principal Investigator & Institution: Corwin, Michael J.; Epidemiology and Biostatistics; Boston University Medical Campus 715 Albany St, 560 Boston, Ma 02118

  Timing: Fiscal Year 2002; Project Start 30-SEP-1991; Project End 31-AUG-2002

  Summary: (Adapted from applicant's description): This is an application for continued participation as the Data Coordinating and Analysis Center in an extended Collaborative Home Infant Monitoring Evaluation (CHIME) Study over the next five years. Each year, approximately 50,000 infants are placed on a home cardiorespiratory (CR) monitor. Monitors are typically prescribed for infants in one of three groups at increased risk for **Sudden Infant Death Syndrome** (SIDS): infants who experience an idiopathic apparent life-threatening event (apnea of infancy, AO1), SIDS siblings, and preterm infants. Despite years of experience, it is not known to what extent monitor use has reduced either infant morbidity or mortality. The CHIME study is designed to address the unresolved questions regarding who has CR events at home, the nature of these events, and their impact on neurodevelopmental outcome. We propose a 5-year extension of the CHIME study in order to complete enrollment, follow-up, and data analysis. A total of 2,115 infants will be enrolled: 375 healthy term infants, 330 SIDS siblings, 330 with AO1, and 1,080 preterm infants < 1750 g birth weight. Each infant will receive an overnight polysonogram and will be monitored at home for 4-5 months using a memory monitor developed for the CHIME study. The monitor will store all CR events occurring at home and the associated oxygen saturation and sleep position, will record periodic non-event (normative) intervals, and will continuously record R-R and breath-to-breath intervals. Apneas will be categorized as central, mixed or obstructive by the use of inductance plethysmography, a technique not previously available for home monitoring. Clinical and neurodevelopmental status will be ascertained longitudinally through 1 year of age. The CHIME study will create a comprehensive summary of the full range of CR events occurring in the home. The results will yield important insights regarding underlying mechanisms, antecedent variables predictive of events, appropriate intervention strategies, and the relationship between CR events and neurodevelopmental outcome.

Website: http://crisp.cit.nih.gov/crisp/Crisp_Query.Generate_Screen

- **Project Title: COMPARATIVE CHEMICAL ANATOMY OF THE VENTRAL MEDULLA**

  Principal Investigator & Institution: Filiano, James J.;; Children's Hospital (Boston) Boston, Ma 021155737

  Timing: Fiscal Year 2002

  Summary: The overall hypothesis of the Program Project is that SIDS is due to developmental abnormalities of the ventral medulla that interfere with protective cardiorespiratory responses to potentially life-threatening, but often occurring, events during sleep, such as hypoxia, hypercapnia, and apnea. In the context of the Program Project, Project IV will attempt to characterize the cyto-and chemoarchitecture of the ventral medulla of the piglet and human infant. The over-riding concept of the project is that the ventral medullary surface contains clusters of small neurons that are cytologically and neurochemically homogenous and thus form a unified class of neurons; and that his class of neurons provides a common influence on autonomic modulation, chemoreception, and cardiopulmonary coupling, although the specific role of each cluster of neurons varies in accordance with its specific somatotopic connections. First, we will test the hypothesis that, in the piglet, the small ventral neurons of the raphe pallidus, the most superficial parapyramidal neurons, and the retrotrapezoid neurons, belong to the unified class of neurons as evidenced by being cytoarchitectonically identical and expressing the same neurotransmitters and neurotransmitter receptors. Second, we will test the hypothesis that, based on cytoarchitectonic and chemoarchitectonic criteria, the human arcuate nucleus is homologous to the small ventral neurons of the piglet raphe pallidus, the piglet superficial parapyramidal nucleus, and the piglet retrotrapezoid nucleus. We will employ the traditional approach of comparative neuroanatomy by testing if neurons in both species share common cell morphology, express common receptors and share common immunohistochemical staining characteristics. Morphologic studies will employ Neurobiotin/R and standard staining methods; autoradiographic studies will test for expression for receptors for glutamate, serotonin, GABA, somatostatin, and acetylcholine (muscarinic); immunohistochemical studies will test for expression of choline acetyltransferase, tyrosine hydroxylase, glutamate decarboxylase, glutamate, substance P, cholecystokinin, and thyrotropin releasing hormone. It is goal of Project IV to develop a comparative anatomic framework that will help the physiologic studies in Projects I-III shed light on the potential significance of arcuate nucleus abnormalities reported in SIDS victims. Ultimately, this neuroanatomic framework may be useful to establish a model for SIDS in the developing piglet based on impaired behavioral and ventilatory responses to asphyxial rebreathing induced by dysfunction of the piglet arcuate homologue.

Website: http://crisp.cit.nih.gov/crisp/Crisp_Query.Generate_Screen

- **Project Title: CONTROL OF BREATHING DURING PHYSIOLOGIC CONDITIONS**

Principal Investigator & Institution: Forster, Hubert V.; Professor; Physiology; Medical College of Wisconsin Po Box26509 Milwaukee, Wi 532260509

Timing: Fiscal Year 2002; Project Start 01-JUN-1986; Project End 31-MAY-2005

Summary: Several theories on the neural control of breathing that were based on data from reduced preparations were not supported by our recent findings in awake and asleep goats on the effects of rostral medullary neuronal dysfunction and/or carotid body denervation (CBD). Some findings mimicked the altered breathing found in obstructive sleep apnea (OSA) and congenital central hypoventilation syndrome (CCHS). The mechanisms that mediated these effects are not established, but one likely mechanism is through intracranial chemoreceptors for years thought to exist only near the ventral medullary surface (including the retrotrapezoid nucleus RTN)). However, findings in reduced preparations of chemoreceptors at widespread brain sites have raised questions related to the location and role of chemoreceptors that affect breathing in awake and asleep states and whether brain chemoreceptor sensitivity is altered by CBD. One recently identified site of chemoreception is the medullary raphe nuclei (MRN) whose role in the control of breathing during awake and asleep states remains speculative. Accordingly, to study chemosensitivity and the role of the RTN and MRN in the control of breathing, we will implant microtubules into these nuclei of goats to: a) create a focal acidosis by dialysis of mock cerebrospinal fluid with different PCO2's, or b) induce neuronal dysfunction through injection of glutamate or serotonin receptor antagonists or agonists, or a neurotoxin. Major hypotheses are: 1) focal acidosis (equivalent to that breathing 7 percent inspired CO2, delta brain pH approximately -.05) in the RTN will increase breathing in awake, but not asleep states, while acidosis in the MRN will increase breathing in asleep, but not awake states, 2) at RTN sites where focal acidosis increases breathing, neuronal dysfunction will attenuate whole body CO2 sensitivity, but not alter rest and exercise breathing, 3) neuronal dysfunction in the MRN will attenuate CO2 sensitivity and rest and exercise breathing, 4) during the first 10 days after CBD, the effect of RTN and MRN focal acidosis will be attenuated but 15 plus days after CBD, the effect of focal acidosis will be accentuated. and 5) at most RTN and MRN sites, the acute effects of neurotoxic lesions will be hypoventilation (rest and exercise) and attenuated CO2 sensitivity; the acute effects of these lesions will be greater in CBD than in intact goats, but recovery after lesioning will be greater in intact than in CBD goats. Our unique studies are important because hypotheses generated largely from reduced preparations will be tested in awake and asleep states to enhance the understanding of medullary chemoreceptor contribution to the control of breathing and how abnormalities in this contribution may underlie diseases such as OSA, CCHS, and the **Sudden infant death syndrome.**

Website: http://crisp.cit.nih.gov/crisp/Crisp_Query.Generate_Screen

- **Project Title: CONTROL OF BREATHING IN RECOVERY FROM APNEA**

Principal Investigator & Institution: Thach, Bradley T.; Professor; Pediatrics; Washington University Lindell and Skinker Blvd St. Louis, Mo 63130

Timing: Fiscal Year 2002; Project Start 30-SEP-1977; Project End 31-MAY-2004

Summary: The **Sudden Infant Death Syndrome** (SIDS) remains a leading cause of infant deaths inspite of recent highly successful public health interventions designed to reduce SIDS risks (The U.S. "Back to Sleep" campaign, "BTS"). We propose to study several physiologic and neuro-developmental mechanisms potentially involved in the etiology of SIDS, as well as, pertinent environmental factors. The research will focus on three areas. In the first of these, we plan to study the physiology of recovery from severe hypoxia by gasping (autoresuscitation, AR). These studies will determine if the previously documented developmentally acquired defect in AR, originally described in SWR mice, is present in other inbred strains and species and, furthermore, if underlying mechanisms causing AR failure are similar to those in SWR mice. Additionally, the effects of increased environmental temperature on AR will be evaluated. Also, Home apnea monitor recordings of infants dying suddenly and unexpectedly while being monitored will be studied to determine if there is evidence of attempted AR and if so, potential reasons for its failure. The second part of our studies will be directed to prospectively obtaining data on the case history, death scene and postmortem examination of infant's dying with the diagnoses of SIDS, accidental suffocation and "cause of death undetermined" in the St. Louis metropolitan area. The aim is to determine how many of these deaths are preventable by public acceptance of current "BTS" guidelines and how many might be prevented by future additions or changes in the recommendations to child caretakers. In connection with this study, we will perform special death scene investigations in certain SIDS and accidental suffocation deaths combined with laboratory death scene reconstruction studies in order to determine if additional simple guidelines for parents and child equipment manufactures can be formulated in order to prevent infant deaths. Finally, we will study development of the infant's ability to avoid potentially suffocating environments during sleep, and determine the potential role of the infant's past experience on this development.

Website: http://crisp.cit.nih.gov/crisp/Crisp_Query.Generate_Screen

- **Project Title: DENSE ARRAY EEG FOR NEONATAL SLEEP MONITORING**

  Principal Investigator & Institution: Tucker, Don M.; Ceo/Chief Scientist; Electrical Geodesics, Inc. 1850 Millrace Dr, Ste 3 Eugene, or 97403

  Timing: Fiscal Year 2002; Project Start 01-MAY-2002; Project End 31-OCT-2002

  Summary: (provided by applicant): Electroencephalography is a safe, noninvasive technique for monitoring neonatal brain function. Acute and long-term EEG monitoring of infants has clinical utility for evaluating the effects of hypoxic ischemic insults and detecting the presence of epileptic activity. The information available in neonatal EEG can be greatly enhanced by using an adequate number of electrodes to accurately map the spatial distribution of the EEG without spatial aliasing. The Geodesic Neonatal EEG Brain Monitor will be designed from experimental studies and theoretical simulations of the required sampling density for scalp potentials on the infant head. Dense Array EEG methods will be developed that incorporate the unique features of infant skull anatomy to estimate the potentials in the brain of the infant. The Geodesic Neonatal EEG Brain Monitor system will be adapted for a variety of clinical uses, initially focusing on monitoring brain function in sleep in the Neonatal Intensive Care Unit (NICU). This monitoring will examine both normal and pathological sleep states of the neonate, providing information on the maturation of arousal control in preterm and full term infants that may be important in understanding **sudden infant death syndrome.** PROPOSED COMMERCIAL APPLICATION: Behavioral outcome studies indicate that brain function is often at risk in the neonatal intensive care unit. An inexpensive, high-resolution neonatal brain state monitor could guide medical management to support brain health and therefore improve neurological and psychological outcome in many infants.

  Website: http://crisp.cit.nih.gov/crisp/Crisp_Query.Generate_Screen

- **Project Title: DEVELOPMENT OF HYPOGLOSSAL MOTONEURON PROPERTIES**

  Principal Investigator & Institution: Berger, Albert J.; Professor; Physiology and Biophysics; University of Washington Grant & Contract Services Seattle, Wa 98105

  Timing: Fiscal Year 2002; Project Start 01-JAN-1993; Project End 30-JUN-2006

  Summary: (provided by applicant): Our long-term objective is to understand postnatal development of fast ligand-gated inhibitory (both GABAergic) and glycinergic) synaptic transmission to an important class of respiratory motoneurons, the hypoglossal motoneurons (HM). HMs innervate the tongue and therefore are important in the regulation of upper airway patency. The upper airway is a site of airway obstruction; thus a full understanding of the development of synaptic inhibition to HMs may provide new insights into certain pathologic states, including apnea of prematurity, **Sudden Infant Death Syndrome** and obstructive sleep apnea. The experiments proposed use two different in vitro brainstem slice preparations. In one rat, HMs will be visualized and studied with whole-cell and outside patch recordings in the absence of respiratory rhythm. The other uses the mouse rhythmic medullary slice preparation to study short-time-scale synchronization of inspiratory-phase HM activity. Specific Aim 1 proposes to investigate developmental changes that occur in GABAergic synaptic currents in HMs, as well as in single GABAA receptor channel properties. We hypothesize that developmental changes in GABAergic synaptic transmission are due to changes in properties of this ligand-gated ion channel. Specific Aim 1 proposes to investigate developmental changes and mechanisms for modulation by EtOH of GABAergic synaptic transmission to HMs. We hypothesize that in HMs the potentiation of GABAergic synaptic events by EtOH is due to altered single channel kinetics of GABAA-Rs. Specific Aim 3 proposes to investigate the postnatal developmental changes that occur in GABAA presynaptic receptor inhibition of GABAergic and glycinergic synaptic transmission. We hypothesize that this inhibition is dependent on postnatal age and is significantly enhanced in older HMs. In Specific Aim 4 we propose to investigate, in the rhythmic medullary slice preparation, short-time-scale synchronous HM inspiratory-phase activity, and to determine the role of GABAA-R and glycine-R activation in the postnatal development of this activity. We hypothesize that changes in sub-unit composition of both these receptors and intracellular chloride ion regulation leads to effects upon short-time-scale HM synchronized activity that are developmentally dependent.

Website: http://crisp.cit.nih.gov/crisp/Crisp_Query.Generate_Screen

- **Project Title: DEVELOPMENT OF SLEEP HOMEOSTASIS IN THE DEVELOPING RAT**

Principal Investigator & Institution: Heller, H Craig.; Professor and Chair; Biological Sciences; Stanford University Stanford, Ca 94305

Timing: Fiscal Year 2002; Project Start 03-JUL-1998; Project End 31-MAY-2004

Summary: (Adapted from applicant's abstract): This proposal will investigate the development of homeostatic sleep mechanisms and emergence of distinct arousal states in the neonatal rat. Arousal states cannot be identified by EEG parameters early in postnatal development, thus, arousal states in neonates are defined behaviorally as active sleep (AS) and quiet sleep (QS). AS and QS are generally considered homologous to REM and NREM sleep in adults, however, we found that EEG slow wave activity (SWA) occurs as often during AS as it does in QS at postnatal day 12 (P12). Thus, AS may not be an immature form of adult REM sleep, rather, it may be an undifferentiated state of the nervous system out of which NREM sleep emerges first and REM sleep second. We will test this hypothesis by determining when additional physiological parameters (e.g., respiratory patterns, electro-oculogram (EOG), brain and skin temperatures, and myoclonia) coalesce and form identifiable arousal states. We have developed a system for simultaneous recording of EEG, EMG, and behavioral sleep (by videotape) in neonatal rats continuously from P12 to P30. We found that adult-like responses to sleep deprivation (SD) were not present until P24; prior to that age, SD elicits increases in total sleep time (TST) without affecting the intensity or amount of SWA. From P12-P24, SWA increases progressively beyond adult levels, yet is not affected by SD. Thus, critical components of adult sleep homeostatic mechanisms must be absent prior to P24. Convergent lines of evidence support a role for adenosine in regulating SWA; however, its link to homeostatic mechanisms is unknown. We found that the adenosine A~ receptor agonist, N6-Cyclopentyladenosine (CPA), mimics the effects of SD in both adult and neonatal rats. Furthermore, CPA elicits SWA at ages (P16 and P20) when 3 h of SD have no effect on SWA. Thus, A1 receptors are present and functional but apparently not activated by SD. This proposal will investigate arousal state emergence, development of sleep homeostasis, and adenosinergic regulation of sleep homeostasis in neonatal rats. These studies will contribute significantly toward clinical studies on **sudden infant death syndrome** (SIDS) because they investigate the mechanisms by which arousal and, hence, failure to arouse, from sleep develop.

Website: http://crisp.cit.nih.gov/crisp/Crisp_Query.Generate_Screen

- **Project Title: DEVELOPMENTAL CONTROL OF THE DIAPHRAGM AND UPPER AIRWAYS**

Principal Investigator & Institution: Cameron, William E.; Associate Professor; Physiology and Pharmacology; Oregon Health & Science University Portland, or 972393098

Timing: Fiscal Year 2002; Project Start 01-FEB-1999; Project End 31-JAN-2004

Summary: (Adapted from the applicant's abstract): This proposal will characterize the postnatal development of the genioglossal and phrenic motoneurons, by correlating physiological changes in membrane conductance and spiking properties with changes in anatomy. The strength of respiratory muscle contraction is determined by the number of respiratory motoneurons activated and their rate of discharge. Both the order in which the neurons are activated and their discharge rates are a function of their resting conductance, that is, the number of membrane channels open at any given time. Most membrane channels are controlled by neurotransmitters and/or by the intrinsic electrical state of the cell membrane. The change in the balance of these two processes are most dramatic during postnatal development. The applicant is interested in these processes that occur in the two respiratory motoneurons that affect the performance of the diaphragm and genioglossus. Activation of these two muscles must be coordinated to move air into the lungs with the least effort; this may be particularly relevant to the pathophysiology of **Sudden Infant Death Syndrome** (SIDS). In the past period, the applicant established that glycine significantly contributed to the increase in resting membrane conductance that occurs at 3 weeks, and that these age-related increases in resting conductance result from an increase in the number of open potassium channels. The proposed studies will be performed on genioglossal and phrenic motoneurons in slice preparations of the rat brainstem and spinal cord. Visually identified motoneurons will be studied from four different age groups (1-2, 5-7, 13-15 and 19-22 days) with a combination of patch-clamp recording, three-dimensional neuronal reconstruction and immunocytochemical localization of certain receptors and ion channels. The application will: 1) examine the anatomy and physiology of glycine, GABA, and glutamate neurotransmitter systems at the four stages during postnatal development; 2) identify specific potassium channels that contribute to the increase in membrane conductance and spike characteristics; and 3) explore the intracellular pathways mediating the enhanced potassium conductance.

Website: http://crisp.cit.nih.gov/crisp/Crisp_Query.Generate_Screen

- **Project Title: EFFECTS OF PRENATAL EXPOSURE TO NICOTINE ON PRIMATE LUNG DEVELOPMENT**

Principal Investigator & Institution: Spindel, Eliot R.; Senior Scientist; Oregon Health & Science University Portland, or 972393098

Timing: Fiscal Year 2002

Summary: The deleterious effects of maternal smoking during pregnancy are well established. Maternal smoking is the major preventable cause of intrauterine growth retardation and prematurity. Perhaps less well appreciated, is the recent, strong evidence, that smoking during pregnancy directly and adversely affects lung development. Respiratory problems associated with in utero tobacco exposure include decreased lung function, increased respiratory diseases and increased incidence of **sudden infant death syndrome** (SIDS). Given the unfortunate prevalence of smoking during pregnancy and the resulting serious consequences, it is of major importance to understand the mechanisms underlying smoking-induced changes in the newborn. We have begun to investigate this by administration of nicotine to timed-pregnant rhesus monkeys. In preliminary studies we have demonstrated that exposure of pregnant rhesus monkeys to a nicotine dose consistent with that of smokers alters fetal a irway dev elopment and that related effects can be reproduced in fetal monkey lung organ culture. Immunohistochemistry shows wide expression of nicotinic receptors in developing lung and nicotine appears to alter the pattern of receptor expression. Preliminary data further suggests that some of the effects of nicotine, acting though nicotinic receptors, may be mediated by antagonism of the mitogenic effects of peptide growth factors such as GRP. From these studies will come the first description of the effects of chronic nicotine exposure on lung function, a determination of the extent to which these effects are reversible, and a beginning understanding of the mechanisms underlying these effects. FUNDING Center-supported project PUBLICATIONS Sekhon HS, Jia Y, Kuryatov A, Cole L, Raab R, Whitsett JA, Lindstrom J, Spindel ER. Interaction of nicotine with nicotinic cholinergic receptors in fetal rhesus monkey lung. Soc Neurosci Abstr 24:335, 1998. Sekhon HS, Jia Y, Kuryatov A, Cole L, Raab R, Lindstrom J, Spindel ER. Interaction between gastrin-releasing peptide (GRP) and nicotine in primate lung development. In National Heart Lung and Blood Institute workshop on Molecular Embryology of the Lung (held in Bethesda, MD, June 1, 1998) (abstract).

Website: http://crisp.cit.nih.gov/crisp/Crisp_Query.Generate_Screen

- **Project Title: ELECTRICAL HETEROGENEITY AND CARDIAC ARRHYTHMIAS**

Principal Investigator & Institution: Antzelevitch, Charles;; Masonic Medical Research Laboratory, Inc 2150 Bleeker St Utica, Ny 13501

Timing: Fiscal Year 2002; Project Start 01-MAY-1993; Project End 31-AUG-2005

Summary: Recent studies by our group and others have demonstrated that ventricular myocardium is not homogeneous as previously thought, but is comprised of at least three electrophysiologically and functionally distinct cell types: epicardium, endocardium and a unique population of cells that we termed M cells, displaying characteristics intermediate between those of ventricular myocardial and Purkinje cells. The three cell types differ with respect to early and late repolarization characteristics. These distinctions have been shown to underlie the various waveforms of the ECG and when amplified create the substrate for the development of life-threatening ventricular arrhythmias, including the polymorphic ventricular arrhythmias associated with the long QT and Brugada syndromes. We and others have recently reported that both syndromes may also be responsible for sudden death in children and infants and may contribute at some level to **sudden infant death syndrome** (SIDS). Our basis for understanding the mechanisms involved are hampered by the near total absence of data regarding the developmental aspects of electrical heterogeneity in ventricular myocardium of larger mammals. An urgent need to close this gap in our knowledge is the motivating force and the principal aim of this competing renewal. Our objectives are to define the developmental stages at which these heterogeneities normally arise in the canine heart and to probe how ion channel defects known to contribute to the long QT and Brugada syndromes may intervene to disrupt the normal electrical function of the heart and set the stage for malignant arrhythmias in the early stages of life. Our principal goals are to probe the extent to which electrical heterogeneity exists within the heart at each stage of development, to identify the underlying mechanisms as well as the conditions and interventions that amplify or diminish the intrinsic differences in regional electrical behavior and to examine to what extent transmural electrical heterogeneity is responsible for developmental changes in the ECG. To achieve these goals, we propose to use a multilevel approach designed to provide and integrate voltage clamp and action potential data from isolated myocytes, tissues and arterially perfused canine ventricular wedge preparations. Our long-range goal is to generate information that will contribute to our understanding of the causes for arrhythmic death in infants and young children.

Website: http://crisp.cit.nih.gov/crisp/Crisp_Query.Generate_Screen

- **Project Title: EXPERIENCE-DEPENDENT STRUCTURAL PLASTICITY IN CNS**

Principal Investigator & Institution: Martinez, Joseph L.; Ewing Halsell Professor of Neuroscience; Biology; University of Texas San Antonio San Antonio, Tx 78249

Timing: Fiscal Year 2002; Project Start 30-SEP-1999; Project End 31-AUG-2004

Summary: A major aspiration of the Division of Life Sciences at the University of Texas at San Antonio (UTSA) is t become a national leader in neurobiology research and training of Hispanics in the next ten years, while fulfilling its regional mission to raise the level of educational achievement of people in South Texas. Th major goal of the Specialized Research Program at Minority institutions (SNRP) at UTSA is to conduct cutting edge collaborative neuroscience research with NIH health relevance, to enhance neuroscience research a he collaborating institutions, and to further the development of an vigorous academic milieu with the strengthening of an existing neuroscience seminar series. The SNRP will inspire students, and minority students in particular, to pursue research careers in neuroscience. A strong External Advisory Committee was chosen to guide the SNRP. All are members of the National Academy of Sciences and one is a Nobel Prize winner. The theme of the SNRP proposals is that experience-dependent changes in neuron morphology alter CNS function in important and exciting ways. For Derrick the addition of new neurons, as in neurogenesis, is measured in new neuron's response to long term potentiation and learning. For Gdovin the developmental changes in neurons or neuron assemblies, are measured in respiratory pace maker cells o pattern generators. For LeBaron changes in extracellular matrix proteins are measured in synaptic plasticity, as in the maintenance of long term potentiation. All of the projects have strong health relevance. Gdovin's collaborator is the James Leiter, Chief, Pulmonary and Critical Care at Dartmouth Medical School, and increased understanding of the development of respiratory oscillators and pacemakers in vertebrates has the potential to impact **Sudden Infant Death Syndrome** in humans. Derrick's collaborator is Bruce McEwen a Rockefeller University, and increased understanding of the mechanisms of neurogenesis in adult vertebrae brain has the potential to impact a large number of debilitating diseases in humans including any loss o unction due to trauma or disease, such as in Parkinson's Disease. LeBaron's collaborator is Joe L. Martinez, r. at UTSA, and increased understanding of how the brain stores information at a cellular level has the potential to suggest therapies for loss of memory function, the most dramatic being Alzheimer's Disease.

Website: http://crisp.cit.nih.gov/crisp/Crisp_Query.Generate_Screen

- **Project Title: FAS, SIDS AND STILLBIRTHS IN CAPE TOWN, SOUTH AFRICA**

  Principal Investigator & Institution: Jacobson, Sandra W.; Professor; Psychiatry & Behav Neuroscis; Wayne State University 656 W. Kirby Detroit, Mi 48202

  Timing: Fiscal Year 2003; Project Start 30-SEP-2003; Project End 31-JUL-2006

Summary: (provided by applicant):Sudden infant death syndrome (SIDS) is a leading cause of infant mortality with incidence of about 0.8/1000 live births in the U.S. and considerably higher rates in at-risk populations, including Native Americans and the Cape Coloured (mixed ancestry) community in South Africa. A recent study has implicated prenatal alcohol exposure as an important risk factor for SIDS that warrants further investigation. It has been hypothesized that medullary serotonergic network deficits may be responsible, in part, for some SIDS deaths. For the past 5 years, we have been conducting a prospective, longitudinal study on the effects of prenatal alcohol exposure in the Cape Coloured community in collaboration with researchers from the University of Cape Town School of Medicine. This research has demonstrated our ability to recruit mothers from this community; obtain valid assessments of FAS, prenatal alcohol exposure, maternal alcoholism, smoking and depression, and socioenvironmental and medical risk; and perform state-of-the-art infant neurobehavioral assessments with Cape Town infants. We have found an exceptionally high rate of alcohol abuse and dependence among pregnant women in this population and of FAS among their infants. The high incidence of both SIDS and FAS in this large metropolitan area, the readily accessible maternal heavy drinking population, and our established, productive research collaboration make Cape Town uniquely appropriate as a Comprehensive Clinical Site. The proposed cooperative agreement would expand our ongoing collaboration to include researchers in pathology and obstetrics. The aims are (1) to conduct an assessment of the incidence of SIDS and stillbirths in Cape Town, using contemporary diagnostic criteria and procedures, including neuropathological examinations of SIDS victims and controls; (2) to test the hypothesis that prenatal binge drinking increases the risk of SIDS and to evaluate that risk in relation to risks associated with prenatal maternal smoking, preterm birth, infant gender and sleeping position, seasonal variation, parental education, and maternal depression; (3) to test the hypothesis that certain moderator variables-- years of drinking, severity of maternal alcohol abuse and dependence, lower maternal weight and prenatal smoking, and the absence of an ADH2*2 allelo will increase the risk of SIDS in alcohol-exposed infants; and (4) to examine whether heavily alcohol-exposed neonates will exhibit alterations in autonomic nervous system behaviors similar to those described in SIDS victims, which are known to be regulated by the medullary serotonergic system, including arousal, cardiorespiratory reflex integration, and sleep/wake patterns. This research has the potential to improve our understanding of neurophysiological mechanisms involved in SIDS and to contribute to developing interventions for mothers and infants whose behaviors indicate that they are at risk for this adverse outcome.

Website: http://crisp.cit.nih.gov/crisp/Crisp_Query.Generate_Screen

- **Project Title: FETAL NEURODEVELOPMENT--EFFECTS OF NICOTINE AND HYPOXIA**

Principal Investigator & Institution: Stark, Raymond I.; Professor; Columbia University Health Sciences Po Box 49 New York, Ny 10032

Timing: Fiscal Year 2002

Summary: Prenatal exposure to nicotine through maternal smoking leads to alterations in fetal responses related to arousal and cardiorespiratory control far beyond the period of exposure. The drug pets fetuses at increased risk for growth restriction, prematurity, perinatal complications and after birth, for the **Sudden Infant Death Syndrome,** behavioral and learning disabilities, and attention deficit disorders; while the adolescent female offspring may be at increased risk for becoming smokers themselves. By hypoxia and direct effects of nicotine on fetal neurodevelopment have been implicated as mechanisms for this array of consequences. Our overall hypothesis is that excessive and untimely stimulation of fetal nicotinic receptors by nicotine induces wide ranging structural and functional changes in the developing nervous system leading to alterations in central regulatory mechanisms controlling autonomic and behavioral functions. While fetal regulatory mechanisms adapt to chronic nicotine exposure to maintain a relatively "normal" physiology, hypoxic stress will reveal deficiencies in physiologic competence. These structural functional alterations, established in utero produce a "vulnerable" newborn who will have a life long risk for stress related pathologies. To test these hypotheses, we will compare key markers of neurophysiologic function (coordinated fetal states, response to hypoxia and baroreceptor gain) in nicotine exposed fetuses with controls and relate their functional impairments to structural differences in brainstem and forebrain arousal and cardiorespiratory centers. Studies are carried out in a unique chronically instrumented baboon model. The homologies in neurodevelopment between the human and baboon fetus make knowledge gained from this research relevant to identifying high risk fetuses and infants.

Website: http://crisp.cit.nih.gov/crisp/Crisp_Query.Generate_Screen

- **Project   Title: GENE   THERAPY   FOR   LUNG   AND CARDIOVASCULAR DISEASE**

Principal Investigator & Institution: Muzyczka, Nicholas; Professor; Molecular Genetics & Microbiol; University of Florida Gainesville, Fl 32611

Timing: Fiscal Year 2002; Project Start 30-SEP-1997; Project End 31-AUG-2003

Summary: The long-range goal of this Program Project is to develop viral vector-based gene transfer strategies for treating genetic aqnd acquired cardiopulmonary disorders. To this end, a group of investigators with diverse, yet complementary, interdisciplinary interests and expertise and expertise has established an integrated research effort that is underscored by a common interest in practical applications of gene therapy. A major focus of the Program is the development of improved methods for gene transfer using recombinant AAV (rAAV) and lentivirus vectors. Project 3 (Muzyczka) will focus on the basic changing viral tropism through the insertion of foreign ligands into the capsid gene. Project 4 (Chang) will investigate ways of improving lentiviral vector yields and study the biodistribution of lentiviruses. Along with the vector development components, there is an emphasis on solving practical issues related to gene therapy for diseases of the heart and muscle. Project 2 (Flotte) focuses on genetic disorders of beta-oxidation of fatty acids within the mitochondria. Disorders of mitochondrial fatty acid oxidation (FAO) as a group represents a relatively common class of metabolic disorders, the most common of which typically present with either **Sudden Infant Death Syndrome** (SIDS) or with a combined cardiac and skeletal myopathy. The recent development of rAAV vectors for highly efficient transduction of hepatocytes and myofibers present new tools for the study of FAO disorders and project 2 will focus on short-chain acyl CoA dehydrogenase (SCAD) and long chain acyl CoA dehydrogenase (LCAD) defects, whose deficiency results in myopathy. Project 1 (Byrne) will focus on a deficiency in the lysosomal enzyme, acid alpha-glucosidase (GAA). This enzyme deficiency leads to glycogen accumulation in lysosomes of striated muscle, and in the infantile form, affected infants die of heart failure within the first year of life. Project 1 will focus on the development of alternative rAAV serotypes and targeted vectors to improve the efficiency and distribution of gene delivery for this disease. In addition, outcomes of vector distribution and biochemical effect will be tested by new MRI/MRS techniques. To assist the projects, the Program has established a Vector Core Laboratory and a Pathology Core. The Vector Core will supply vectors of uniform and reproducible quality6 to all subprojects, and investigated improved methods of generating rAAV.

The Pathology Core (Core C) will carry out biodistribution and toxicology studies for all subprojects. Finally, an Administrative Core (Core A) will insure centralized fiscal management and oversight for the subprojects. The Cores will also serve as a mechanism to insure rapid exchange of information among all subprojects.

Website: http://crisp.cit.nih.gov/crisp/Crisp_Query.Generate_Screen

- **Project Title: GENETIC DETERMINANTS OF SUDDEN CARDIAC DEATH**

Principal Investigator & Institution: Albert, Christine M.;; Brigham and Women's Hospital 75 Francis Street Boston, Ma 02115

Timing: Fiscal Year 2003; Project Start 05-JUL-2003; Project End 30 JUN-2007

Summary: (provided by applicant): Sudden cardiac death (SCD) affects 400,000 individuals each year in the U.S. alone. Over half have no evidence of heart disease prior to death, and our ability to identify those at risk and therefore prevent SCD is poor. Mutations in cardiac ion channel genes including SCN5A, KVLQT1, HERG, KCNE1, KCNE2, and RyR2 have been implicated in monogenic traits with a high risk of SCD, such as the long-QT, Brugada, **sudden infant death syndrome,** and catecholaminergic polymorphic ventricular tachycardia. Alterations in ion channel function can result in life-threatening ventricular arrhythmias in diverse disease states. Therefore, sequence variants in these genes that alter function or transcription of these ion channels may confer a predisposition to ventricular arrhythmia and SCD in broader populations. This research program proposes to determine if sequence variants in the above candidate genes are associated with an increased risk of SCD in apparently healthy populations. Cases of SCD will be assembled from five NIH-funded prospective cohorts with a total of 106,314 individuals with existent blood samples. All cohorts are exceptionally wellcharacterized with respect to environmental exposures and have collected medical records on cardiovascular endpoints. We will characterize all coding sequence variation and selected non-coding sequence variation among 100 cases and controls from these cohorts. Using these novel markers, we will define the haplotype block structure (SNPs in linkage disequilibrium) for the six genes. We will then employ a nested case-control design and conditional logistic regression to test for associations between haplotypes (haplotype tag SNPs) in both coding and non-coding regions and SCD risk. We will also test directly for associations between single loci that may have functional significance and SCD risk. An estimated 600 cases of well-documented SCD will be confirmed over the first three years of the grant period, and these cases will be matched on age, sex, ethnicity, and geographic location to two control subjects from the same cohort. In addition, based upon known sex-differences in the phenotypic expression of the candidate genes in the primary arrhythmic disorders, we will specifically examine sex-differences in the risk of SCD associated with sequence variation in these genes. The findings generated will have substantial implications for our understanding of the SCD syndrome and risk stratification in the general population.

Website: http://crisp.cit.nih.gov/crisp/Crisp_Query.Generate_Screen

- **Project Title: GENETIC MOUSE MODELING OF MEDULLARY SEROTONERGIC DEVELOPMENT**

Principal Investigator & Institution: Dymecki, Susan M.;; Children's Hospital (Boston) Boston, Ma 021155737

Timing: Fiscal Year 2003; Project Start 07-JUL-2003; Project End 31-MAR-2008

Summary: Penetrating investigations into the pathogenesis of neurological SIDS have implicated a developmental defect in the medullary serotonergic (5-HT) system, defined as an interrelated group of 5-HT and non-5-HT neurons centered around the medullary raphe. Unfortunately, littte is known about the molecules during differentiation of these neurons and how their development is affected by environmental SIDS risk factors -information that is critical for determining the etiology of SIDS. To help fill this void, studies proposed in Project 6 focus on testing in mice the hypotheses that neurons of the medullary 5-HT system come from the rhombic lip; that their identities are specified, at least in part, as precursor cells in the rhombic tip, and that abnormalities in these early specification events underlie the medullary dysfunction associated with SIDS. In aim 1, we use a unique set of generic tools to establish that neurons of the medullary 5-HT system come from the rhombic lip; indeed, our preliminary fate maps indicate this is the case. We extend these analyses to characterize the dispersion of 5-HT system neurons from the rhombic lip and map their acquisition of different neurochemical identities. In most neuroepithetia, including the rhombic lip, the potential to give rise to different neuron types appears to change over time, with restrictive events occurring in the dividing progenitor cells themselves. Thus, at distinct developmental stages a given neuroepithelium is multipotent but not equipotent, presumably due in part to temporal changes in intrinsic regulators. To identify such regulators in the rhombic lip, in aim 2, we perform whole-genome expression studies of rhombic lip tissue at sequential developmental stages corresponding to its peak production times of different brainstem neurons. By comparing mRNA profiles across time points, we will identify gene sets associated with neuron subtype production. To further sift from these gene sets the best candidate regulators for future functional studies, we perform similar analyses on tissue from mice null for Pax6, a transcription factor required for producing a subset of rhombic-lip derivatives and an established regulator of CNS fate. From this, we identify mRNAs dependent on Pax6 and which may be important for a subset of 5-HT-system specification events. In aim3, we determine if prenatal exposure to nicotine (a major component of cigarette smoke and proven neuroteratogen) alters development of the 5-HT system in ways that may explain the increased risk for SIDS following maternal smoking. Completion of these aims will provide a comprehensive molecular basis for delineating brainstem development and for identifying mechanisms underlying SIDS.

Website: http://crisp.cit.nih.gov/crisp/Crisp_Query.Generate_Screen

- **Project Title: HYPERTHERMIC RESPONSE OF THE RESPIRATORY NEURAL NETWORK**

Principal Investigator & Institution. Tryba, Andrew K.; Organismal Biology and Anatomy; University of Chicago 5801 S Ellis Ave Chicago, Il 60637

Timing: Fiscal Year 2002; Project Start 01-JUN-2002

Summary: (Applicant's abstract): Breathing is modulated as the result of changes in the internal and external environment (e.g. ionic concentration, pH, pCO2 and temperature) and the behavioral state of the animal. In response to these challenges, respiratory neural network activity is modified to affect the timing and intensity of respiratory events. While these changes are specific to respiration, the issue of how neural networks adapt a behavior during environmental changes is of interest to those studying many motor systems. In mammals, hyperthermia causes an initial increase in respiration frequency (RF) that serves to enhance heat loss through evaporative cooling, but heat loss mechanisms are not always effective. For example, hyperthermia associated with conditions such as fever and heat-stroke may lead to cardiac arrest, cessation of breathing (apnea) and death. In fact, hyperthermia is a major risk factor for **sudden infant death syndrome.** Despite these implications, little is known about the neural mechanisms underlying the temperature-induced changes in respiratory activity. In this proposal: 1) I will determine the effects of hyperthermia on respiratory activity generated in the isolated brain-stem respiratory neural network. The response of the pre- Botzinger Complex (pBC) respiratory network to hyperthermia will be characterized by integrating population pBC neural activity and quantifying changes in RF. 2) I will use patch-clamp recordings from pBC neurons to test whether changes in RF during hypothermia result from modulation of pacemaker neurons or the emergent properties of the respiratory neural network. 3) I will also use patch-clamp recordings from pBC neurons to examine if membrane properties and/or synaptic inputs in respiratory pacemaker neurons are modulated during hypothermia.

Website: http://crisp.cit.nih.gov/crisp/Crisp_Query.Generate_Screen

- **Project Title: HYPOXIA AND CONTROL OF FETAL BREATHING MOVEMENTS**

  Principal Investigator & Institution: Koos, Brian J.; Professor; Obstetrics and Gynecology; University of California Los Angeles 10920 Wilshire Blvd., Suite 1200 Los Angeles, Ca 90024

  Timing: Fiscal Year 2002; Project Start 01-AUG-1985; Project End 30-NOV-2003

  Summary: Hypoxia abolishes fetal breathing (FB) through a direct effect of low P02 on the brain. We have recently shown that the parafascicular nuclear complex (Pf) in the thalamus is critically involved in hypoxic depression of FB, leading to a new paradigm regarding the neural substrate mediating hypoxic inhibition. The proposed studies in fetal sheep have four goals: 1) To determine the role of Pf in the second- phase reduction in ventilation in newborns, which undoubtedly involves the same central mechanism that mediates hypoxic inhibition of FB. Hypoxic inhibition of FB will be abolished by selectively destroying fetal Pf neurons with subsequent testing of newborn respiratory responses to hypoxia. The large size of the near-term fetal sheep brain will greatly facilitate the identification of the neural substrate mediating ventilatory "roll off" during hypoxia in the newborn. 2) To identify the Pf neural pathways involved in inhibition of FB. The lipophilic dye DiI will enable anterograde and retrograde labelling of fiber tracts which will determine the connections of these cells and thus help establish the neural network involved in hypoxic inhibition. Distinct advantages of DiI include its applicability to postmortem tissue and optimum efficiency in perinatal brains. 3) To determine the mechanism of hypoxic inhibition. Increased brain adenosine (ADO) concentrations, derived from hydrolysis of extracellular adenine nucleotides, mediate hypoxic inhibition of FB. Microdialysis with a novel inhibitor of extracellular ATPase will establish whether extracellular ATP is an essential precursor for the hypoxia-induced rise in ADO. 4) To identify the locus of ADO receptors that mediate hypoxic inhibition of FB. ADO receptor agonists and antagonists will be microinjected into Pf to determine whether ADO A1 or A2 receptors in or proximate to this sector inhibit FB during hypoxia. Hypoxic inhibition appears to be part of a survival mechanism whereby O2 that would otherwise be used for breathing is made available to vital organs, especially the heart and brain; thus it has relevance to hypoxia-induced perinatal brain damage. Such injury may predispose infants to **Sudden Infant Death Syndrome** (SIDS) by increasing the depressing effects of hypoxia on ventilation and by altering sleep state regulation of breathing postnatally. Thus, these studies on hypoxic inhibition should provide insight into mechanisms of SIDS and enhance our understanding of the clinically important transition of neural control of respiration in the perinatal period.

Website: http://crisp.cit.nih.gov/crisp/Crisp_Query.Generate_Screen

- **Project Title: HYPOXIC EFFECTS ON MAMMALIAN RESPIRATORY NEURAL NETWORK**

Principal Investigator & Institution: Ramirez, Jan M.; Associate Professor; None; University of Chicago 5801 S Ellis Ave Chicago, Il 60637

Timing: Fiscal Year 2003; Project Start 07-DEC-1998; Project End 31-JAN-2007

Summary: (provided by applicant): The **sudden infant death syndrome** (SIDS) remains the leading cause of postnatal infant mortality in the USA. Increasing evidence indicates that SIDS is due to a failure of autoresuscitation, which is a protective brainstem response to asphyxia or severe hypoxia. An essential mechanism for autoresuscitation is gasping, a respiratory motor pattern which is distinct from the normal respiration occurring in normoxia. However, despite considerable relevance, the question how gasping is generated by the nervous system remains largely unknown. Transections at the pontomedullary junction transforms the motor pattern for normal respiration into gasping (Lumsden, 1923), which suggested to some researchers that different forms of breathing are generated by separate "centers" and that gasping is generated in the medulla. Using a slice preparation from the medulla of mice we demonstrated that the isolated respiratory network in the pre-Botzinger complex (PBC) generates not only one, but three forms of fictive respiratory activities with striking similarities to normal respiratory, sigh and gasping activity. Like in vivo, these three activities are generated in a stereotypic manner during the response to anoxia: An initial augmentation in the frequency of normal respiratory and sigh activities is followed by a depression and the generation of gasping. Our network characterization indicates that all three activities are generated by the reconfiguration of the same neuronal network located within the PBC. The proposed research aims at examining the cellular mechanisms that lead to the reconfiguration of the respiratory network. We specifically test the hypothesis that the transition from normal respiratory activity into gasping is associated with a change in the organization of the respiratory network: In normal respiratory activity pacemaker neurons are fully integrated in a network of inhibitory and excitatory non-pacemaker neurons. In gasping most nonpacemaker and calcium-dependent pacemaker neurons inactivate and only a small population of pacemaker neurons remains active that become essential for rhythm generation. We propose three Aims to examine this hypothesis: Aim 1 compares the synaptic modulation of pacemaker and non-pacemaker neurons, Aim 2 investigates the differential modulation of ion channel properties in pacemaker and non-pacemaker neurons and Aim 3 proposes connectivity experiments to directly test the anoxia-induced changes in the network organization. By bridging different levels of integration the proposed research will lead to a better understanding of the neuronal mechanisms that underlie normal respiratory and gasping activities. Understanding how anoxia leads to the reconfiguration of neuronal network activity is of great general interest as every year numerous victims suffer brain damage from hypoxic insults. In the context of SIDS, our research may ultimately lead to a better understanding why certain infants fail to autoresuscitate.

Website: http://crisp.cit.nih.gov/crisp/Crisp_Query.Generate_Screen

- **Project Title: INFLUENCE OF THE VENTRAL MEDULLA ON REFLEX RESPONES TO STIMULATION**

Principal Investigator & Institution: Leiter, James C.;; Children's Hospital (Boston) Boston, Ma 021155737

Timing: Fiscal Year 2002

Summary: We propose that the **sudden infant death syndrome** (SIDS) results when an infant when a neuronal vulnerability is exposed to an exogenous stressor at a critical time in development. The arcuate nucleus in humans, and homologous structures in the piglet- the retrotrapezoid nucleus, parapyramidal neurons, caudal raphe and chemoreceptor regions along the rostral and caudal surface of the ventral medulla-are possible sites of neuronal vulnerability. The exogenous stressor may be stimulation of facial or upper airway receptors or compression of the chest. These exogenous stressors inhibit respiration and may promote cardiovascular instability, but normal protective responses arising from asphyxia (hypoxia and hypercapnia) oppose the effect of these stressors, increase breathing, stabilize blood pressure, promote arousal, which alleviates inhibitory influences on respiration and may lead to postural changes that relieve asphyxia. Disruption of the arcuate neurons or the piglet homologue diminishes or eliminates protective responses, permits the unfettered actions of stimuli inhibiting respiration and may make a fatal outcome more likely. Specific Aim 1: In the decerebrate piglet at different developmental ages, we will examine the effect of lesions in the piglet homologue of the arcuate nucleus on ventilatory and cardiovascular responses (phrenic nerve activity, heart rate and blood pressure) during stimulation of the trigeminal or superior laryngeal nerve or stimulation of a now intercostal nerve during hypercapnia or hypoxia. Specific Aim 2: In decerebrate piglets at the developmental age most susceptible to disruption of protective responses we will examine the role of muscarinic, ionotropic glutamate and thyrotropin releasing hormone receptors in brainstem regions homologous to the arcuate nucleus on ventilatory and cardiovascular responses as in Specific Aim 1. Specific Aim 3: We will examine the effect of chronic lesions in the homologue of the arcuate nucleus on ventilatory and cardiovascular responses during stimulation of the trigeminal, superior laryngeal and intercostal nerves in unanesthetized piglets during room air exposure, hypercapnia or hypoxia during wakefulness and sleep (NREM and REM).

Website: http://crisp.cit.nih.gov/crisp/Crisp_Query.Generate_Screen

- **Project Title: INTERMOUNTAIN CHILD HEALTH SERVICES RESEARCH CONSORTIUM**

Principal Investigator & Institution: Young, Paul C.; Pediatrics; University of Utah Salt Lake City, Ut 84102

Timing: Fiscal Year 2003; Project Start 30-SEP-2001; Project End 29-SEP-2006

Summary: (provided by applicant): The goal of the Intermountain Consortium for Child Health Services Research is to launch nationally competitive research in Utah and the Intermountain West to inform the design and delivery of optimal care for children, especially those with special health care needs. The Consortium will achieve this goal by building upon the investments and accomplishments of its first two years of development. Our new objectives include completing critical components of infrastructure building, adding to the current pool of investigators through faculty development and recruitment, and conducting research projects leading to significant extramural funding. By the end of the funding period, the applicants will have a substantial and sustainable infrastructure, new key personnel, and a pool of experienced mentors, advisors, and collaborators. Their 5-year vision is that of an effective pediatric health services research program and an environment that facilitates vibrant exchange between research and practice. Our specific aims for the next three years are to: 1) Expand the

Intermountain Consortium for Child Health Services Research and strengthen relationships among partners; 2) Create a Research Resource Office to coordinate and integrate health services research, clinical research, and projects designed to translate research into practice; 3) Increase the number of independent, productive health services researchers in the Intermountain West by training and supporting existing faculty and by recruiting additional faculty with training in health services research; and 4) Complete two individual pilot research projects. Two Faculty Development Scholars will lead these studies. The first, "Measurement and Prevalence of Deformational Plagiocephaly", will validate a measure and determine the prevalence of a rapidly increasing phenomenon, flattening of the head in infancy associated with positioning to prevent **sudden infant death syndrome.** The second, "Use and Allocation of Home Health Care Services", will provide an analysis of pediatric home health care for children with special health care needs. These projects will provide publishable, preliminary data for grant applications for a collaborative intervention study and for a career development award.

Website: http://crisp.cit.nih.gov/crisp/Crisp_Query.Generate_Screen

- **Project Title: INTRACELLULAR PH RESPONSES OF CENTRAL CHEMORECEPTORS**

Principal Investigator & Institution: Putnam, Robert W.; Professor; Physiology and Biophysics; Wright State University Colonel Glenn Hwy Dayton, Oh 45435

Timing: Fiscal Year 2002; Project Start 01-JUL-1997; Project End 31-JUL-2005

Summary: Increased CO_2 (hypercapnia) is a major stimulus for increased respiration and blood pressure. This pathway for cardiorespiratory control involves specialized central neurons, called chemosensitive neurons, that sense hypercapnia, but the cellular mechanisms that transduce hypercapnia into an increased neuronal firing rate are not well understood. Our work will involve the study of individual neurons from at least two chemosensitive brainstem areas (locus coeruleus and either nucleus tractus solitarius or ventrolateral medulla) and at least one nonchemosensitive area (either inferior olive or hypoglossal nucleus) using slices from neonatal rat brains. Simultaneous measurements of neuronal membrane potential (Vm) and intracellular pH (pHi) will be achieved using perforated patch recordings or whole cell recordings (WCR) combined with pH- sensitive fluorescent dyes and fluorescence imaging microscopy. Our first aim is to identify the signal pathways that transduce hypercapnia into an increased firing rate. It will consist of 4 separate aims: i) study the roles of molecular CO2, external pH (pHO) and pHi as the proximate signal of chemoreception by exposing neurons to solutions that vary in each of these parameters; ii) examine the phenomenon of "washout", whereby the Vm response to hypercapnia is lost during WCR measurements, to see if additional signal molecules (e.g. Cai, polyamines or carbonic anhydrase) are also involved in chemoreception; iii) study the "hypoxia paradox" (hypoxia-induced acidification does not appear to increase firing rate in chemosensitive neurons) to see if it is due to the lack of additional signal molecules; and iv) study the changes in the Vm and pHi response to hypercapnia in chemosensitive neurons from rats with reduced chemosensitivity (induced by chronic exposure to hypercapnia). Our second aim is to study the effects of the signals, identified in Aim 1, on various K+ channels and determine the role of each of these channels in modifying the shape of the action potential and neuronal firing rate. Three K+ channels will be studied: i) inward rectifying K+ channels, important in determining the slope of the interspike depolarization and thereby the firing rate of the neuron; ii) Ca2+-activated K+ channels, important in determining the shape of the action potential and the magnitude of the after hyperpolarization; and iii) TWIK-related acid sensitive K+ channels (TASK), important in determining the resting Vm. This work should indicate the precise nature of the proximate signal of chemosensitivity, elucidate the way in which hypercapnic stimuli affect various K+ channels and give insight into how these effects are integrated to result in the final neuronal response. Further, by comparing the findings in neurons from 2 chemosensitive areas, our findings should help clarify why there are numerous chemosensitive regions in the brainstem. These studies will contribute to our understanding of respiratory diseases thought to be due in part to central chemoreceptor dysfunction, such as **sudden infant death syndrome** (SIDS) and central alveolar hypoventilation syndromes.

Website: http://crisp.cit.nih.gov/crisp/Crisp_Query.Generate_Screen

- **Project Title: MECHANISM OF CARDIORESPIRATORY RHYTHM IN NEONATES**

Principal Investigator & Institution: Mendelowitz, David S.; Professor; Pharmacology; George Washington University 2121 I St Nw Washington, Dc 20052

Timing: Fiscal Year 2002; Project Start 01-APR-1998; Project End 31-MAR-2007

Summary: (Provided By Applicant) The neural control of the cardiovascular and respiratory systems is highly interrelated. During each respiratory cycle, the heart beats more rapidly in inspiration and slows during post-inspiration, which is referred to as respiratory sinus arrhythmia. This cardio-respiratory interaction occurs within the central nervous system and is mediated largely, if not entirely, via the parasympathetic innervation of the heart. Respiratory sinus arrhythmia is diminished in many disease states and it has been speculated that an abnormality of cardio-respiratory control may be involved in **sudden infant death syndrome** (SIDS). This proposal is a logical extension of the results obtained during the previous funding period and will build a unifying framework that identifies the neurons and mechanisms responsible for respiratory modulation of cardiac parasympathetic vagal activity. We will use a novel in-vitro preparation that maintains rhythmic respiratory activity with an innovative transsynaptic virus that evokes expression of green fluorescent protein (GFP) that identifies neurons that project to cardiac vagal neurons in-vitro without altering their electrophysiological properties. Specifically, we will test whether cardiac vagal neurons are inhibited during inspiration by an increased frequency of inhibitory GABAergic inputs, and that the increased GABA frequency is mediated by activation of presynaptic nicotinic receptors. We will also test the hypothesis that cardiac vagal neurons are directly excited during post-inspiration via electrical synapses which can be abolished by gap junction blockers. Furthermore, we will identify and characterize the rhythmic respiratory activity of the neurons that synapse upon, and make gap junction contacts with, cardiac vagal neurons. This work will not only address hypotheses fundamental to understanding the basis and mechanisms of cardiorespiratory rhythms in the neonatal rat that originate in the medulla, but will also suggest which receptors and processes could be altered in diseases of the cardiorespiratory system such as SIDS.

Website: http://crisp.cit.nih.gov/crisp/Crisp_Query.Generate_Screen

- **Project Title: MEDULLARY MECHANISMS OF HYPOXIC RESPIRATORY EXCITATION**

Principal Investigator & Institution: Solomon, Irene C.; Assistant Professor; Physiology and Biophysics; State University New York Stony Brook Stony Brook, Ny 11794

Timing: Fiscal Year 2002; Project Start 01-SEP-2000; Project End 31-JUL-2004

Summary: (Applicant's abstract): Severe brain hypoxia results in respiratory and sympathetic excitation. Respiratory excitation takes the form of gasping which is characterized by an abrupt onset, short duration, high amplitude burst of activity, associated exclusively with inspiratory discharge. Survival during hypoxia exposures appears to be critically dependent upon this integrated cardiorespiratory reflex which has been referred to as "autoresuscitation", and is associated with rapid reoxygenation of arterial blood and restoration of blood pressure. Failure to gasp has been proposed as a potential cause of **sudden infant death syndrome.** The principle hypothesis of this proposal is that the putative respiratory pacemaker is located in the pre-Botzinger complex (the proposed locus of respiratory rhythm generation; pre-BotC), is hypoxia chemosensitive, and when released from strong GABAergic inhibition, exhibits chemosensitivity to systemic hypoxia over the range associated with chemoreception of the carotid bodies. Additionally, we propose that both disinhibition of GABA" ?receptors and direct hypoxic excitation of neurons (i.e., hypoxic chemosensitivity) located in the pre-BotC play complimentary roles in the genesis of hypoxia related gasping. The goal of the experiments proposed in this application is to examine the roles of direct hypoxic excitation of pre-BotC neurons, GABAergic disinhibition of pre-BotC neurons, and ionotropic excitatory amino acid (EAA) receptor activation of pre-BotC neurons as potential mechanisms for the respiratory excitation seen during gasping in response to severe brain hypoxia. Microinjection of neurotransmitter agonists and antagonists in conjunction with whole nerve and medullary single unit extracellular recordings will be used. Experiments will be conducted in both decerebrate and chloralose-anesthetized, vagotomized, deafferented, paralyzed, and ventilated cats. The specific aims are: (1) test whether pre-inspiratory (I-driver) neurons located in the pre-BotC are activated by focal hypoxia, and whether focal hypoxia phase shifts and synchronizes other respiratory-modulated subtypes or respiratory neurons located in the pre-BotC to a gasp-synchronous discharge, (2) test whether pre-inspiratory (I-driver) neurons located in the pre-BotC are activated during severe systemic hypoxia phase shifts and synchronizes other inspiratory-modulated subtypes of respiratory neurons located in the pre-BotC to a gasp-synchronous discharge, (3) test whether GABA" -mediated disinhibition neurons located in the pre-BotC plays a facilitatory role in the production of respiratory excitation seen during hypoxia, and (4) test whether ionotropic EAA receptor activation of neurons located in the pre-BotC plays a modulatory role in the respiratory excitation seen during hypoxia-induced gasping.

Website: http://crisp.cit.nih.gov/crisp/Crisp_Query.Generate_Screen

- **Project Title: MEDULLARY SEROTONERGIC INVOLVEMENT IN SLEEP, THERMOREG**

Principal Investigator & Institution: Darnall, Robert A.; Professor; Children's Hospital (Boston) Boston, Ma 021155737

Timing: Fiscal Year 2003; Project Start 07-JUL-2003; Project End 31-MAR-2008

Summary: The important findings that a substantial subset of SIDS infants have decreases in serotonin receptor binding the ventral medulla form the basis for the hypothesis that abnormalities in the 'medullary 5-HT system' play an important rote in SIDS. Neurons in this region participate in widespread autonomic functions including cardiorespiratory control, thermoregutation, and based on recent new information from our laboratory, sleep. The overall aim of this proposal is to investigate the roles of phenotypically specific neurons in the medullary 5-HT system on sleep homeostasis, responses to a thermal stress, and on cardiorespiratory variability. Our strategy will be to use novel neurochemicals to locally inhibit or destroy serotonergic neurons and/or neurons expressing the 5-HT(1A), NK1, or m1 muscarinic receptor in chronically instrumented piglets. 8-OH DPAT will be used to selectively activate 5-HT(1A) autoreceptors on 5-HT neurons, and 5,7-DHT or the neurotoxin saporin conjugated to an antibody to the serotonin transporter protein (SERT-SAP) will be used to selectively destroy serotonergic neurons. Analogous methods will be usedto inhibit or destroy neurons expressing the NK1 or m1 muscarinic receptor with SP-SAP or a powerful toxin obtained from the venom of the green mamba highly selective for m1 muscarinic receptors (m1-toxin1). We will evaluate the effects of these specific 'lesions' on sleep architecture in piglets using EEG wavelet analysis and behavioral observations during short (6 hr) plethysmograph recordings, and long (12-24 hr) recordings in their natural habitat (with the sow and siblings) using telemetry. We will also evaluate responses to thermal stresses focusing on shivering and non-shivering thermogenesis, skin blood flow, and hyperpnea. Finally, we will use the sensitive techniques of fractal analysis to evaluate the complexity of cardiorespiratory variability, the decrease in which is associated with decreased ability of a control system to respond to a perturbation. Indeed, infants who subsequently die of SIDS have decreases in heart rate variability. Lesions will be made in the midline and lateral columns and all areas simultaneously to test the hypothesis that neurons are organized in a functionally specific manner. We hypothesize that the medullary 5-HT system is a major site for the integration of cardiorespiratory, thermoregulatory, and sleep and arousal mechanisms, and that abnormalities in this region could produce local or widespread effects that might contribute to sudden death.

Website: http://crisp.cit.nih.gov/crisp/Crisp_Query.Generate_Screen

- **Project Title: MOLECULAR STRUCTURE OF THE 900 KD BOTULINUM NEUROTOXIN COMPLEX**

Principal Investigator & Institution: Stevens, Raymond C.;; University of Calif-Lawrenc Berkeley Lab Lawrence Berkeley National Laboratory Berkeley, Ca 94720

Timing: Fiscal Year 2002; Project Start 01-JUL-2001; Project End 30-JUN-2002

Summary: Botulinum neurotoxin complex serotype A is a 900 kiloDalton (kDa) protein produced as one of eight serotypes (A-G) by the anaerobic bacterium Clostridium botulinum. Among the most potent biological toxins known to man, botulinum neurotoxin causes inhibition of synaptic vesicle release at the neuromuscular junction resulting in flaccid paralysis and ultimately death. Botulinum neurotoxin type A (BoNT/A) is a potent disease agent in both food-borne botulism and **Sudden Infant Death Syndrome** (SIDS), an established biological weapon, and a novel therapeutic in the treatment of involuntary muscle disorders. Previously, we have determined the 3-D structure of the 150 kDNA neurotoxin component of the 900 kDa complex by x-ray crystallography. We have also completed antibody mapping experiments to determine how the 150 kDa neurotoxin is bound into the 900 kDa toxin complex. We have conducted a series of biophysical stability experiments in order to understand how the two assemblies (150 kDa toxin and 750 kDa non-toxic component) combine and stabilize the 900 kDa complex. Lastly, based on the work above, and preliminary electron microscopy work, we are designing an alternative vaccine strategy for botulism. Current vaccine programs for botulism are not very effective. The preliminary objective of this proposal is to obtain a three- dimensional structure of the 900 kDa botulinum neurotoxin complex, and understand how the neurotoxin component fits into the complex. To accomplish this goal, we will use a 2-D crystals of the 900 kDa complex to conduct 3-D image reconstruction experiments. We have already obtained 2-D crystals of the 900 kDa complex to conduct 3-D image reconstruction experiments. We have already obtained 2-D crystals of the 900 kDa complex that diffract weakly to 14 Angstroms resolution in negative strain, and a density projection map has been produced at 30 Angstroms resolution. Based on the crystal quality and the frequency with which defects were observed in the crystals used in our earlier investigation, it appears as though much higher quality crystals can be obtained. Specifically, our transfer technique is presently crude due to our new venture into this area of research, and several suggestions have been made by other program project members on how to improve our transfer techniques. We are also investigating alternative buffer conditions to help stabilize the protein further. Once optimization of the 2-D crystals has been completed, we will complete the negative stain work at the maximum resolution possible using data collection in a tilt series followed by 3-D image reconstruction. This work will be followed by attempting higher resolution studies with cryo-techniques. We will crystallize the 900 kDa complex in the presence of scFv antibody molecules that have a high affinity for exposed regions of the neurotoxin when bound to the 900 kDn complex.

Website: http://crisp.cit.nih.gov/crisp/Crisp_Query.Generate_Screen

- **Project Title: MONITORING A SIDS MODEL IN NEONATAL SWINE**

Principal Investigator & Institution: Sica, Anthony L.; Physiology and Pharmacology; Suny Downstate Medical Center 450 Clarkson Ave New York, Ny 11203

Timing: Fiscal Year 2002; Project Start 30-SEP-1991; Project End 30-JUN-2004

Summary: The long-term objective of the proposed research is to evaluate the role of cardiac mechanisms in the etiology of sudden death in the **Sudden Infant Death Syndrome** (SIDS). Thus this project is directly related to a problem in infant survival and health. The specific aims of the proposed research are designed to test the hypothesis that a developmental anomaly in cardiac innervation could reduce ventricular electrical stability and favor the onset of sudden cardiac death. The research design and surgical methods have been worked out in the previous grant period; newborn swine with surgically induced imbalance in cardiac autonomic innervation will be continuously monitored (24 hrs.) throughout eight postnatal weeks. Those surviving and similarly surgically prepared littermates will be tested (at ages 2,4,6,8 wks) for cardiovascular responses to: (i) hypoxia, (ii) hypercapnia, (iii) stimulation of cardiopulmonary receptors, and (iv) alterations in baroreceptor afferent inputs. Results obtained from study of these possible precipitating factors should reveal the increased susceptibility of the neonate at risk for sudden death. Sleep is the predominant behavioral state of the neonate and ontogeny of EEG sleep in neonates can be monitored by serial EEG recordings. We plan to examine ECG recordings as a function of state determined by VCR tapes of behavior, diaphragmatic EMG and EEG, and correlate these variables against both age and type of denervation. Nonlinear analysis of heart rate variability in infants has revealed an increase in complexity with maturation and our own results included similar findings in piglets. This grant proposal would pursue these findings and the effects of selected cardiac denervation on this complexity, correlating results with sudden death in denervated piglets. Such studies should confirm our working hypothesis regarding the importance of cardiac innervation in the etiology of sudden death in infants. We are, therefore, postulating an abnormality at the effector level, i.e., at the cardiac level, specifically: maturation of the normal innervation of the heart and its reflex control.

Website: http://crisp.cit.nih.gov/crisp/Crisp_Query.Generate_Screen

- **Project Title: MU OPIOID RECEPTOR REGULATION IN NEONATAL BRAINSTEM**

Principal Investigator & Institution: Olsen, George D.; Professor; Physiology and Pharmacology; Oregon Health & Science University Portland, or 972393098

Timing: Fiscal Year 2003; Project Start 15-DEC-1993; Project End 31-MAR-2007

Summary: (provided by applicant): The long-term goal of the proposed research is to understand mechanisms by which chronic in utero morphine and methadone exposure affect regulation and function of mu opioid receptors (MOR) in respiratory control areas of newborn brainstem. Respiratory depression is induced by endogenous opioid peptides and exogenous opioids that activate MOR. A critical brainstem site for these effects is the nucleus tractus solitarius (NTS), which integrates sensory signals and drives respiratory muscles. Profound disturbance of neonatal breathing is a well-documented consequence of maternal opioid abuse. These neonates exhibit withdrawal hyperventilation and an increased incidence of **sudden infant death syndrome** (SIDS). The proposed studies are essential for understanding normal respiratory development, drug-induced changes, and effective treatment of pregnant heroin addicts and methadone maintained patients. The exact role of NTS MOR in neonatal congenital narcotic dependence and these respiratory disturbances is unknown. For anatomical, physiological, and pharmacological reasons, the guinea pig is a superb model for study of maternal opioid abuse. Guinea pig kappa opioid receptor has been cloned, but only partial sequences of MOR and delta opioid receptors have been available. However, our laboratory has recently determined the complete guinea pig MOR cDNA sequence. Availability of this sequence will enable us to define for the first time guinea pig MOR pharmacology, and systematically compare it to human and mouse MOR. Research is guided by four hypotheses: 1) guinea pig MOR is functionally similar to human MOR with respect to mu agonist efficacy, binding kinetics, and activation of G-protein, but different from murine MOR; 2) methadone induces respiratory depression and is equipotent to, but of longer duration than morphine in the neonatal guinea pig; 3) chronic in utero morphine and methadone exposure results in increased functional MOR on the cell surface, but decreases the coupling efficiency of MOR with G-proteins in the NTS; 4) chronic in utero morphine and methadone exposure up-regulates MOR mRNA in the NTS. Hypotheses are explored through four specific aims: 1) to compare mu agonist selectivity and potency, and development of cellular tolerance for guinea pig, human and murine MOR each expressed in stably transfected CHO cells; 2) to prove that the respiratory effects of methadone are similar to morphine in the neonatal guinea pig; 3) to study the effects of morphine and methadone on guinea pig MOR in NTS of brainstem sections from guinea pig neonates exposed in utero; and 4) to quantitate MOR mRNA in NTS from guinea pig neonates exposed to morphine and methadone in utero. These studies will provide developmental information on guinea pig NTS MOR following chronic in utero opioid exposure.

Website: http://crisp.cit.nih.gov/crisp/Crisp_Query.Generate_Screen

- **Project Title: NEUROCHEMICAL ORGANIZATION OF CENTRAL CHEMOSENSORY NEURONS**

Principal Investigator & Institution: Pete, Gina M.;; Howard University Washington, Dc 20059

Timing: Fiscal Year 2002

Summary: This proposal consists of research focused on: 1) the central neurochemical organization of sensory neurons that triggers integrated respiratory responses to changes in $CO_2/H+$, 2) the receptor systems of these neurons, activation of which may modulate their response to $CO_2/H+$ signal, and 3) their connectivity with respiratory output neurons such as hypoglossal motor cells. Recently, it has been shown that expression of immediate-early genes are sensitive, inducible, and broadly applicable markers for neurons activated by extracellular stimuli. In the proposed studies, we will use expression of c-fos gene encoded protein (cFos) to identify neurons activated by hypercapnia, in order to investigate neurotransmitter content and receptor systems of these cells. The connectivity of chemosensory neurons with the respiratory-related motoneuron pools will be determined by combining retrograde tracer technique with cFos immunohistochemistry. The data derived from these studies will provide basic information related to the central chemosensory network, neurochemical organization, and chemical nature of communications between chemosensitive ells and brainstem output neurons. These results will have indirect bearing on the understanding of neurochemical mechanisms underlying centrally mediated respiratory and cardiovascular dysfunctions, as might occur in idiopathic alveolar hypoventilation, sleep apnea and **sudden infant death syndrome.**

Website: http://crisp.cit.nih.gov/crisp/Crisp_Query.Generate_Screen

- **Project Title: NEURONAL DETERMINANTS OF RESPIRATORY RHYTHMOGENESIS**

Principal Investigator & Institution: Butera, Robert J.; Electrical and Computer Engr; Georgia Institute of Technology 505 Tenth St. Nw Atlanta, Ga 303320420

Timing: Fiscal Year 2002; Project Start 01-MAY-2001; Project End 30-APR-2004

Summary: (Applicant's abstract): The neuronal circuitry underlying respiratory rhythm genesis is a complex system with complex neuronal dynamics involving various neuronal populations within the mammalian brainstem. This rhythm persists in reduced in vitro preparations, including the en bloc brainstem-spinal cord and the transverse slice. While these reduced preparations have greatly advanced the study of respiratory rhythm genesis at the cellular level, the neuronal dynamics of even these reduced preparations are not completely understood. The objective of this particular application is to fully understand mechanisms for respiratory rhythm genesis in both in vitro and in vivo preparations; our particular approach is the use of computational models and quantitative data analysis techniques. We hypothesize that the aspiratory phase of the respiratory rhythm is generated by neurons in the pre-Botzinger complex (pBc) that display adaptive ion channel properties, and that this population interacts via excitatory and inhibitory connections with other respiratory regions to produce the complete respiratory rhythm in vivo. We further hypothesize that the nature of the excitatory synaptic connectivity within the pBc not only coordinates the aspiratory phase but also makes the respiratory rhythm more robust in the presence of cell-to-cell variability and external disturbances. Our specific aims are 1) determine how intrinsic ion channel properties and extrinsic synaptic input regulate burst frequency and duration and action potential firing rates of aspiratory pBc neurons; 2) determine how cellular heterogeneity and synaptic properties affect the synchronization and stability of the respiratory rhythm; and 3) determine the role of pacemaker-based and network-based modes of respiratory rhythm generation by extending our model to consider the en bloc brainstem spinal cord preparation. This research will increase our understanding of basic cellular and synaptic mechanisms underlying respiratory rhythm generation and may ultimately lead to new pharmacological techniques for clinical intervention and prophylaxis for such disorders as **sudden**

Infant death syndrome, sleep apnea and apnea of prematurity, central alveolar syndrome, and other forms of respiratory control failure.

Website: http://crisp.cit.nih.gov/crisp/Crisp_Query.Generate_Screen

- **Project Title: NICOTINE INDUCED NEUROPLASTICITY IN THE CAROTID BODY**

Principal Investigator & Institution: Gauda, Estelle B.; Associate Professor; Pediatrics; Johns Hopkins University 3400 N Charles St Baltimore, Md 21218

Timing: Fiscal Year 2002; Project Start 01-APR-2001; Project End 31-JAN-2005

Summary: (Scanned from the applicant's description): Nicotine, a major component of tobacco smoke, is a neuroteratogen that binds to nicotinic cholinergic receptors on catecholamine-containing neurons and induces neuroplasticity. Catecholaminergic systems are vulnerable to the effects of prenatal exposure to nicotine since these systems develop early in ontogeny and have trophic influences on the development of multiple neuronal networks. Perturbations in neurotransmission in dopaminergic and noradrenergic neurons in the central nervous system induced by nicotine exposure are associated with postnatal morbidities which include, impaired cognitive function, attention deficit disorders and abnormalities in locomotion. Prenatal nicotine exposure also affects maturation of adrenal chromaffin cells resulting in altered stress responses. We present data that prenatal nicotine exposure increases catecholaminergic traits in peripheral arterial chemoreceptors that are involved in cardiorespiratory control. An increase in inhibitory catecholaminergic traits in peripheral arterial chemoreceptors may in part account for the striking epidemologic association between prenatal exposure to tobacco smoke and **sudden infant death syndrome** (SIDS). Infants born to smoking mothers have depressed hypoxic arousal responses, reduced respiratory drive, and blunted ventilatory responses to hypoxia. Similarly, animals exposed prenatally to nicotine have abnormalities in hypoxic ventilation, delayed autoresuscitation and increased mortality with exposure to hypoxia. Comparable to nigrostriatal neurons and adrenal chromaffin cells, peripheral arterial chemoreceptors are rich in catecholamines and express nicotinic receptors. Plasticity of neurons in the central nervous system induced by nicotine exposure involves regulation of catecholaminergic traits mediated by cAMP/calcium and the neurotrophins, basic fibroblast growth factor (bFGF) and brain-derived nerve growth factor (BDNF). Our preliminary data show that prenatal nicotine increases tyrosine hydroxylase (TH) mRNA expression, the rate-limiting enzyme for catecholamine synthesis, in peripheral arterial chemoreceptors. However, the mechanism for this effect is unknown. Yet, it is known that the expression of catecholaminergic traits in peripheral arterial chemoreceptors during development is neurotrophin dependent. In the current proposal, we hypothesize that nicotine exposure during development up-regulates catecholaminergic systems in peripheral arterial chemoreceptors via cAMP/calcium mechanisms and the induction of neurotrophins. Thus, using an in vitro rat model of peripheral arterial chemoreceptors, the goals of this proposal are to 1) determine the plasticity of peripheral arterial chemoreceptors induced by late fetal and early postnatal nicotine exposure and 2), elucidate the cellular and molecular mechanisms involved in this plasticity.

Website: http://crisp.cit.nih.gov/crisp/Crisp_Query.Generate_Screen

- **Project Title: NORTHERN PLAINS PRENATAL AND INFANT HEALTH CONSORTIUM**

Principal Investigator & Institution: Elliott, Amy J.; Pediatrics; University of South Dakota 414 E Clark St Vermillion, Sd 57069

Timing: Fiscal Year 2003; Project Start 26-SEP-2003; Project End 31-JUL-2006

Summary: (provided by applicant): The 'Northern Plains Prenatal and Infant Health Consortium' is comprised of three institutions that each have existing links to communities across South and North Dakota and an Advisory Board with representatives from numerous community agencies and disciplines. The primary purpose behind the formation of this consortium is to provide a structure in which collaborative research projects can be conducted to clarify the role prenatal alcohol exposure plays in fetal death, stillbirth, and **sudden infant death syndrome.** Deciphering the impact of prenatal alcohol exposure on fetal/infant mortality and development will require the input of individuals from a variety of disciplines, in addition to input regarding community needs and concerns. The Northern Plains Consortium is committed to participating in the multidisciplinary steering committee that will result from this RFA and will work in a cooperative manner with the other Comprehensive Clinical Sites, the Developmental Biology and Pathology Center, the Data Coordinating and Analysis Center, and the NIH to design protocols that can be implemented across numerous clinical sites. It is hoped that this collaborative effort will result in answers that will decrease fetal and infant mortality rates, thereby improving child health in the communities we serve. The primary goal for Phase I of this project will be to formalize the collaborative relationships, with both the Steering Committee and the Northern Plains Advisory Board, which will serve as the basis for conducting multi-site research projects. These relationships will be formed through meetings which will occur 4 times in the first year for the Steering Committee and twice with the Advisory Board. We will meet with our advisory board twice each year, coincident with the bi-annual meetings of the Aberdeen Area Perinatal Infant Mortality Review Committee (PIMR). These meetings will lead to the creation of the collaborative structure and processes through which research projects suitable for multi-site implementation will be designed. Furthermore, the Advisory Board, which contains many community leaders, will help develop ways to strengthen the functional community partnerships that will be necessary to successfully carry out this research agenda. A final goal will be to refine the design of a potential pilot study that draws upon our expertise in the areas of exposure assessment and measurement of physiologic function during the fetal and early newborn period.

Website: http://crisp.cit.nih.gov/crisp/Crisp_Query.Generate_Screen

- **Project Title: PERINATAL ASSESSMENT OF AT RISK POPULATIONS**

Principal Investigator & Institution: Fifer, William P.; Professor; New York State Psychiatric Institute 1051 Riverside Dr New York, Ny 10032

Timing: Fiscal Year 2002; Project Start 30-SEP-1994; Project End 30-APR-2004

Summary: (adapted from investigator's abstract) The long-term objectives of this proposal are to elucidate physiologic mechanisms that underlie the **Sudden Infant Death Syndrome,** and to develop age-appropriate, non-invasive tests that will identify infants who are at the greatest risk for SIDS. These tests focus on assessments of peripheral and central mechanisms involved in the integrated control of cardiac, blood pressure, and respiratory function. Subjects are the fetuses and infants of mothers from a low-socioeconomic status population in New York City and from a rural Native American population on the Pine Ridge Reservation in South Dakota, which is at unusually high risk for SIDS. The proposed studies begin with measurements made during late gestation. Assessments then continue through infancy to document the physiologic changes that coincide with the period of maximal risk for SIDS. These postnatal studies incorporate measurements made during sleep under basal conditions as well as during head-up and head-down tilting. The principal dependent variables are heart rate and several indices of heart rate variability, respiratory rate and variability, body temperature, and electrocortical activity and beat-to-beat blood pressure. Five experiments will address the following aims; Patterns of developmental change in cardiorespiratory activity measured from the late fetal period through infancy will distinguish groups of infants at increased risk for SIDS How postnatal development of heart rate, blood pressure and respiratory responses to the challenge of head-up and head-down tilting will be altered in groups of infants at increased risk for SIDS Physiologic responses to tilt are dependent upon sleep state and this dependency may change with age Blood pressure decreases to head-up tilt are larger in the prone sleeping position Head-up tilting will induce cortical activation which will be diminished during the period of greatest vulnerability to SIDS Respiratory and heart rate responses to tilt will be diminished in the morning hours and Responses to tilt will vary with time after feeding.

Website: http://crisp.cit.nih.gov/crisp/Crisp_Query.Generate_Screen

- **Project Title: PHYSIOLOGICAL DEVELOPMENT IN SIDS**

  Principal Investigator & Institution: Harper, Ronald M.; Professor; Neurobiology; University of California Los Angeles 10920 Wilshire Blvd., Suite 1200 Los Angeles, Ca 90024

  Timing: Fiscal Year 2002; Project Start 01-DEC-1986; Project End 30-JUN-2004

  Summary: The objective is to identify brain structures which mediate controlling influences on breathing and blood pressure during waking and quiet sleep, and thus to assist determination of the mechanisms of failure in the **Sudden Infant Death syndrome** (SIDS). Blood oxygen level dependent (BOLD) functional magnetic resonance imaging will be used to visualize neural activity in 1) twenty-two patients with Congenital Central Hypoventilation Syndrome (CCHS), a disorder characterized by absence of central chemoreception, loss of breathing drive during sleep, impaired breathing responses to hyperthermia, and occasional waking hypotonia; 2) twnety-two Prader-Walli patients, who show diminished peripheral, but intact central chemoreception; and 3) twenty-two age- and gender-matched controls. Images will be acquired during baseline, and during hyperoxic, hypercapnic, hypoxic, inspiratory loading, hyperthermic, paced breathing and passive motion challenges, and during cold pressor application, while respiratory measures, heart rate and variability, non-invasive blood pressure, and an index of sympathetic outflow (sweating" are collected. Brain images from baseline conditions will be compare to images collected during experimental challenges in waking for all three groups, and in quiet sleep for CCHS and control subjects. The extent of activation and time course of changes in activated brain regions during challenges will be compared between groups. The timing of signal changes in different brain sites will be correlated with physiological changes accompanying the challengers. The studies have the potential to reveal the rain sites underlying breathing and blood pressure control, and the potential mechanisms of failure in SIDS.

Website: http://crisp.cit.nih.gov/crisp/Crisp_Query.Generate_Screen

- **Project Title: POSTNATAL RESETTING OF CAROTID CHEMORECEPTOR SENSITIVITY**

Principal Investigator & Institution: Carroll, John L.; Associate Professor; Arkansas Children's Hospital Res Inst Research Institute Little Rock, Ar 72202

Timing: Fiscal Year 2002; Project Start 01-AUG-1995; Project End 31-AUG-2004

Summary: The main sensors of arterial oxygen (02) tension are the carotid bodies (CB). Although they are critically important during infancy, they are not fully developed at birth, and take time to mature. The site of O2 sensing is believed to be the type I cell, which depolarizes in response to hypoxia, leading to Ca2+ influx through calcium channels, a rise in intracellular calcium and release of neurotransmitters which are thought to stimulate carotid sinus nerve endings. We previously reported that the type I cell calcium response to hypoxia matures after birth, and our recent studies suggest that several aspects of this cascade change after birth, as follows: (a) depolarization of type I cells by hypoxia is minimal in cells from newborns and increases with age; (b)the O2-sensitivity of a background K+ conductance is small in cells from newborns and increases with age; and (c) calcium currents of immature, but not mature, type cells are inhibited 50% by hypoxia. The proposed work will test the hypothesis that developmental changes in the O2-sensitivity of a background "leak" K+ conductance account, in part, for postnatal maturation of carotid chemoreceptor O2 sensitivity. In addition, we will determine whether (1) background K+ conductance is carried by one major background K+ channel type, the O2 sensitivity of which increases with age; or (2) background K+ conductance in type I cells is carried by at least 2 channel types, one O2-sensitive and one non-O2-sensitive, and development involves a change in the ratio of the O2-sensitive to non-O2-sensitive channels. We will also seek to understand whether developmental shifts occur in 0a-sensitive calcium channels during maturation. The results will answer important questions about the mechanisms underlying postnatal development of carotid chemoreceptor function. The ultimate goal of the proposed studies is to understand how the carotid chemoreceptors mature and how development is modulated, so that a number of potentially life threatening disorders such as asthma, bronchopulmonary dysplasia, apnea and **sudden infant death syndrome** (SIDS) can be better treated or prevented.

Website: http://crisp.cit.nih.gov/crisp/Crisp_Query.Generate_Screen

- **Project Title: PREDICTING LIFE-THREATENING EVENTS IN CHIME INFANT DATA**

Principal Investigator & Institution: Schuckers, Stephanie C.; Electrical and Computer Engr; Clarkson University Division of Research Potsdam, Ny 136995630

Timing: Fiscal Year 2002; Project Start 27-JUL-2002; Project End 30-JUN-2004

Summary: (provided by applicant): **Sudden infant death syndrome** (SIDS) is the sudden death of an infant under one year old without any apparent warning signs. It is the leading cause of death of infants between the age of one month and one year in the developed countries. Previous studies have indicated that SIDS victims may suffer from cardiorespiratory failure, which reflects immaturity of autonomic nervous system (ANS) control. Heart variability (HRV) has been shown to be a noninvasive and inexpensive way to assess the ANS. Increased heart rate and decreased heart rate variability have been observed in SIDS victims. While it is unclear whether there is a relationship between SIDS and infants who have apparent life-threatening events (ALTE) like apnea and bradycardia, there is a desire to gain a better understanding of the nature of ALTE, their frequency and severity, and the ability of home monitors to detect events and provide an alarm. The Collaborative Home Infant Monitoring Evaluation (CHIME) study group, formed by NIH, sought to study these issues through the collection of a massive clinical database, which includes physiological, signals from 529 infants recorded in polysomnographic (PSG) studies. The infants were then studied several months using a home monitor which recorded life-threatening events. A classification is available regarding which infants had verified, apparent life-threatening events. Given the wealth of information linking SIDS and heart rate variability (HRV), we desire to investigate whether heart rate variability is effective predictor for life-threatening events. This research will investigate whether HRV can differentiate infants at risk for future apparent life-threatening events (FALTE). First statistical methods will be used to determine if there is significant difference in HRV between normal and FALTE infant groups. Next, the major goal is to design a method to classify infants using HRV, exploring various prediction models including logistic regression, decision tree, and neural networks. The relationship between HRV parameters and all the affected factors will also be studied to provide a clearer understanding of the parameters, and to help determine how to use HRV as a classifier. Successful prediction of infants with future apparent life-threatening events could have clinical significance and provide physicians with an opportunity for treatment.

Website: http://crisp.cit.nih.gov/crisp/Crisp_Query.Generate_Screen

- **Project Title: PROFILING THE NEEDS OF DYING CHILDREN**

Principal Investigator & Institution: Feudtner, John C.;; Children's Hospital of Philadelphia 34Th St and Civic Ctr Blvd Philadelphia, Pa 191044399

Timing: Fiscal Year 2002; Project Start 01-AUG-2000; Project End 31-JUL-2005

Summary: Addressing the needs of dying children- a benchmark of societal compassion and a gauge of health care quality-rises as a challenge for the 21st century. As deaths due to injury, prematurity, and **sudden infant death syndrome** are prevented, the remaining deaths may be increasingly associated with chronic conditions. I hypothesize that deaths attributable to complex chronic conditions (CCCs) constitute an increasing proportion of all pediatric deaths, both at a population level and more specifically among patients cared for by children's hospitals, and that the prolongation of life has led to a rising prevalence of these conditions. Furthermore, I postulate that quality of care and support for these dying children and their families deteriorates over the last two years of life, with declining continuity of care and untimely referral to hospice and other social support services. This five-year research plan will profile the needs of dying children specifically aiming to: 1. Determine whether the prevalence of terminal congenital CCCs is rising in the national population. 2. Measure the change in prevalence of children with terminal CCCs in tertiary children's hospitals, thereby assessing the magnitude of need for hospital-based pediatric palliative care services. 3. Test whether the 'intensity' of medical care increases in the 30-day interval prior to the day on which death compared to the preceding 23 month interval, so as to improve clinicians prognostic inferences regarding likelihood of death. 4. Examine two markers of quality of care of children with CCCs by: Testing whether the continuity of care deteriorates in the last two years of life for children with CCCs; and 5. Examining the timing of referral to hospice. This research seeks to improve the care and health policy for dying children in three ways. First, evidence of a 'epidemiological transition' in pediatric mortality-from mostly accidental and sudden death to deaths that occur somewhat inevitably with a longer yet unpredictable dying process-would motivate the redesign of pediatric health care services and physician training at both the regional and national level. Second, this research will produce several techniques to monitor health utilization data for indicators of the quality of care provided to terminally ill children. Finally, the results of these studies will ultimately inform the development and trial of a longitudinal needs assessment program for children with complex chronic conditions. These studies of the epidemiology of pediatric death and the needs of dying children will help enhance the individual care provided to these children and their families as well as broader policy. They will also foster the development of the applicant's research skills so as to become an independent researcher addressing the needs of children with complex chronic conditions.

Website: http://crisp.cit.nih.gov/crisp/Crisp_Query.Generate_Screen

- **Project Title: PROTECTIVE RESPONSES AND BRAINSTEM ANALYSIS IN SUDDEN INFANT DEATH SYNDROME**

  Principal Investigator & Institution: Kinney, Hannah C.; Associate Professor; Children's Hospital (Boston) Boston, Ma 021155737

  Timing: Fiscal Year 2002

  Summary: The overall hypothesis of the program project is that the **sudden infant death syndrome** (SIDS), or a subset of SIDS, is due to developmental abnormalities of the ventral medulla in the brainstem that interfere with normal protective responses to potentially life-threatening, but often occurring, events during sleep, such as hypoxia, hypercapnia, and apnea. Recently we reported neurotransmitter receptor binding deficiencies in SIDS victims in the arcuate nucleus, a region considered homologous to neurons located on the ventral medullary surface in cats that are responsible for the protective responses to hypercapnia and asphyxia. A lesion in the arcuate nucleus could be the only defect in SIDS victims, or a group of SIDS victims. Given the multiple and complex brainstem circuits that underlie protective response to hypoxia, hypercapnia, and apnea, however, a lesion in the arcuate nucleus could be but one of a group of disorders in brainstem protective responses, or alternatively, a central link in a chain of brainstem abnormalities that result in sudden infant death. In this project, we will test the hypothesis that neurotransmitter receptor binding abnormalities in the arcuate nucleus are part of a complex of neurochemical abnormalities in brainstem components related to protective responses to hypoxia, hypercapnia, and apnea. Our Specific Aims are: 1) To determine if there are neurochemical differences between SIDS and age-matched control brainstems in sites related to protective responses, e.g., in the caudal raphe; and 2) To determine if the putative abnormality in neurotransmitter receptor binding in sites related to protective responses correlate with abnormal 3H-kainate binding to kainate receptors in the arcuate nucleus in the same SIDS cases. Quantitative tissue receptor autoradiography will be used. This project would advance our understanding of the role of the brainstem in the pathogenesis of sudden death in SIDS victims.

Website: http://crisp.cit.nih.gov/crisp/Crisp_Query.Generate_Screen

- **Project Title: PROTECTIVE VENTILATORY RESPONSES TO HYPOXIA**

Principal Investigator & Institution: St. John, Walter; Professor; Children's Hospital (Boston) Boston, Ma 021155737

Timing: Fiscal Year 2002; Project Start 01-APR-2002; Project End 31-MAR-2003

Summary: The protective response to hypoxia is organized in two layers. With initial exposure, eupneic ventilation increase. In severe hypoxia, eupnea is replaced by gasping, which promotes "autoresuscitation." The eupneic ventilatory response to hypoxia changes with development. In the newborn, ventilation rises and then falls. With age, the hypoxia-induced augmentation becomes more sustained. We hypothesize that hypoxia- induced ventilatory depression results from activation of a mesencephalic- pontine "central oxygen detector." Piglets will be studied. We will identify the region containing the "central oxygen detector." Hypoxia-induced depressions of ventilation will be attenuated if neurons of this central oxygen are destroyed. Neuronal activities of this detector will be characterized. These activities are hypothesized to increased during depressions of phrenic activity in hypoxia or during localized hypoxia by applications of sodium cyanide. We will then examine the role of neurons in the ventral medulla in hypoxia-induced ventilatory depressions and in the neurogenesis of gasping. These ventral medullary neuronal activities may provide a generalized tonic input for ventilatory activity. Yet gasping will not be altered since the mechanisms underlying the neurogenesis of eupnea and gasping differ fundamentally. In unanesthetized piglets, ventilatory activity will be recorded during wakefulness and sleep. We hypothesize that apneic episodes will be recorded following ablation of neurons in the medullary gasping center and those in the ventral medulla. Our results will have profound implications as to the mechanisms of apnea and the **sudden infant death syndrome.** Mechanisms of central apnea may be elucidated by our studies of the "direct" influence of hypoxia on the brainstem ventilatory control system, of the role of ventral medullary mechanisms in this hypoxia-induced depression and the role of medullary gasping mechanisms in the control of eupnea.

Website: http://crisp.cit.nih.gov/crisp/Crisp_Query.Generate_Screen

- **Project Title: REGULATION OF CAROTID BODY AFFERENT DEVELOPMENT**

Principal Investigator & Institution: Katz, David M.; Associate Professor; Neurosciences; Case Western Reserve University 10900 Euclid Ave Cleveland, Oh 44106

Timing: Fiscal Year 2002; Project Start 01-JUL-1989; Project End 30-JUN-2004

Summary: The proposed research seeks to define the role of neuronal growth factors in development of chemoafferent neurons and peripheral chemoreflexes in rats and mice. Chemoafferent neurons in the petrosal are the afferent link between the carotid body and central autonomic pathways and thereby play a pivotal role in regulating chemoreceptor control of cardiorespiratory function. Until recently, relatively little was known about mechanisms that underlie development of the chemoafferent pathway, despite evidence that derangements of chemoreflex maturation may contribute to developmental disorders of cardiorespiratory control, including **Sudden Infant Death Syndrome** and hypoventilation and apneic syndromes in neonates and infants. This continuation proposal is based on our recent discovery that Brain-Derived Neurotrophic Factor (BDNF), a member of the neurotrophin family of neuronal growth factors, is expressed in the fetal carotid body and is required for survival of chemoafferent neurons and development of peripheral chemoreflexes. The proposed studies are designed to further define the role of BDNF in development of chemoreflex function and to elucidate the role of Glial Cell Line-Derived Neurotrophic Factor (GDNF), a newly discovered growth factor in the developing chemoafferent pathway. To approach these issues, the proposed research seeks to define growth factor influences on chemoafferent development and chemoreflex maturation, using rat fetuses and neonates, as well as genetically engineered mice lacking functional growth factor alleles. Specifically, we plan to define 1) Growth factor regulation of chemoafferent survival and differentiation, in vivo and in vitro, 2) Growth factor regulation of chemoreflex development, using plethysmographic recording in intact animals, 3) Regulation of chemoafferent survival by oxygen availability in vivo, and 4) The role of endogenous BDNF in chemoafferent neurons. By defining growth factor regulation of chemoafferent pathway development, the proposed research aims to shed light on cellular and molecular mechanisms relevant to understanding and improved management of hypoventilation and apnea syndromes in neonates and infants. Already, molecular genetic studies have identified bdnf and gdnf as candidate genes for at least one developmental disorder of breathing, Congenital Central

Hypoventilation Syndrome. In addition, by elucidating how oxygen availability regulates chemoafferent survival after birth, these studies are designed to provide insight into potential links between supplemental oxygen therapy and delayed maturation of peripheral chemoreflexes in preterm infants. Moreover, it is hoped that defining development of this system will, in turn, create a model of growth factor function and regulation that is applicable to the nervous system as a whole.

Website: http://crisp.cit.nih.gov/crisp/Crisp_Query.Generate_Screen

- **Project Title: RESPIRATORY PATTERN GENERATION STUDIED IN VITRO**

Principal Investigator & Institution: Feldman, Jack L.; Chairman; Neurobiology; University of California Los Angeles 10920 Wilshire Blvd., Suite 1200 Los Angeles, Ca 90024

Timing: Fiscal Year 2002; Project Start 01-JUL-1988; Project End 30-JUN-2004

Summary: The brain is vigilant in control of breathing, regulating blood O_2 and CO_3 over an order of magnitude range in metabolic demand, wide ranges of posture and body movements, compromises in muscle or cardiopulmonary function, from birth till death without lapses beyond a few minutes. This grant continues our effort to determine the sites and mechanisms underlying the nervous system generation and modulation of breathing rhythm. Determination of these properties is critical for understanding pathologies where ventilatory failure results from dysfunction of nervous system, including such diseases as apnea of prematurity, congenital central hypoventilation, central alveolar hypoventilation, sleep apnea and, perhaps, **sudden infant death syndrome.** Significant progress in identifying critical sites and cellular mechanisms involved in the generation of the respiratory rhythm followed the development of novel in vitro preparations. These preparations generate a respiratory-related rhythm, and their exploitation led to two hypotheses that are the focus of this application: SITE HYPOTHESIS: The preBotzinger Complex (preBotC) contains the kernel for respiratory rhythm generation. The preBotC is the limited portion of the ventrolateral respiratory column necessary and sufficient for in vitro neonatal rodent medullary slice preparations to generate respiratory-related motor nerve output. We discovered that the anatomical extent of the preBotC in rodent is demarked by neurons expressing Neurokinin 1 receptors. Two goals of this project are to use this information to: i) test the SITE HYPOTHESIS, and; ii) identify the preBotC in neonatal and adult human brain. RHYTHMOGENESIS HYPOTHESIS: Endogenous bursting, i.e., pacemaker(-like), neurons in the preBotC are the cellular kernel for respiratory rhythm. There are three questions that must be answered to understand the generation of the respiratory rhythm: i) Which neurons are necessary and/or sufficient for the rhythm?; ii) By what mechanism do these neurons generate the rhythm?; How is the rhythm modulated? Of the various neurons which are candidates for this role, we propose a population of neurons called Type-1. Two additional goals are to:) test whether Type- 1 neurons are required for generation of respiratory rhythm, and; ii) determine the synaptic interactions amongst preBotC neurons that define the respiratory rhythm generating network.

Website: http://crisp.cit.nih.gov/crisp/Crisp_Query.Generate_Screen

- **Project Title: SIDS DATA COORDINATING AND ANALYSIS CENTER**

Principal Investigator & Institution: Dukes, Kimberly A.;; Dm-Stat, Inc. 407 Rear Mystic Ave, Unit 11A Medford, Ma 02155

Timing: Fiscal Year 2003; Project Start 30-SEP-2003; Project End 31-JUL-2006

Summary: (provided by applicant): In multi-center studies or collaborative projects, a centralized Data Coordinating and Analysis Center (DCAC) with strong leadership, organization and analytic skills is critical to the success of the project. DMSTAT, Inc. proposes to serve as the DCAC for the multi-disciplinary research network on prenatal alcohol exposure and **sudden infant death syndrome** (SIDS) that will be established through responses to RFA HD- 03-004. DM-STAT has a proven track record of success as the designated DCAC on NICHD and NIAAA sponsored multi-center trials and collaborations. Our goal is to make life easier for participating staff so that they can focus on their areas of expertise. To achieve that goal, DM-STAT will create and maintain a study-wide infrastructure to support the activities of and facilitate information sharing between members of the Network, including the NICHD, NIAAA, and governing boards. This infrastructure will revolve around a Network website containing administrative and data management components. The website will provide instant access to all project documentation and materials, data management reports, statistical analysis summaries, and will provide a forum (the Meeting Center) for sharing ideas and issues. The first phase (of two phases) calls for formalizing a collaborative structure between, Comprehensive Clinical Sites (CCS), Developmental Biology and Pathology Center(s) (DBPC) and the DCAC to investigate the relationship between prenatal alcohol exposure and the risk for **sudden infant death syndrome** (SIDS) and adverse pregnancy outcomes (e.g., stillbirth and fetal alcohol syndrome (FAS)). In addition, the Network will investigate social and behavioral factors that may be related to a woman's decision to drink alcohol during pregnancy and lactation. Phase I will require development of testable hypotheses, pilot testing of the core and site-specific protocols and producing an executive summary with recommendations based upon the results of these pilot studies in order to assess feasibility and justification for Phase II. DM-STAT will provide leadership and guidance to the network with respect to study design, protocol development, data management and statistical analysis. With a cohesive Network in place, DM-STAT will then be responsible for coordinating safe and consistent implementation of the core protocol, monitoring key indicators of quality, and performing analysis of pilot data. DM-STAT is committed to quality; it is the focal point of everything we do. We are proactive as opposed to reactive, innovative in streamlining and organizing processes and procedures, able to educate and communicate with study staff at all levels, and we are passionate and committed to getting the job done right the first time. We believe that DM-STAT is best positioned to serve the needs of this Network in an efficient and effective manner.

Website: http://crisp.cit.nih.gov/crisp/Crisp_Query.Generate_Screen

- **Project Title: STACHYBOTRYS INDUCED HEMORRHAGE IN THE DEVELOPING LUNG**

Principal Investigator & Institution: Dearborn, Dorr G.; Associate Professor of Biochemistry; Pediatrics; Case Western Reserve University 10900 Euclid Ave Cleveland, Oh 44106

Timing: Fiscal Year 2002; Project Start 05-FEB-1999; Project End 31-JAN-2004

Summary: Over the past 4 years in Cleveland, Ohio there have been 34 cases of pulmonary hemorrhage and hemosiderosis in young infants. To date, ten infants have died. A CDC case-controlled study found an association with water damaged homes and the toxigenic fungus called Stachybotrys atra which requires water-saturated cellulose to grow. The spores of this fungus do not germinate in the lung, but do not contain very potent mycotoxins which appear to be particularly toxic to the rapidly developing lungs of young infants. Secondary stresses, e.g. environmental tobacco smoke, appear to be important triggers for overt hemorrhage. Concern that there may be a large number of undetected infants with the disorder ted to examination of all infant coroner cases, which revealed six **sudden infant death syndrome** cases with major amounts of pulmonary hemosiderin-laden macrophages, indicating extensive hemosiderosis existing prior to death. All of these infants lived in the same contiguous area as the majority of the hemosiderosis patients. This disorder may extend beyond Cleveland, since toxigenic fungi are widespread. We are aware of 122 infants with idiopathic pulmonary hemorrhage in this country in the past 4 years. The purpose of this proposal is to establish an original rat pup model for Stachybotrymycotoxicosis which can be used to understand the developmental pathophysiology by which fungal spores induces hemorrhage, address practical problems in clinical care, and foster public health prevention. This model uses tracheal instillation of toxic Stachybotrys spores in neonatal to weanling rats to initiate the pathologic process. Specific aim 1 will evaluate dose response to Stachybotrys spore inhalation, critical age of vulnerability, histopathology, inflammatory mediator response, and change in lung function during injury and recovery. Specific aim 2 will explore the vulnerability of pulmonary capillaries to leakage in the Stachybotrys exposed pups in vivo and in vitro, specific stress triggers of hemorrhage, and efficacy of anti-inflammatory therapy. Specific aim 3 will develop and test biochemical markers for Stachybotrys exposure including toxins and antibody production. The experiments in this proposal will provide fundamental new information on Stachybotrys exposure applicable to detection and treatment of this new disorder.

Website: http://crisp.cit.nih.gov/crisp/Crisp_Query.Generate_Screen

- **Project Title: THE UPPER AIRWAY AND THE SUDDEN INFANT DEATH SYNDROME**

Principal Investigator & Institution: Bartlett, Donald; Professor and Chair; Physiology; Dartmouth College 11 Rope Ferry Rd. #6210 Hanover, Nh 03755

Timing: Fiscal Year 2003; Project Start 01-APR-2003; Project End 31-MAR-2007

Summary: (provided by applicant): Despite recent progress in its prevention, the **Sudden Infant Death Syndrome** (SIDS) remains the most frequent cause of infant mortality between the ages of one month and one year in the United States. A striking epidemiological finding is that more victims than expected are found in the prone position, often with the face in the bedclothes. Campaigns to encourage putting infants to sleep on their backs have led to a gratifying reduction in the incidence of SIDS in several countries, yet the influence of posture remains mysterious. This project will use decerebrate neonatal piglets to explore the possibility that the risk of prone sleeping is determined by reflex responses involving the upper airway, and that these responses may be aggravated by CO_2 in the upper airway (from re-breathing), by abnormalities of the ventral medulla (for which there is evidence in some SIDS victims), or from elevated body temperature (for which there is epidemiologic evidence and an intriguing report of a study in puppies). We will examine the influence of each of these conditions on three upper airway reflex responses: the "diving" response, the laryngeal chemo reflex and the load-compensating reflex response to upper airway obstruction. Our general hypothesis is that some combination of conditions and stimuli will exaggerate the reflex interruption of breathing, possibly contributing to the pathogenesis of SIDS.

Website: http://crisp.cit.nih.gov/crisp/Crisp_Query.Generate_Screen

- **Project Title: TRIGEMINAL AUTONOMIC INTERACTIONS**

    Principal Investigator & Institution: Mcculloch, Paul F.; Physiology; Midwestern University 555 31St St Downers Grove, Il 605151235

    Timing: Fiscal Year 2002; Project Start 30-SEP-2002; Project End 29-SEP-2004

    Summary: (provided by applicant): The long-term goal of this application to establish the mechanisms and circuitry by which signals from the upper respiratory tract integrate within the brainstem to produce reflex autonomic responses. Stimulation of the upper respiratory tract can produce an intense functional reorganization of the cardiovascular and respiratory systems. This reflex includes central apnea, parasympathetic bradycardia and sympathetically mediated vasoconstriction. Initiation of this response results from stimulation of trigeminal receptors that innervate the face and nasal passages. This autonomic response is primarily a defensive reflex, and is only elicited when a potentially life threatening external stimulus is presented. Because an animal is in imminent danger during such an event, homeostatic control, such as the maintenance or arterial blood pressure, should no longer be primary objective of the animal?s autonomic nervous system. In this situation a defensive reflex should temporarily become more powerful than a homeostatic reflex. It is hypothesized that stimulation of the trigeminal inhibits the baroreflex at the level of the nucleus tractus solitarius (NTS). The objectives of this proposal are to determine 1) the response of brainstem trigeminal neurons during nasal stimulation; 2) the relationship between the trigeminal system and secondary brainstem neurons located in the NTS and rostral ventrolateral medulla (RVLM); and 3) if trigeminal stimulation inhibits second-order barosensitive NTS neurons. It is expected that extracellular recordings will determine that neurons located within the superficial laminae of the trigeminal medullary dorsal horn (MDH) respond to nasal stimulation with an increase in firing rate that positively correlates with the cardiorespiratory changes elicited by the nasal stimulation. It is also expected that electrical stimulation of the NTS and RVLM will antidromically stimulate these same MDH neurons. This would determine that these nuclei are part of the brainstem circuitry of this response. Finally, it is expected that extracellular recordings will determine that trigeminal stimulation inhibits barosensitive neurons within the NTS, thus inhibiting the brainstem baroreflex pathway. This would indicate that a defensive reflex (upper respiratory tract stimulation) can inhibit a homeostatic reflex (arterial baroreflex). This proposal has clinical implications because it investigates the relationship between a defensive reflex and a homeostatic reflex, and explores the mechanisms of integrative cardiorespiratory control within the brainstem. Also, stimulation of the upper respiratory tract may be a casual factor in **Sudden Infant Death Syndrome** (SIDS). Some infants at risk for SIDS present autonomic dysfunction and abnormalities of respiratory and/or cardiovascular control mechanisms, especially after stimulation of the upper respiratory tract. Having a better understanding of brainstem cardiorespiratory integration might provide a neurological basis for the etiology of SIDS.

Website: http://crisp.cit.nih.gov/crisp/Crisp_Query.Generate_Screen

- **Project Title: VENTRAL MEDULLA, BREATHING, AND CENTRAL CHEMORECEPTION**

Principal Investigator & Institution: Nattie, Eugene E.; Professor of Physiology; Children's Hospital (Boston) Boston, Ma 021155737

Timing: Fiscal Year 2002

Summary: We proposed that SIDS results from abnormalities in the ventral medulla that interfere with normal protective cardiorespiratory reflexes. In this project we shall disrupt experimentally in piglets, at two developmental times, the homologue of the human arcuate nucleus found to be abnormal in SIDS victims. This homologue is proposed to contain the retrotrapezoid nucleus (RTN) and parapyramidal regions, the medullary raphe region, and the central chemoreceptor regions of the caudal ventrolateral medulla. In adult animals, disruption of the RTN/parapyramidal and raphe regions is known to diminish respiratory output and the sensitivity of the respiratory response to increased carbon dioxide. The magnitude of the effects is greater in anesthesia. Denervation of peripheral chemoreceptors magnifies the deleterious effects of this disruption in adult animals; when performed in newborn animals with intact brainstem function, it results in hypoventilation, more frequent apneas, and death. We shall, in the decerebrate piglet with and without intact carotid bodies, alter arcuate homologue function by microinjection of 1) an excitatory amino acid neurotoxin to produce lesions, and 2) muscarinic and ionotropic glutamate agonists/antagonists, and thyrotropin releasing-hormone. Phrenic nerve output and blood pressure in the baseline state and their responses to hypercapnia and asphyxia will be measured. In the unanesthetized chronic piglet preparations with and without intact carotid bodies, we will examine the effect of arcuate homologue lesions on breathing and blood pressure during natural wakefulness and sleep and on the responses to hypercapnia and asphyxia. Our goal is to examine the relative roles of arcuate homologue neurons and carotid body inputs on breathing and blood pressure in the absence of anesthesia and in natural sleep and wakefulness. In respect to the Triple Risk Model for SIDS pathogenesis, we are 1) experimentally creating a vulnerability by means of our lesions or injections, at 2) two separate developmental ages, and 3) examining, as exogenous stresses, responses to hypercapnia and asphyxia in wakefulness and sleep with and without afferent input from the carotid body.

Website: http://crisp.cit.nih.gov/crisp/Crisp_Query.Generate_Screen

E-Journals: PubMed Central[16]

PubMed Central (PMC) is a digital archive of life sciences journal literature developed and managed by the National Center for Biotechnology Information (NCBI) at the U.S. National Library of Medicine (NLM).[17] Access to this growing archive of e-journals is free and unrestricted.[18] To search, go to **http://www.ncbi.nlm.nih.gov/entrez/query.fcgi?db=Pmc**, and type "sudden infant death syndrome" (or synonyms) into the search box. This search gives you access to full-text articles. The following is a sample of items found for sudden infant death syndrome in the PubMed Central database:

- **Babies sleeping with parents: case-control study of factors influencing the risk of the sudden infant death syndrome.** by Blair PS, Fleming PJ, Smith IJ, Platt MW, Young J, Nadin P, Berry PJ, Golding J.; 1999 Dec 4; http://www.pubmedcentral.gov/articlerender.fcgi?tool=pmcentrez&arti d=28288

---

[16] Adapted from the National Library of Medicine: **http://www.pubmedcentral.nih.gov/about/intro.html**.

[17] With PubMed Central, NCBI is taking the lead in preservation and maintenance of open access to electronic literature, just as NLM has done for decades with printed biomedical literature. PubMed Central aims to become a world-class library of the digital age.

[18] The value of PubMed Central, in addition to its role as an archive, lies the availability of data from diverse sources stored in a common format in a single repository. Many journals already have online publishing operations, and there is a growing tendency to publish material online only, to the exclusion of print.

- **Facial structure in the sudden infant death syndrome: case-control study.** by Rees K, Wright A, Keeling JW, Douglas NJ.; 1998 Jul 18; http://www.pubmedcentral.gov/articlerender.fcgi?tool=pmcentrez&artid=28609

- **Functional and Developmental Studies of the Peripheral Arterial Chemoreceptors in Rat: Effects of Nicotine and Possible Relation to Sudden Infant Death Syndrome.** by Holgert H, Hokfelt T, Hertzberg T, Lagercrantz H.; 1995 Aug 1; http://www.pubmedcentral.gov/articlerender.fcgi?tool=pmcentrez&rendertype=abstract&artid=41382

- **Used infant mattresses and sudden infant death syndrome in Scotland: case-control study.** by Tappin D, Brooke H, Ecob R, Gibson A.; 2002 Nov 2; http://www.pubmedcentral.gov/articlerender.fcgi?tool=pmcentrez&artid=131017

The National Library of Medicine: PubMed

One of the quickest and most comprehensive ways to find academic studies in both English and other languages is to use PubMed, maintained by the National Library of Medicine. The advantage of PubMed over previously mentioned sources is that it covers a greater number of domestic and foreign references. It is also free to the public.[19] If the publisher has a Web site that offers full text of its journals, PubMed will provide links to that site, as well as to sites offering other related data. User registration, a subscription fee, or some other type of fee may be required to access the full text of articles in some journals.

To generate your own bibliography of studies dealing with sudden infant death syndrome, simply go to the PubMed Web site at **www.ncbi.nlm.nih.gov/pubmed**. Type "sudden infant death syndrome" (or synonyms) into the search box, and click "Go." The following is the type of output you can expect from PubMed for "sudden infant death syndrome" (hyperlinks lead to article summaries):

---

[19] PubMed was developed by the National Center for Biotechnology Information (NCBI) at the National Library of Medicine (NLM) at the National Institutes of Health (NIH). The PubMed database was developed in conjunction with publishers of biomedical literature as a search tool for accessing literature citations and linking to full-text journal articles at Web sites of participating publishers. Publishers that participate in PubMed supply NLM with their citations electronically prior to or at the time of publication.

- A case of murder and the BMJ. Was it truly murder or sudden infant death syndrome?
  Author(s): Lowry RB.
  Source: Bmj (Clinical Research Ed.). 2002 May 4; 324(7345): 1096-7.
  http://www.ncbi.nlm.nih.gov/entrez/query.fcgi?cmd=Retrieve&db=pubmed&dopt=Abstract&list_uids=11993496

- A comparison of respiratory symptoms and inflammation in sudden infant death syndrome and in accidental or inflicted infant death.
  Author(s): Krous HF, Nadeau JM, Silva PD, Blackbourne BD.
  Source: The American Journal of Forensic Medicine and Pathology : Official Publication of the National Association of Medical Examiners. 2003 March; 24(1): 1-8.
  http://www.ncbi.nlm.nih.gov/entrez/query.fcgi?cmd=Retrieve&db=pubmed&dopt=Abstract&list_uids=12604990

- A comparison of the effects of parental risk markers on pre- and perinatal variables in multiple patient cohorts with fetal alcohol syndrome, autism, Tourette syndrome, and sudden infant death syndrome: an enviromic analysis.
  Author(s): Klug MG, Burd L, Kerbeshian J, Benz B, Martsolf JT.
  Source: Neurotoxicology and Teratology. 2003 November-December; 25(6): 707-17.
  http://www.ncbi.nlm.nih.gov/entrez/query.fcgi?cmd=Retrieve&db=pubmed&dopt=Abstract&list_uids=14624970

- A serotonin malfunction hypothesis by finding clear mutual relationships between several risk factors and symptoms associated with sudden infant death syndrome.
  Author(s): Okado N, Narita M, Narita N.
  Source: Medical Hypotheses. 2002 March; 58(3): 232-6.
  http://www.ncbi.nlm.nih.gov/entrez/query.fcgi?cmd=Retrieve&db=pubmed&dopt=Abstract&list_uids=12018976

- A study on how to increase the sudden infant death syndrome (SIDS) autopsy rate.
  Author(s): Matoba R.
  Source: Forensic Science International. 2002 September 14; 130 Suppl: S104-8.
  http://www.ncbi.nlm.nih.gov/entrez/query.fcgi?cmd=Retrieve&db=pubmed&dopt=Abstract&list_uids=12350311

- **A triple-risk model for the sudden infant death syndrome (SIDS) and the apparent life-threatening episode (ALTE): the stressed magnesium deficient weanling rat.**
  Author(s): Caddell JL.
  Source: Magnes Res. 2001 September; 14(3): 227-38.
  http://www.ncbi.nlm.nih.gov/entrez/query.fcgi?cmd=Retrieve&db=pubmed&dopt=Abstract&list_uids=11599557

- **Addendum: Distinguishing Sudden Infant Death Syndrome From Child Abuse Fatalities.**
  Author(s): American Academy of Pediatrics. Committee on Child Abuse and Neglect.
  Source: Pediatrics. 2001 September; 108(3): 812.
  http://www.ncbi.nlm.nih.gov/entrez/query.fcgi?cmd=Retrieve&db=pubmed&dopt=Abstract&list_uids=11547803

- **Adult hemoglobin levels at birth and risk of sudden infant death syndrome.**
  Author(s): Richardson DB, Wing S, Lorey F, Hertz-Picciotto I.
  Source: Archives of Pediatrics & Adolescent Medicine. 2004 April; 158(4): 366-71.
  http://www.ncbi.nlm.nih.gov/entrez/query.fcgi?cmd=Retrieve&db=pubmed&dopt=Abstract&list_uids=15066877

- **Age at death, season, and day of death as indicators of the effect of the back to sleep program on sudden infant death syndrome in the United States, 1992-1999.**
  Author(s): Malloy MH, Freeman DH.
  Source: Archives of Pediatrics & Adolescent Medicine. 2004 April; 158(4): 359-65.
  http://www.ncbi.nlm.nih.gov/entrez/query.fcgi?cmd=Retrieve&db=pubmed&dopt=Abstract&list_uids=15066876

- **Air pollution and sudden infant death syndrome.**
  Author(s): Koehler SA.
  Source: Pediatrics. 1996 October; 98(4 Pt 1): 796-8.
  http://www.ncbi.nlm.nih.gov/entrez/query.fcgi?cmd=Retrieve&db=pubmed&dopt=Abstract&list_uids=8885969

- **Alpha2-adrenergic receptor subtype alterations in the brainstem in the sudden infant death syndrome.**
  Author(s): Ozawa Y, Takashima S, Tada H.
  Source: Early Human Development. 2003 December; 75 Suppl: S129-38.
  http://www.ncbi.nlm.nih.gov/entrez/query.fcgi?cmd=Retrieve&db=pubmed&dopt=Abstract&list_uids=14693399

- **An analysis of sudden infant death syndrome in aboriginal infants.**
  Author(s): Alessandri LM, Read AW, Burton PR, Stanley FJ.
  Source: Early Human Development. 1996 July 19; 45(3): 235-44.
  http://www.ncbi.nlm.nih.gov/entrez/query.fcgi?cmd=Retrieve&db=pubmed&dopt=Abstract&list_uids=8855397

- **An assessment of behavioural characteristics in infants who died of sudden infant death syndrome using the Early Infancy Temperament Questionnaire.**
  Author(s): Kelmanson IA.
  Source: Acta Paediatrica (Oslo, Norway : 1992). 1996 August; 85(8): 977-80.
  http://www.ncbi.nlm.nih.gov/entrez/query.fcgi?cmd=Retrieve&db=pubmed&dopt=Abstract&list_uids=8863882

- **Analysis of the mitochondrial genome in sudden infant death syndrome.**
  Author(s): Divne AM, Rasten-Almqvist P, Rajs J, Gyllensten U, Allen M.
  Source: Acta Paediatrica (Oslo, Norway : 1992). 2003; 92(3): 386-8.
  http://www.ncbi.nlm.nih.gov/entrez/query.fcgi?cmd=Retrieve&db=pubmed&dopt=Abstract&list_uids=12725556

- **Apnea, sudden infant death syndrome, and home monitoring.**
  Author(s): Committee on Fetus and Newborn. American Academy of Pediatrics.
  Source: Pediatrics. 2003 April; 111(4 Pt 1): 914-7.
  http://www.ncbi.nlm.nih.gov/entrez/query.fcgi?cmd=Retrieve&db=pubmed&dopt=Abstract&list_uids=12671135

- **Are risk factors for sudden infant death syndrome different at night?**
  Author(s): Williams SM, Mitchell EA, Taylor BJ.
  Source: Archives of Disease in Childhood. 2002 October; 87(4): 274-8.
  http://www.ncbi.nlm.nih.gov/entrez/query.fcgi?cmd=Retrieve&db=pubmed&dopt=Abstract&list_uids=12243991

- **Are substitutions in the first hypervariable region of the mitochondrial DNA displacement-loop in sudden infant death syndrome due to maternal inheritance?**
  Author(s): Arnestad M, Opdal SH, Musse MA, Vege A, Rognum TO.
  Source: Acta Paediatrica (Oslo, Norway : 1992). 2002; 91(10): 1060-4.
  http://www.ncbi.nlm.nih.gov/entrez/query.fcgi?cmd=Retrieve&db=pubmed&dopt=Abstract&list_uids=12434891

- **Association between sudden infant death syndrome and prone sleep position, bed sharing, and sleeping outside an infant crib in Alaska.**
  Author(s): Gessner BD, Ives GC, Perham-Hester KA.
  Source: Pediatrics. 2001 October; 108(4): 923-7.
  http://www.ncbi.nlm.nih.gov/entrez/query.fcgi?cmd=Retrieve&db=pubmed&dopt=Abstract&list_uids=11581445

- **Association of the serotonin transporter gene with sudden infant death syndrome: a haplotype analysis.**
  Author(s): Weese-Mayer DE, Zhou L, Berry-Kravis EM, Maher BS, Silvestri JM, Marazita ML.
  Source: American Journal of Medical Genetics. 2003 October 15; 122A(3): 238-45.
  http://www.ncbi.nlm.nih.gov/entrez/query.fcgi?cmd=Retrieve&db=pubmed&dopt=Abstract&list_uids=12966525

- **Awareness of sudden infant death syndrome risk factors among mothers of Pacific infants in New Zealand.**
  Author(s): Paterson J, Tukuitonga C, Butler S, Williams M.
  Source: N Z Med J. 2002 February 8; 115(1147): 33-5.
  http://www.ncbi.nlm.nih.gov/entrez/query.fcgi?cmd=Retrieve&db=pubmed&dopt=Abstract&list_uids=11942511

- **Babies sleeping with parents and sudden infant death syndrome. Down with smoking and babies sleeping in separate rooms.**
  Author(s): Mermer CA.
  Source: Bmj (Clinical Research Ed.). 2000 October 21; 321(7267): 1019; Author Reply 1020.
  http://www.ncbi.nlm.nih.gov/entrez/query.fcgi?cmd=Retrieve&db=pubmed&dopt=Abstract&list_uids=11203210

- **Babies sleeping with parents and sudden infant death syndrome. Invoking sudden infant death syndrome in cosleeping may be misleading.**
  Author(s): Carter N, Rutty GN.
  Source: Bmj (Clinical Research Ed.). 2000 October 21; 321(7267): 1019; Author Reply 1020.
  http://www.ncbi.nlm.nih.gov/entrez/query.fcgi?cmd=Retrieve&db=pubmed&dopt=Abstract&list_uids=11039984

- **Babies sleeping with parents and sudden infant death syndrome. Smoking may be residual confounder in bed sharing.**
  Author(s): Ezeonyeji A, Jewitt S, Poyser L, Stadward T.
  Source: Bmj (Clinical Research Ed.). 2000 October 21; 321(7267): 1019-20.
  http://www.ncbi.nlm.nih.gov/entrez/query.fcgi?cmd=Retrieve&db=pubmed&dopt=Abstract&list_uids=11203209

- **Babies sleeping with parents: case-control study of factors influencing the risk of the sudden infant death syndrome. CESDI SUDI research group.**
  Author(s): Blair PS, Fleming PJ, Smith IJ, Platt MW, Young J, Nadin P, Berry PJ, Golding J.
  Source: Bmj (Clinical Research Ed.). 1999 December 4; 319(7223): 1457-61.
  http://www.ncbi.nlm.nih.gov/entrez/query.fcgi?cmd=Retrieve&db=pubmed&dopt=Abstract&list_uids=10582925

- **Bed sharing and the sudden infant death syndrome.**
  Author(s): Klonoff-Cohen H, Edelstein SL.
  Source: Bmj (Clinical Research Ed.). 1995 November 11; 311(7015): 1269-72.
  http://www.ncbi.nlm.nih.gov/entrez/query.fcgi?cmd=Retrieve&db=pubmed&dopt=Abstract&list_uids=7496236

- **Bedding and sleeping position in the sudden infant death syndrome.**
  Author(s): Fleming P, Berry J, Gilbert R, Rudd P.
  Source: Bmj (Clinical Research Ed.). 1990 October 13; 301(6756): 871-2.
  http://www.ncbi.nlm.nih.gov/entrez/query.fcgi?cmd=Retrieve&db=pubmed&dopt=Abstract&list_uids=2282429

- **Bedsharing and sudden infant death syndrome (SIDS) in Scotland, UK.**
  Author(s): Tappin D, Brooke H, Ecob R.
  Source: Lancet. 2004 March 20; 363(9413): 994.
  http://www.ncbi.nlm.nih.gov/entrez/query.fcgi?cmd=Retrieve&db=pubmed&dopt=Abstract&list_uids=15043979

- **Biovolatilization of antimony and sudden infant death syndrome (SIDS).**
  Author(s): Jenkins RO, Craig PJ, Goessler W, Irgolic KJ.
  Source: Human & Experimental Toxicology. 1998 April; 17(4): 231-8.
  http://www.ncbi.nlm.nih.gov/entrez/query.fcgi?cmd=Retrieve&db=pubmed&dopt=Abstract&list_uids=9617636

- **Birth weight- and gestational age-specific sudden infant death syndrome mortality: United States, 1991 versus 1995.**
  Author(s): Malloy MH, Freeman DH Jr.
  Source: Pediatrics. 2000 June; 105(6): 1227-31.
  http://www.ncbi.nlm.nih.gov/entrez/query.fcgi?cmd=Retrieve&db=pubmed&dopt=Abstract&list_uids=10835061

- **Blood ferritin concentrations in newborn infants and the sudden infant death syndrome.**
  Author(s): Raha-Chowdhury R, Moore CA, Bradley D, Henley R, Worwood M.
  Source: Journal of Clinical Pathology. 1996 February; 49(2): 168-70.
  http://www.ncbi.nlm.nih.gov/entrez/query.fcgi?cmd=Retrieve&db=pubmed&dopt=Abstract&list_uids=8655686

- **Bottle feeding and the sudden infant death syndrome.**
  Author(s): Mitchell EA, Stewart AW, Ford RP.
  Source: Bmj (Clinical Research Ed.). 1995 July 8; 311(6997): 122-3.
  http://www.ncbi.nlm.nih.gov/entrez/query.fcgi?cmd=Retrieve&db=pubmed&dopt=Abstract&list_uids=7613372

- **Bottle feeding and the sudden infant death syndrome. Study was not large enough to show effect.**
  Author(s): Tappin DM.
  Source: Bmj (Clinical Research Ed.). 1995 April 22; 310(6986): 1070; Author Reply 1071.
  http://www.ncbi.nlm.nih.gov/entrez/query.fcgi?cmd=Retrieve&db=pubmed&dopt=Abstract&list_uids=7728081

- **Bottle feeding and the sudden infant death syndrome. Type of formula was not specified.**
  Author(s): Walker-Smith JA.
  Source: Bmj (Clinical Research Ed.). 1995 April 22; 310(6986): 1070; Author Reply 1071.
  http://www.ncbi.nlm.nih.gov/entrez/query.fcgi?cmd=Retrieve&db=pubmed&dopt=Abstract&list_uids=7728082

- **Brain stem gliosis in the victims of sudden infant death syndrome (SIDS): a sign of retarded maturation?**
  Author(s): Kelmanson IA.
  Source: Zentralbl Pathol. 1995 April; 140(6): 449-52.
  http://www.ncbi.nlm.nih.gov/entrez/query.fcgi?cmd=Retrieve&db=pubmed&dopt=Abstract&list_uids=7756248

- **Brain stem lesions in the sudden infant death syndrome: variability in the hypoplasia of the arcuate nucleus.**
  Author(s): Matturri L, Biondo B, Suarez-Mier MP, Rossi L.
  Source: Acta Neuropathologica. 2002 July; 104(1): 12-20. Epub 2002 March 14.
  http://www.ncbi.nlm.nih.gov/entrez/query.fcgi?cmd=Retrieve&db=pubmed&dopt=Abstract&list_uids=12070659

- **Brain stem nuclei in sudden infant death syndrome (SIDS): volumes, neuronal numbers and positions.**
  Author(s): Lamont P, Murray N, Halliday G, Hilton J, Pamphlett R.
  Source: Neuropathology and Applied Neurobiology. 1995 June; 21(3): 262-8.
  http://www.ncbi.nlm.nih.gov/entrez/query.fcgi?cmd=Retrieve&db=pubmed&dopt=Abstract&list_uids=7477735

- **Brain weight and sudden infant death syndrome.**
  Author(s): Falck G, Rajs J.
  Source: Journal of Child Neurology. 1995 March; 10(2): 123-6.
  http://www.ncbi.nlm.nih.gov/entrez/query.fcgi?cmd=Retrieve&db=pubmed&dopt=Abstract&list_uids=7782602

- **Brainstem 3H-nicotine receptor binding in the sudden infant death syndrome.**
  Author(s): Nachmanoff DB, Panigrahy A, Filiano JJ, Mandell F, Sleeper LA, Valdes-Dapena M, Krous HF, White WF, Kinney HC.
  Source: Journal of Neuropathology and Experimental Neurology. 1998 November; 57(11): 1018-25.
  http://www.ncbi.nlm.nih.gov/entrez/query.fcgi?cmd=Retrieve&db=pubmed&dopt=Abstract&list_uids=9825938

- **Breast feeding and the sudden infant death syndrome in Scandinavia, 1992-95.**
  Author(s): Alm B, Wennergren G, Norvenius SG, Skjaerven R, Lagercrantz H, Helweg-Larsen K, Irgens LM.
  Source: Archives of Disease in Childhood. 2002 June; 86(6): 400-2.
  http://www.ncbi.nlm.nih.gov/entrez/query.fcgi?cmd=Retrieve&db=pubmed&dopt=Abstract&list_uids=12023166

- **Bronchus-associated lymphoid tissue (BALT) in the lungs of children who had died from sudden infant death syndrome and other causes.**
  Author(s): Tschernig T, Kleemann WJ, Pabst R.
  Source: Thorax. 1995 June; 50(6): 658-60.
  http://www.ncbi.nlm.nih.gov/entrez/query.fcgi?cmd=Retrieve&db=pubmed&dopt=Abstract&list_uids=7638809

- **Cardiac sodium channel gene mutations and sudden infant death syndrome: confirmation of proof of concept?**
  Author(s): Towbin JA, Ackerman MJ.
  Source: Circulation. 2001 September 4; 104(10): 1092-3.
  http://www.ncbi.nlm.nih.gov/entrez/query.fcgi?cmd=Retrieve&db=pubmed&dopt=Abstract&list_uids=11535560

- **Cerebral c-jun expression mapping in sudden infant death syndrome.**
  Author(s): Rickert CH, Zahiragic L, Nolte KW, Bajanowski T, Brinkmann B, Paulus W.
  Source: Acta Neuropathologica. 2004 February; 107(2): 119-26. Epub 2003 November 06.
  http://www.ncbi.nlm.nih.gov/entrez/query.fcgi?cmd=Retrieve&db=pubmed&dopt=Abstract&list_uids=14605833

- Changes in the epidemiological pattern of sudden infant death syndrome in southeast Norway, 1984-1998: implications for future prevention and research.
  Author(s): Arnestad M, Andersen M, Vege A, Rognum TO.
  Source: Archives of Disease in Childhood. 2001 August; 85(2): 108-15.
  http://www.ncbi.nlm.nih.gov/entrez/query.fcgi?cmd=Retrieve&db=pubmed&dopt=Abstract&list_uids=11466184

- Changes in the epidemiology of sudden infant death syndrome in Sweden 1973-1996.
  Author(s): Alm B, Norvenius SG, Wennergren G, Skjaerven R, Oyen N, Milerad J, Wennborg M, Kjaerbeck J, Helweg-Larsen K, Irgens LM; Nordic Epidemiological SIDS Study.
  Source: Archives of Disease in Childhood. 2001 January; 84(1): 24-30.
  http://www.ncbi.nlm.nih.gov/entrez/query.fcgi?cmd=Retrieve&db=pubmed&dopt=Abstract&list_uids=11124779

- Chlamydia and sudden infant death syndrome. A study of 166 SIDS and 30 control cases.
  Author(s): Lundemose JB, Lundemose AG, Gregersen M, Helweg-Larsen K, Simonsen J.
  Source: International Journal of Legal Medicine. 1990 December; 104(1): 3-7.
  http://www.ncbi.nlm.nih.gov/entrez/query.fcgi?cmd=Retrieve&db=pubmed&dopt=Abstract&list_uids=11453089

- Circadian variations in sudden infant death syndrome: associations with maternal smoking, sleeping position and infections. The Nordic Epidemiological SIDS Study.
  Author(s): Daltveit AK, Irgens LM, Oyen N, Skjaerven R, Markestad T, Wennergren G.
  Source: Acta Paediatrica (Oslo, Norway : 1992). 2003 September; 92(9): 1007-13.
  http://www.ncbi.nlm.nih.gov/entrez/query.fcgi?cmd=Retrieve&db=pubmed&dopt=Abstract&list_uids=14599060

- **Clinicopathological correlation between brainstem gliosis using GFAP as a marker and sleep apnea in the sudden infant death syndrome.**
  Author(s): Sawaguchi T, Patricia F, Kadhim H, Groswasser J, Sottiaux M, Nishida H, Kahn A.
  Source: Early Human Development. 2003 December; 75 Suppl: S3-11.
  http://www.ncbi.nlm.nih.gov/entrez/query.fcgi?cmd=Retrieve&db=pubmed&dopt=Abstract&list_uids=14693386

- **Comment on "Whole blood levels of dodecanoic acid, a routinely detectable forensic marker for a genetic disease often misdiagnosed as sudden infant death syndrome (SIDS): MCAD deficiency".**
  Author(s): Ross KF, Guileyardo JM, Bennett MJ, Barnard JJ.
  Source: The American Journal of Forensic Medicine and Pathology : Official Publication of the National Association of Medical Examiners. 1996 December; 17(4): 349-50.
  http://www.ncbi.nlm.nih.gov/entrez/query.fcgi?cmd=Retrieve&db=pubmed&dopt=Abstract&list_uids=8947364

- **Comparative analysis of differences by gender in sudden infant death syndrome in Hungary and Japan.**
  Author(s): Toro K, Sawaguchi T, Sawaguchi A, Rozsa S, Sotonyi P.
  Source: Forensic Science International. 2001 April 15; 118(1): 15-9.
  http://www.ncbi.nlm.nih.gov/entrez/query.fcgi?cmd=Retrieve&db=pubmed&dopt=Abstract&list_uids=11343850

- **Comparative epidemiology of sudden infant death syndrome and sudden intrauterine unexplained death.**
  Author(s): Froen JF, Arnestad M, Vege A, Irgens LM, Rognum TO, Saugstad OD, Stray-Pedersen B.
  Source: Archives of Disease in Childhood. Fetal and Neonatal Edition. 2002 September; 87(2): F118-21.
  http://www.ncbi.nlm.nih.gov/entrez/query.fcgi?cmd=Retrieve&db=pubmed&dopt=Abstract&list_uids=12193518

- **Comparative evaluation of diagnostic guidelines for sudden infant death syndrome (SIDS) in Japan.**
  Author(s): Sawaguchi T, Sawaguchi A, Matoba R.
  Source: Forensic Science International. 2002 September 14; 130 Suppl: S65-70.
  http://www.ncbi.nlm.nih.gov/entrez/query.fcgi?cmd=Retrieve&db=pubmed&dopt=Abstract&list_uids=12350304

- **Confounding in the study of pacifier use in sudden infant death syndrome.**
  Author(s): Schlaud M, Poets CF.
  Source: European Journal of Pediatrics. 2000 July; 159(7): 542-3.
  http://www.ncbi.nlm.nih.gov/entrez/query.fcgi?cmd=Retrieve&db=pubmed&dopt=Abstract&list_uids=10923233

- **Considering suffocatory abuse and Munchausen by proxy in the evaluation of children experiencing apparent life-threatening events and sudden infant death syndrome.**
  Author(s): Truman TL, Ayoub CC.
  Source: Child Maltreatment. 2002 May; 7(2): 138-48.
  http://www.ncbi.nlm.nih.gov/entrez/query.fcgi?cmd=Retrieve&db=pubmed&dopt=Abstract&list_uids=12020070

- **Co-sleeping and sudden infant death syndrome.**
  Author(s): Mitchell EA.
  Source: Lancet. 1996 November 30; 348(9040): 1466.
  http://www.ncbi.nlm.nih.gov/entrez/query.fcgi?cmd=Retrieve&db=pubmed&dopt=Abstract&list_uids=8942773

- **Cost-effectiveness and implications of newborn screening for prolongation of QT interval for the prevention of sudden infant death syndrome.**
  Author(s): Zupancic JA, Triedman JK, Alexander M, Walsh EP, Richardson DK, Berul CI.
  Source: The Journal of Pediatrics. 2000 April; 136(4): 481-9.
  http://www.ncbi.nlm.nih.gov/entrez/query.fcgi?cmd=Retrieve&db=pubmed&dopt=Abstract&list_uids=10753246

- **Could Pneumocystis carinii have a role in sudden infant death syndrome?**
  Author(s): Orellana C.
  Source: Lancet. 2001 July 7; 358(9275): 43.
  http://www.ncbi.nlm.nih.gov/entrez/query.fcgi?cmd=Retrieve&db=pubmed&dopt=Abstract&list_uids=11454387

- **Coxsackie B3 myocarditis in 4 cases of suspected sudden infant death syndrome: diagnosis by immunohistochemical and molecular-pathologic investigations.**
  Author(s): Dettmeyer R, Baasner A, Schlamann M, Haag C, Madea B.
  Source: Pathology, Research and Practice. 2002; 198(10): 689-96.
  http://www.ncbi.nlm.nih.gov/entrez/query.fcgi?cmd=Retrieve&db=pubmed&dopt=Abstract&list_uids=12498225

- **Curliated Escherichia coli, soluble curlin and the sudden infant death syndrome (SIDS).**
  Author(s): Goldwater PN, Bettelheim KA.
  Source: Journal of Medical Microbiology. 2002 November; 51(11): 1009-12.
  http://www.ncbi.nlm.nih.gov/entrez/query.fcgi?cmd=Retrieve&db=pubmed&dopt=Abstract&list_uids=12448686

- **Cytochrome P-450 expression in sudden infant death syndrome.**
  Author(s): Treluyer JM, Cheron G, Sonnier M, Cresteil T.
  Source: Biochemical Pharmacology. 1996 August 9; 52(3): 497-504.
  http://www.ncbi.nlm.nih.gov/entrez/query.fcgi?cmd=Retrieve&db=pubmed&dopt=Abstract&list_uids=8687505

- **Cytokines in sudden infant death syndrome.**
  Author(s): Waters KA.
  Source: Lancet. Neurology. 2004 February; 3(2): 81. Review.
  http://www.ncbi.nlm.nih.gov/entrez/query.fcgi?cmd=Retrieve&db=pubmed&dopt=Abstract&list_uids=14746996

- **Debate on cot death. In 1994, 29% of suspicious deaths were officially recorded as due to sudden infant death syndrome.**
  Author(s): Reder P, Duncan S.
  Source: Bmj (Clinical Research Ed.). 2000 January 29; 320(7230): 311.
  http://www.ncbi.nlm.nih.gov/entrez/query.fcgi?cmd=Retrieve&db=pubmed&dopt=Abstract&list_uids=10722290

- **Decreased autonomic responses to obstructive sleep events in future victims of sudden infant death syndrome.**
  Author(s): Franco P, Szliwowski H, Dramaix M, Kahn A.
  Source: Pediatric Research. 1999 July; 46(1): 33-9.
  http://www.ncbi.nlm.nih.gov/entrez/query.fcgi?cmd=Retrieve&db=pubmed&dopt=Abstract&list_uids=10400131

- **Decreased kainate receptor binding in the arcuate nucleus of the sudden infant death syndrome.**
  Author(s): Panigrahy A, Filiano JJ, Sleeper LA, Mandell F, Valdes-Dapena M, Krous HF, Rava LA, White WF, Kinney HC.
  Source: Journal of Neuropathology and Experimental Neurology. 1997 November; 56(11): 1253-61.
  http://www.ncbi.nlm.nih.gov/entrez/query.fcgi?cmd=Retrieve&db=pubmed&dopt=Abstract&list_uids=9370236

- **Decreased serotonergic receptor binding in rhombic lip-derived regions of the medulla oblongata in the sudden infant death syndrome.**
  Author(s): Panigrahy A, Filiano J, Sleeper LA, Mandell F, Valdes-Dapena M, Krous HF, Rava LA, Foley E, White WF, Kinney HC.
  Source: Journal of Neuropathology and Experimental Neurology. 2000 May; 59(5): 377-84.
  http://www.ncbi.nlm.nih.gov/entrez/query.fcgi?cmd=Retrieve&db=pubmed&dopt=Abstract&list_uids=10888367

- **Deficient heat shock protein expression: a potential mechanism for the sudden infant death syndrome.**
  Author(s): Gozal D.
  Source: Medical Hypotheses. 1996 January; 46(1): 52-4.
  http://www.ncbi.nlm.nih.gov/entrez/query.fcgi?cmd=Retrieve&db=pubmed&dopt=Abstract&list_uids=8746129

- **Deficient hypoxia awakening response in infants of smoking mothers: possible relationship to sudden infant death syndrome.**
  Author(s): Lewis KW, Bosque EM.
  Source: The Journal of Pediatrics. 1995 November; 127(5): 691-9.
  http://www.ncbi.nlm.nih.gov/entrez/query.fcgi?cmd=Retrieve&db=pubmed&dopt=Abstract&list_uids=7472818

- **Defining the sudden infant death syndrome.**
  Author(s): Beckwith JB.
  Source: Archives of Pediatrics & Adolescent Medicine. 2003 March; 157(3): 286-90. Review.
  http://www.ncbi.nlm.nih.gov/entrez/query.fcgi?cmd=Retrieve&db=pubmed&dopt=Abstract&list_uids=12622679

- **Delayed central nervous system myelination in the sudden infant death syndrome.**
  Author(s): Kinney HC, Brody BA, Finkelstein DM, Vawter GF, Mandell F, Gilles FH.
  Source: Journal of Neuropathology and Experimental Neurology. 1991 January; 50(1): 29-48.
  http://www.ncbi.nlm.nih.gov/entrez/query.fcgi?cmd=Retrieve&db=pubmed&dopt=Abstract&list_uids=1985152

- **Delayed neuronal maturation of the medullary arcuate nucleus in sudden infant death syndrome.**
  Author(s): Biondo B, Lavezzi A, Tosi D, Turconi P, Matturri L.
  Source: Acta Neuropathologica. 2003 December; 106(6): 545-51. Epub 2003 September 12.
  http://www.ncbi.nlm.nih.gov/entrez/query.fcgi?cmd=Retrieve&db=pubmed&dopt=Abstract&list_uids=13680277

- **Deprivation and sudden infant death syndrome.**
  Author(s): Mitchell EA, Stewart AW, Crampton P, Salmond C.
  Source: Social Science & Medicine (1982). 2000 July; 51(1): 147-50.
  http://www.ncbi.nlm.nih.gov/entrez/query.fcgi?cmd=Retrieve&db=pubmed&dopt=Abstract&list_uids=10817477

- **Detection of pyrogenic toxins of Staphylococcus aureus in sudden infant death syndrome.**
  Author(s): Zorgani A, Essery SD, Madani OA, Bentley AJ, James VS, MacKenzie DA, Keeling JW, Rambaud C, Hilton J, Blackwell CC, Weir DM, Busuttil A.
  Source: Fems Immunology and Medical Microbiology. 1999 August 1; 25(1-2): 103-8.
  http://www.ncbi.nlm.nih.gov/entrez/query.fcgi?cmd=Retrieve&db=pubmed&dopt=Abstract&list_uids=10443497

- **Developmental and environmental factors that enhance binding of Bordetella pertussis to human epithelial cells in relation to sudden infant death syndrome (SIDS).**
  Author(s): Saadi AT, Blackwell CC, Essery SD, Raza MW, el Ahmer OR, MacKenzie DA, James VS, Weir DM, Ogilvie MM, Elton RA, Busuttil A, Keeling JW.
  Source: Fems Immunology and Medical Microbiology. 1996 November; 16(1): 51-9.
  http://www.ncbi.nlm.nih.gov/entrez/query.fcgi?cmd=Retrieve&db=pubmed&dopt=Abstract&list_uids=8954353

- **Developmental characteristics of apnea in infants who succumb to sudden infant death syndrome.**
  Author(s): Kato I, Groswasser J, Franco P, Scaillet S, Kelmanson I, Togari H, Kahn A.
  Source: American Journal of Respiratory and Critical Care Medicine. 2001 October 15; 164(8 Pt 1): 1464-9.
  http://www.ncbi.nlm.nih.gov/entrez/query.fcgi?cmd=Retrieve&db=pubmed&dopt=Abstract&list_uids=11704597

- **Developmental neurotransmitter pathology in the brainstem of sudden infant death syndrome: a review and sleep position.**
  Author(s): Ozawa Y, Takashima S.
  Source: Forensic Science International. 2002 September 14; 130 Suppl: S53-9.
  http://www.ncbi.nlm.nih.gov/entrez/query.fcgi?cmd=Retrieve&db=pubmed&dopt=Abstract&list_uids=12350301

- **Dicyclomine in the sudden infant death syndrome (SIDS)--a cause of death or an incidental finding?**
  Author(s): Randall B, Gerry G, Rance F.
  Source: J Forensic Sci. 1986 October; 31(4): 1470-4.
  http://www.ncbi.nlm.nih.gov/entrez/query.fcgi?cmd=Retrieve&db=pubmed&dopt=Abstract&list_uids=3783112

- **Do differences in the prevalence of risk factors explain the higher mortality from sudden infant death syndrome in New Zealand compared with the UK?**
  Author(s): Mitchell EA, Esmail A, Jones DR, Clements M.
  Source: N Z Med J. 1996 September 27; 109(1030): 352-5.
  http://www.ncbi.nlm.nih.gov/entrez/query.fcgi?cmd=Retrieve&db=pubmed&dopt=Abstract&list_uids=8890859

- **Does circadian variation in risk factors for sudden infant death syndrome (SIDS) suggest there are two (or more) SIDS subtypes?**
  Author(s): Mitchell EA, Williams SM.
  Source: Acta Paediatrica (Oslo, Norway : 1992). 2003 September; 92(9): 991-3.
  http://www.ncbi.nlm.nih.gov/entrez/query.fcgi?cmd=Retrieve&db=pubmed&dopt=Abstract&list_uids=14599054

- **DPT-OPV immunization and sudden infant death syndrome.**
  Author(s): John TJ.
  Source: Indian Pediatrics. 1997 November; 34(11): 1045-6.
  http://www.ncbi.nlm.nih.gov/entrez/query.fcgi?cmd=Retrieve&db=pubmed&dopt=Abstract&list_uids=9567540

- **Dummy sucking and sudden infant death syndrome (SIDS)**
  Author(s): Cozzi F, Cardi E, Cozzi DA.
  Source: European Journal of Pediatrics. 1998 November; 157(11): 952.
  http://www.ncbi.nlm.nih.gov/entrez/query.fcgi?cmd=Retrieve&db=pubmed&dopt=Abstract&list_uids=9835447

- **Dynamics of respiratory patterning in normal infants and infants who subsequently died of the sudden infant death syndrome.**
  Author(s): Schechtman VL, Lee MY, Wilson AJ, Harper RM.
  Source: Pediatric Research. 1996 October; 40(4): 571-7.
  http://www.ncbi.nlm.nih.gov/entrez/query.fcgi?cmd=Retrieve&db=pubmed&dopt=Abstract&list_uids=8888285

- **Effect of a sudden infant death syndrome risk reduction education program on risk factor compliance and information sources in primarily black urban communities.**
  Author(s): Rasinski KA, Kuby A, Bzdusek SA, Silvestri JM, Weese-Mayer DE.
  Source: Pediatrics. 2003 April; 111(4 Pt 1): E347-54.
  http://www.ncbi.nlm.nih.gov/entrez/query.fcgi?cmd=Retrieve&db=pubmed&dopt=Abstract&list_uids=12671150

- Effect of prenatal cocaine on respiration, heart rate, and sudden infant death syndrome.
  Author(s): Silvestri JM, Long JM, Weese-Mayer DE, Barkov GA.
  Source: Pediatric Pulmonology. 1991; 11(4): 328-34.
  http://www.ncbi.nlm.nih.gov/entrez/query.fcgi?cmd=Retrieve&db=pubmed&dopt=Abstract&list_uids=1758757

- **Effect of time post mortem on the concentration of endotoxin in rat organs: implications for sudden infant death syndrome (SIDS).**
  Author(s): Sayers NM, Crawley BA, Humphries K, Drucker DB, Oppenheim BA, Hunt LP, Morris JA, Telford DR.
  Source: Fems Immunology and Medical Microbiology. 1999 August 1; 25(1-2): 125-30.
  http://www.ncbi.nlm.nih.gov/entrez/query.fcgi?cmd=Retrieve&db=pubmed&dopt=Abstract&list_uids=10443500

- **Elevated serum concentrations of beta-tryptase, but not alpha-tryptase, in Sudden Infant Death Syndrome (SIDS). An investigation of anaphylactic mechanisms.**
  Author(s): Buckley MG, Variend S, Walls AF.
  Source: Clinical and Experimental Allergy : Journal of the British Society for Allergy and Clinical Immunology. 2001 November; 31(11): 1696-704.
  http://www.ncbi.nlm.nih.gov/entrez/query.fcgi?cmd=Retrieve&db=pubmed&dopt=Abstract&list_uids=11696045

- **Endotoxin in blood and tissue in the sudden infant death syndrome.**
  Author(s): Crawley BA, Morris JA, Drucker DB, Barson AJ, Morris J, Knox WF, Oppenheim BA.
  Source: Fems Immunology and Medical Microbiology. 1999 August 1; 25(1-2): 131-5.
  http://www.ncbi.nlm.nih.gov/entrez/query.fcgi?cmd=Retrieve&db=pubmed&dopt=Abstract&list_uids=10443501

- **Enhanced reactivity of Alz-50 antibody in brains of sudden infant death syndrome victims versus brains with lethal hypoxic/ischemic injury. Diagnostic significance after application of the ImmunoMax technique on routine paraffin material.**
  Author(s): Oehmichen M, Theuerkauf I, Bajanowski T, Merz H, Meissner C.
  Source: Acta Neuropathologica. 1998 March; 95(3): 280-6.
  http://www.ncbi.nlm.nih.gov/entrez/query.fcgi?cmd=Retrieve&db=pubmed&dopt=Abstract&list_uids=9542593

- **Environment of infants during sleep and risk of the sudden infant death syndrome: results of 1993-5 case-control study for confidential inquiry into stillbirths and deaths in infancy. Confidential Enquiry into Stillbirths and Deaths Regional Coordinators and Researchers.**
  Author(s): Fleming PJ, Blair PS, Bacon C, Bensley D, Smith I, Taylor E, Berry J, Golding J, Tripp J.
  Source: Bmj (Clinical Research Ed.). 1996 July 27; 313(7051): 191-5.
  http://www.ncbi.nlm.nih.gov/entrez/query.fcgi?cmd=Retrieve&db=pubmed&dopt=Abstract&list_uids=8696193

- **Enzyme-linked immunoassay for respiratory syncytial virus is not predictive of bronchiolitis in sudden infant death syndrome.**
  Author(s): Parham DM, Cheng R, Schutze GE, Dilday B, Nelson R, Erickson S, Kokes C, Peretti F, Sturner WQ.
  Source: Pediatric and Developmental Pathology : the Official Journal of the Society for Pediatric Pathology and the Paediatric Pathology Society. 1998 September-October; 1(5): 375-9.
  http://www.ncbi.nlm.nih.gov/entrez/query.fcgi?cmd=Retrieve&db=pubmed&dopt=Abstract&list_uids=9688761

- **Epidemiological investigation of sudden infant death syndrome infants--recommendations for future studies.**
  Author(s): Blair P, Fleming P.
  Source: Child: Care, Health and Development. 2002 September; 28 Suppl 1: 49-54.
  http://www.ncbi.nlm.nih.gov/entrez/query.fcgi?cmd=Retrieve&db=pubmed&dopt=Abstract&list_uids=12515441

- **Epidemiology of intrathoracic petechial hemorrhages in sudden infant death syndrome.**
  Author(s): Becroft DM, Thompson JM, Mitchell EA.
  Source: Pediatric and Developmental Pathology : the Official Journal of the Society for Pediatric Pathology and the Paediatric Pathology Society. 1998 May-June; 1(3): 200-9.
  http://www.ncbi.nlm.nih.gov/entrez/query.fcgi?cmd=Retrieve&db=pubmed&dopt=Abstract&list_uids=10463279

- **Epidemiology of sudden infant death syndrome (SIDS) in the Tyrol before and after an intervention campaign.**
  Author(s): Kiechl-Kohlendorfer U, Peglow UP, Kiechl S, Oberaigner W, Sperl W.
  Source: Wiener Klinische Wochenschrift. 2001 January 15; 113(1-2): 27-32.
  http://www.ncbi.nlm.nih.gov/entrez/query.fcgi?cmd=Retrieve&db=pubmed&dopt=Abstract&list_uids=11233464

- **Estimation of mean nuclear volume of neocortical neurons in sudden infant death syndrome cases using the nucleator estimator technique.**
  Author(s): Ansari T, Sibbons PD, Howard CV.
  Source: Biology of the Neonate. 2001 July; 80(1): 48-52.
  http://www.ncbi.nlm.nih.gov/entrez/query.fcgi?cmd=Retrieve&db=pubmed&dopt=Abstract&list_uids=11474149

- **Estimation of the incidence of sudden infant death syndrome in Korea: using the capture-recapture method.**
  Author(s): Ha M, Yoon SJ, Lee HY, Goh UY, Kim CH, Lee YS.
  Source: Paediatric and Perinatal Epidemiology. 2004 March; 18(2): 138-42.
  http://www.ncbi.nlm.nih.gov/entrez/query.fcgi?cmd=Retrieve&db=pubmed&dopt=Abstract&list_uids=14996254

- **Ethnic differences in incidence of sudden infant death syndrome in Birmingham.**
  Author(s): Kyle D, Sunderland R, Stonehouse M, Cummins C, Ross O.
  Source: Archives of Disease in Childhood. 1990 August; 65(8): 830-3.
  http://www.ncbi.nlm.nih.gov/entrez/query.fcgi?cmd=Retrieve&db=pubmed&dopt=Abstract&list_uids=2400217

- **Evidence for a genetic component in sudden infant death syndrome.**
  Author(s): Gordon AE, MacKenzie DA, El Ahmer OR, Al Madani OM, Braun JM, Weir DM, Busuttil A, Blackwell CC.
  Source: Child: Care, Health and Development. 2002 September; 28 Suppl 1: 27-9.
  http://www.ncbi.nlm.nih.gov/entrez/query.fcgi?cmd=Retrieve&db=pubmed&dopt=Abstract&list_uids=12515435

- **Evidence for retarded kidney growth in sudden infant death syndrome.**
  Author(s): Kelmanson IA.
  Source: Pediatric Nephrology (Berlin, Germany). 1996 December; 10(6): 683-6.
  http://www.ncbi.nlm.nih.gov/entrez/query.fcgi?cmd=Retrieve&db=pubmed&dopt=Abstract&list_uids=8971878

- **Exacerbation of bacterial toxicity to infant ferrets by influenza virus: possible role in sudden infant death syndrome.**
  Author(s): Jakeman KJ, Rushton DI, Smith H, Sweet C.
  Source: The Journal of Infectious Diseases. 1991 January; 163(1): 35-40. Erratum In: J Infect Dis 1991 July; 164(1): 232.
  http://www.ncbi.nlm.nih.gov/entrez/query.fcgi?cmd=Retrieve&db=pubmed&dopt=Abstract&list_uids=1984474

- **Exposure of piglet coronary arterial muscle cells to low concentrations of Mg^{2+} found in blood of ischemic heart disease patients result in rapid elevation of cytosolic Ca^{2+}: relevance to sudden infant death syndrome.**
  Author(s): Altura BM, Zhang A, Altura BT.
  Source: European Journal of Pharmacology. 1997 November 5; 338(2): R7-9.
  http://www.ncbi.nlm.nih.gov/entrez/query.fcgi?cmd=Retrieve&db=pubmed&dopt=Abstract&list_uids=9456006

- **Exposure to cigarette smoke, a major risk factor for sudden infant death syndrome: effects of cigarette smoke on inflammatory responses to viral infection and bacterial toxins.**
  Author(s): Raza MW, Essery SD, Elton RA, Weir DM, Busuttil A, Blackwell C.
  Source: Fems Immunology and Medical Microbiology. 1999 August 1; 25(1-2): 145-54.
  http://www.ncbi.nlm.nih.gov/entrez/query.fcgi?cmd=Retrieve&db=pubmed&dopt=Abstract&list_uids=10443503

- **Extramedullary hematopoiesis in the liver in sudden infant death syndrome.**
  Author(s): Gilbert-Barness EF, Kenison K, Giulian G, Chandra S.
  Source: Archives of Pathology & Laboratory Medicine. 1991 March; 115(3): 226-9.
  http://www.ncbi.nlm.nih.gov/entrez/query.fcgi?cmd=Retrieve&db=pubmed&dopt=Abstract&list_uids=2001157

- **Facial structure in the sudden infant death syndrome: case-control study.**
  Author(s): Rees K, Wright A, Keeling JW, Douglas NJ.
  Source: Bmj (Clinical Research Ed.). 1998 July 18; 317(7152): 179-80.
  http://www.ncbi.nlm.nih.gov/entrez/query.fcgi?cmd=Retrieve&db=pubmed&dopt=Abstract&list_uids=9665897

- **Factors enhancing adherence of toxigenic Staphylococcus aureus to epithelial cells and their possible role in sudden infant death syndrome.**
  Author(s): Saadi AT, Blackwell CC, Raza MW, James VS, Stewart J, Elton RA, Weir DM.
  Source: Epidemiology and Infection. 1993 June; 110(3): 507-17.
  http://www.ncbi.nlm.nih.gov/entrez/query.fcgi?cmd=Retrieve&db=pubmed&dopt=Abstract&list_uids=8519316

- **Factors potentiating the risk of sudden infant death syndrome associated with the prone position.**
  Author(s): Ponsonby AL, Dwyer T, Gibbons LE, Cochrane JA, Wang YG.
  Source: The New England Journal of Medicine. 1993 August 5; 329(6): 377-82.
  http://www.ncbi.nlm.nih.gov/entrez/query.fcgi?cmd=Retrieve&db=pubmed&dopt=Abstract&list_uids=8326970

- **Factors relating to the infant's last sleep environment in sudden infant death syndrome in the Republic of Ireland.**
  Author(s): McGarvey C, McDonnell M, Chong A, O'Regan M, Matthews T.
  Source: Archives of Disease in Childhood. 2003 December; 88(12): 1058-64.
  http://www.ncbi.nlm.nih.gov/entrez/query.fcgi?cmd=Retrieve&db=pubmed&dopt=Abstract&list_uids=14670769

- **Familial predisposition and cosegregation analysis of adult obstructive sleep apnea and the sudden infant death syndrome.**
  Author(s): Gislason T, Johannsson JH, Haraldsson A, Olafsdottir BR, Jonsdottir H, Kong A, Frigge ML, Jonsdottir GM, Hakonarson H, Gulcher J, Stefansson K.
  Source: American Journal of Respiratory and Critical Care Medicine. 2002 September 15; 166(6): 833-8.
  http://www.ncbi.nlm.nih.gov/entrez/query.fcgi?cmd=Retrieve&db=pubmed&dopt=Abstract&list_uids=12231493

- **Fatal child abuse and sudden infant death syndrome (SIDS): a critical diagnostic decision.**
  Author(s): Beeber B, Cunningham N.
  Source: Pediatrics. 1994 March; 93(3): 539-40.
  http://www.ncbi.nlm.nih.gov/entrez/query.fcgi?cmd=Retrieve&db=pubmed&dopt=Abstract&list_uids=8115231

- **Fatal child abuse and sudden infant death syndrome: a critical diagnostic decision.**
  Author(s): Reece RM.
  Source: Pediatrics. 1993 February; 91(2): 423-9.
  http://www.ncbi.nlm.nih.gov/entrez/query.fcgi?cmd=Retrieve&db=pubmed&dopt=Abstract&list_uids=8424022

- **Febrile convulsions and sudden infant death syndrome.**
  Author(s): Vestergaard M, Basso O, Henriksen TB, Ostergaard J, Olsen J.
  Source: Archives of Disease in Childhood. 2002 February; 86(2): 125-6.
  http://www.ncbi.nlm.nih.gov/entrez/query.fcgi?cmd=Retrieve&db=pubmed&dopt=Abstract&list_uids=11827907

- **Fetal behaviour and the sudden infant death syndrome (SIDS).**
  Author(s): Smoleniec J, James D.
  Source: Archives of Disease in Childhood. Fetal and Neonatal Edition. 1995 May; 72(3): F168-71.
  http://www.ncbi.nlm.nih.gov/entrez/query.fcgi?cmd=Retrieve&db=pubmed&dopt=Abstract&list_uids=7796231

- **Fetal growth retardation in sudden infant death syndrome (SIDS) babies and their siblings.**
  Author(s): Oyen N, Skjaerven R, Little RE, Wilcox AJ.
  Source: American Journal of Epidemiology. 1995 July 1; 142(1): 84-90.
  http://www.ncbi.nlm.nih.gov/entrez/query.fcgi?cmd=Retrieve&db=pubmed&dopt=Abstract&list_uids=7785678

- **Fetal hemoglobin and sudden infant death syndrome.**
  Author(s): Gilbert-Barness E, Kenison K, Carver J.
  Source: Archives of Pathology & Laboratory Medicine. 1993 February; 117(2): 177-9.
  http://www.ncbi.nlm.nih.gov/entrez/query.fcgi?cmd=Retrieve&db=pubmed&dopt=Abstract&list_uids=7678955

- **Fetal hemoglobin levels in sudden infant death syndrome.**
  Author(s): Perry GW, Vargas-Cuba R, Vertes RP.
  Source: Archives of Pathology & Laboratory Medicine. 1997 October; 121(10): 1048-54.
  http://www.ncbi.nlm.nih.gov/entrez/query.fcgi?cmd=Retrieve&db=pubmed&dopt=Abstract&list_uids=9341583

- **Fetal hemoglobin synthesis determined by gamma-mRNA/gamma-mRNA + beta-mRNA quantitation in infants at risk for sudden infant death syndrome being monitored at home for apnea.**
  Author(s): Bard H, Cote A, Praud JP, Infante-Rivard C, Gagnon C.
  Source: Pediatrics. 2003 October; 112(4): E285.
  http://www.ncbi.nlm.nih.gov/entrez/query.fcgi?cmd=Retrieve&db=pubmed&dopt=Abstract&list_uids=14523213

- **Finding the failure mechanism in Sudden Infant Death Syndrome.**
  Author(s): Harper RM, Bandler R.
  Source: Nature Medicine. 1998 February; 4(2): 157-8.
  http://www.ncbi.nlm.nih.gov/entrez/query.fcgi?cmd=Retrieve&db=pubmed&dopt=Abstract&list_uids=9461186

- **Foundation is helping carers to reduce risk of sudden infant death syndrome.**
  Author(s): Deri-Bowen A.
  Source: Bmj (Clinical Research Ed.). 2001 February 24; 322(7284): 491.
  http://www.ncbi.nlm.nih.gov/entrez/query.fcgi?cmd=Retrieve&db=pubmed&dopt=Abstract&list_uids=11222433

- **Frequency of 985A-to-G mutation in medium-chain acyl-CoA dehydrogenase gene among patients with sudden infant death syndrome, Reye syndrome, severe motor and intellectual disabilities and healthy newborns in Japan.**
  Author(s): Nagao M.
  Source: Acta Paediatr Jpn. 1996 August; 38(4): 304-7.
  http://www.ncbi.nlm.nih.gov/entrez/query.fcgi?cmd=Retrieve&db=pubmed&dopt=Abstract&list_uids=8840534

- **From epidemiology to physiology and pathology: apnea and arousal deficient theories in sudden infant death syndrome (SIDS)--with particular reference to hypoxic brainstem gliosis.**
  Author(s): Sawaguchi T, Franco P, Kato I, Shimizu S, Kadhim H, Groswasser J, Sottiaux M, Togari H, Kobayashi M, Takashima S, Nishida H, Sawaguchi A, Kahn A.
  Source: Forensic Science International. 2002 September 14; 130 Suppl: S21-9.
  http://www.ncbi.nlm.nih.gov/entrez/query.fcgi?cmd=Retrieve&db=pubmed&dopt=Abstract&list_uids=12350297

- **From physiology to pathology: arousal deficiency theory in sudden infant death syndrome (SIDS)--with reference to apoptosis and neuronal plasticity.**
  Author(s): Sawaguchi T, Franco P, Kato I, Shimizu S, Kadhim H, Groswasser J, Sottiaux M, Togari H, Kobayashi M, Takashima S, Nishida H, Sawaguchi A, Kahn A.
  Source: Forensic Science International. 2002 September 14; 130 Suppl: S37-43.
  http://www.ncbi.nlm.nih.gov/entrez/query.fcgi?cmd=Retrieve&db=pubmed&dopt=Abstract&list_uids=12350299

- **Functional and developmental studies of the peripheral arterial chemoreceptors in rat: effects of nicotine and possible relation to sudden infant death syndrome.**
  Author(s): Holgert H, Hokfelt T, Hertzberg T, Lagercrantz H.
  Source: Proceedings of the National Academy of Sciences of the United States of America. 1995 August 1; 92(16): 7575-9.
  http://www.ncbi.nlm.nih.gov/entrez/query.fcgi?cmd=Retrieve&db=pubmed&dopt=Abstract&list_uids=7638233

- Fungal volatilization of arsenic and antimony and the sudden infant death syndrome.
  Author(s): Pearce RB, Callow ME, Macaskie LE.
  Source: Fems Microbiology Letters. 1998 January 15; 158(2): 261-5.
  http://www.ncbi.nlm.nih.gov/entrez/query.fcgi?cmd=Retrieve&db=pubmed&dopt=Abstract&list_uids=9465397

- Gastric secretion in infants. Application to the study of sudden infant death syndrome and apparently life-threatening events.
  Author(s): Mouterde O, Dacher JN, Basuyau JP, Mallet E.
  Source: Biology of the Neonate. 1992; 62(1): 15-22.
  http://www.ncbi.nlm.nih.gov/entrez/query.fcgi?cmd=Retrieve&db=pubmed&dopt=Abstract&list_uids=1391271

- Gastroesophageal reflux and sudden infant death syndrome.
  Author(s): Byard RW, Moore L.
  Source: Pediatr Pathol. 1993 January-February; 13(1): 53-7.
  http://www.ncbi.nlm.nih.gov/entrez/query.fcgi?cmd=Retrieve&db=pubmed&dopt=Abstract&list_uids=8474951

- Gastroesophageal reflux, as measured by 24-hour pH monitoring, in 509 healthy infants screened for risk of sudden infant death syndrome.
  Author(s): Vandenplas Y, Goyvaerts H, Helven R, Sacre L.
  Source: Pediatrics. 1991 October; 88(4): 834-40.
  http://www.ncbi.nlm.nih.gov/entrez/query.fcgi?cmd=Retrieve&db=pubmed&dopt=Abstract&list_uids=1896295

- Gastro-oesophageal reflux in near-miss sudden infant death syndrome or suspected recurrent aspiration.
  Author(s): MacFadyen UM, Hendry GM, Simpson H.
  Source: Archives of Disease in Childhood. 1983 February; 58(2): 87-91.
  http://www.ncbi.nlm.nih.gov/entrez/query.fcgi?cmd=Retrieve&db=pubmed&dopt=Abstract&list_uids=6830303

- Gender and the sudden infant death syndrome. New Zealand Cot Death Study Group.
  Author(s): Mitchell EA, Stewart AW.
  Source: Acta Paediatrica (Oslo, Norway : 1992). 1997 August; 86(8): 854-6.
  http://www.ncbi.nlm.nih.gov/entrez/query.fcgi?cmd=Retrieve&db=pubmed&dopt=Abstract&list_uids=9307167

- **Gender differences in parental psychological distress following perinatal death or sudden infant death syndrome.**
  Author(s): Vance JC, Boyle FM, Najman JM, Thearle MJ.
  Source: The British Journal of Psychiatry; the Journal of Mental Science. 1995 December; 167(6): 806-11.
  http://www.ncbi.nlm.nih.gov/entrez/query.fcgi?cmd=Retrieve&db=pubmed&dopt=Abstract&list_uids=8829751

- **Generalized view of the origins of the sudden infant death syndrome.**
  Author(s): Vorontsov IM, Kelmanson IA.
  Source: Medical Hypotheses. 1990 November; 33(3): 187-92. Review.
  http://www.ncbi.nlm.nih.gov/entrez/query.fcgi?cmd=Retrieve&db=pubmed&dopt=Abstract&list_uids=2292983

- **Geophysical variables and behavior: LXXXII. A strong association between sudden infant death syndrome and increments of global geomagnetic activity--possible support for the melatonin hypothesis.**
  Author(s): O'Connor RP, Persinger MA.
  Source: Percept Mot Skills. 1997 April; 84(2): 395-402.
  http://www.ncbi.nlm.nih.gov/entrez/query.fcgi?cmd=Retrieve&db=pubmed&dopt=Abstract&list_uids=9106826

- **Glomerulosclerosis in the sudden infant death syndrome.**
  Author(s): Valdes-Dapena M, Hoffman HJ, Froelich C, Requeira O.
  Source: Pediatr Pathol. 1990; 10(1-2): 273-9.
  http://www.ncbi.nlm.nih.gov/entrez/query.fcgi?cmd=Retrieve&db=pubmed&dopt=Abstract&list_uids=2315230

- **Gluconeogenic enzymes in fibroblasts from infants dying of the sudden infant death syndrome (SIDS).**
  Author(s): Sumbilla CM, Zielke HR, Krause BL, Ozand PT.
  Source: European Journal of Pediatrics. 1983 June-July; 140(3): 276-7.
  http://www.ncbi.nlm.nih.gov/entrez/query.fcgi?cmd=Retrieve&db=pubmed&dopt=Abstract&list_uids=6628449

- **Growth and the sudden infant death syndrome.**
  Author(s): Williams SM, Scragg R, Mitchell EA, Taylor BJ.
  Source: Acta Paediatrica (Oslo, Norway : 1992). 1996 November; 85(11): 1284-9.
  http://www.ncbi.nlm.nih.gov/entrez/query.fcgi?cmd=Retrieve&db=pubmed&dopt=Abstract&list_uids=8955453

- **Guidance on preventing sudden infant death syndrome.**
  Author(s): Kenyon S.
  Source: Community Nurse. 2000 October; 6(9): S9-10. Review. No Abstract Available.
  http://www.ncbi.nlm.nih.gov/entrez/query.fcgi?cmd=Retrieve&db=pubmed&dopt=Abstract&list_uids=11982157

- **Has changing diagnostic preference been responsible for the recent fall in incidence of sudden infant death syndrome in South Australia?**
  Author(s): Byard RW, Beal SM.
  Source: Journal of Paediatrics and Child Health. 1995 June; 31(3): 197-9.
  http://www.ncbi.nlm.nih.gov/entrez/query.fcgi?cmd=Retrieve&db=pubmed&dopt=Abstract&list_uids=7669379

- **Hazards in the epidemiological study of sudden infant death syndrome.**
  Author(s): Meadow SR.
  Source: Archives of Disease in Childhood. 2003 May; 88(5): 460-1.
  http://www.ncbi.nlm.nih.gov/entrez/query.fcgi?cmd=Retrieve&db=pubmed&dopt=Abstract&list_uids=12716730

- **Heart rate variability and sudden infant death syndrome.**
  Author(s): Perticone F, Ceravolo R, Maio R, Cosco C, Mattioli PL.
  Source: Pacing and Clinical Electrophysiology : Pace. 1990 December; 13(12 Pt 2): 2096-9.
  http://www.ncbi.nlm.nih.gov/entrez/query.fcgi?cmd=Retrieve&db=pubmed&dopt=Abstract&list_uids=1704600

- **Heart weight in infants--a comparison between sudden infant death syndrome and other causes of death.**
  Author(s): Rasten-Almqvist P, Eksborg S, Rajs J.
  Source: Acta Paediatrica (Oslo, Norway : 1992). 2000 September; 89(9): 1062-7.
  http://www.ncbi.nlm.nih.gov/entrez/query.fcgi?cmd=Retrieve&db=pubmed&dopt=Abstract&list_uids=11071085

- **Heavy caffeine consumption in pregnancy, smoking, and sudden infant death syndrome.**
  Author(s): Leviton A.
  Source: Archives of Disease in Childhood. 1998 September; 79(3): 291.
  http://www.ncbi.nlm.nih.gov/entrez/query.fcgi?cmd=Retrieve&db=pubmed&dopt=Abstract&list_uids=9875035

- **Heavy caffeine intake in pregnancy and sudden infant death syndrome. New Zealand Cot Death Study Group.**
  Author(s): Ford RP, Schluter PJ, Mitchell EA, Taylor BJ, Scragg R, Stewart AW.
  Source: Archives of Disease in Childhood. 1998 January; 78(1): 9-13.
  http://www.ncbi.nlm.nih.gov/entrez/query.fcgi?cmd=Retrieve&db=pu bmed&dopt=Abstract&list_uids=9534669

- **Heavy metals, chlorinated pesticides and polychlorinated biphenyls in sudden infant death syndrome (SIDS).**
  Author(s): Kleemann WJ, Weller JP, Wolf M, Troger HD, Bluthgen A, Heeschen W.
  Source: International Journal of Legal Medicine. 1991 March; 104(2): 71-5.
  http://www.ncbi.nlm.nih.gov/entrez/query.fcgi?cmd=Retrieve&db=pu bmed&dopt=Abstract&list_uids=1905149

- **Helicobacter pylori is not the cause of sudden infant death syndrome (SIDS).**
  Author(s): Ho GY, Windsor HM, Snowball B, Marshall BJ.
  Source: The American Journal of Gastroenterology. 2001 December; 96(12): 3288-94.
  http://www.ncbi.nlm.nih.gov/entrez/query.fcgi?cmd=Retrieve&db=pu bmed&dopt=Abstract&list_uids=11774938

- **High postmortem concentrations of hypoxanthine and urate in the vitreous humor of infants are not confined to cases of sudden infant death syndrome.**
  Author(s): Belonje PC, Wilson GR, Siroka SA.
  Source: South African Medical Journal. Suid-Afrikaanse Tydskrif Vir Geneeskunde. 1996 July; 86(7): 827-8.
  http://www.ncbi.nlm.nih.gov/entrez/query.fcgi?cmd=Retrieve&db=pu bmed&dopt=Abstract&list_uids=8764909

- **Home apnea monitoring and sudden infant death syndrome.**
  Author(s): Malloy MH, Hoffman HJ.
  Source: Preventive Medicine. 1996 November-December; 25(6): 645-9.
  http://www.ncbi.nlm.nih.gov/entrez/query.fcgi?cmd=Retrieve&db=pu bmed&dopt=Abstract&list_uids=8936564

- **Home monitoring for infants at high risk for the sudden infant death syndrome.**
  Author(s): Sivan Y, Kornecki A, Baharav A, Glaser N, Spirer Z.
  Source: Isr J Med Sci. 1997 January; 33(1): 45-9.
  http://www.ncbi.nlm.nih.gov/entrez/query.fcgi?cmd=Retrieve&db=pubmed&dopt=Abstract&list_uids=9203517

- **Housing and sudden infant death syndrome. The New Zealand Cot Death Study Group.**
  Author(s): Schluter PJ, Ford RP, Mitchell EA, Taylor BJ.
  Source: N Z Med J. 1997 July 11; 110(1047): 243-6.
  http://www.ncbi.nlm.nih.gov/entrez/query.fcgi?cmd=Retrieve&db=pubmed&dopt=Abstract&list_uids=9251707

- **How does prone sleeping increase prevalence of sudden infant death syndrome?**
  Author(s): Thach BT.
  Source: Pediatr Pulmonol Suppl. 1997; 16: 115-6. Review. No Abstract Available.
  http://www.ncbi.nlm.nih.gov/entrez/query.fcgi?cmd=Retrieve&db=pubmed&dopt=Abstract&list_uids=9443232

- **Human heat shock protein gene polymorphisms and sudden infant death syndrome.**
  Author(s): Rahim RA, Boyd PA, Ainslie Patrick WJ, Burdon RH.
  Source: Archives of Disease in Childhood. 1996 November; 75(5): 451-2.
  http://www.ncbi.nlm.nih.gov/entrez/query.fcgi?cmd=Retrieve&db=pubmed&dopt=Abstract&list_uids=8957963

- **Hypercapnea and hypoxia challenge tests in infants at risk for sudden infant death syndrome.**
  Author(s): Lindenberg JA, Newcomb JD.
  Source: Am J Dis Child. 1986 May; 140(5): 466-70.
  http://www.ncbi.nlm.nih.gov/entrez/query.fcgi?cmd=Retrieve&db=pubmed&dopt=Abstract&list_uids=3962942

- **Hyperplasia of the aorticopulmonary paraganglia: a new insight into the pathogenesis of sudden infant death syndrome?**
  Author(s): Ramos SG, Matturri L, Biondo B, Ottaviani G, Rossi L.
  Source: Cardiologia. 1998 September; 43(9): 953-8.
  http://www.ncbi.nlm.nih.gov/entrez/query.fcgi?cmd=Retrieve&db=pubmed&dopt=Abstract&list_uids=9859610

- **Hyper-releasability of mast cells in family members of infants with sudden infant death syndrome and apparent life-threatening events.**
  Author(s): Gold Y, Goldberg A, Sivan Y.
  Source: The Journal of Pediatrics. 2000 April; 136(4): 460-5.
  http://www.ncbi.nlm.nih.gov/entrez/query.fcgi?cmd=Retrieve&db=pubmed&dopt=Abstract&list_uids=10753243

- **Hypoxanthine levels in vitreous humor: a study of influencing factors in sudden infant death syndrome.**
  Author(s): Opdal SH, Rognum TO, Vege A, Saugstad OD.
  Source: Pediatric Research. 1998 August; 44(2): 192-6.
  http://www.ncbi.nlm.nih.gov/entrez/query.fcgi?cmd=Retrieve&db=pubmed&dopt=Abstract&list_uids=9702913

- **Hypoxanthine levels in vitreous humor: evidence of hypoxia in most infants who died of sudden infant death syndrome.**
  Author(s): Rognum TO, Saugstad OD.
  Source: Pediatrics. 1991 March; 87(3): 306-10.
  http://www.ncbi.nlm.nih.gov/entrez/query.fcgi?cmd=Retrieve&db=pubmed&dopt=Abstract&list_uids=1796934

- **Hypoxic responses in infants. No known mechanism links hypoxia and sudden infant death syndrome.**
  Author(s): Niermeyer S, Moore LG.
  Source: Bmj (Clinical Research Ed.). 1998 September 5; 317(7159): 675-6; Author Reply 677-8.
  http://www.ncbi.nlm.nih.gov/entrez/query.fcgi?cmd=Retrieve&db=pubmed&dopt=Abstract&list_uids=9758493

- **Identification of Pneumocystis carinii in the lungs of infants dying of sudden infant death syndrome.**
  Author(s): Morgan DJ, Vargas SL, Reyes-Mugica M, Walterspiel JN, Carver W, Gigliotti F.
  Source: The Pediatric Infectious Disease Journal. 2001 March; 20(3): 306-9.
  http://www.ncbi.nlm.nih.gov/entrez/query.fcgi?cmd=Retrieve&db=pubmed&dopt=Abstract&list_uids=11303835

- **Immune and inflammatory responses in sudden infant death syndrome.**
  Author(s): Forsyth KD.
  Source: Fems Immunology and Medical Microbiology. 1999 August 1; 25(1-2): 79-83. Review.
  http://www.ncbi.nlm.nih.gov/entrez/query.fcgi?cmd=Retrieve&db=pubmed&dopt=Abstract&list_uids=10443494

- **Immunohistochemical techniques improve the diagnosis of myocarditis in cases of suspected sudden infant death syndrome (SIDS).**
  Author(s): Dettmeyer R, Schlamann M, Madea B.
  Source: Forensic Science International. 1999 November 1; 105(2): 83-94.
  http://www.ncbi.nlm.nih.gov/entrez/query.fcgi?cmd=Retrieve&db=pubmed&dopt=Abstract&list_uids=10605078

- **Immunological evidence for a bacterial toxin aetiology in sudden infant death syndrome.**
  Author(s): Siarakas S, Brown AJ, Murrell WG.
  Source: Fems Immunology and Medical Microbiology. 1999 August 1; 25(1-2): 37-50.
  http://www.ncbi.nlm.nih.gov/entrez/query.fcgi?cmd=Retrieve&db=pubmed&dopt=Abstract&list_uids=10443490

- **Impaired arousals and sudden infant death syndrome: preexisting neural injury?**
  Author(s): Harper RM.
  Source: American Journal of Respiratory and Critical Care Medicine. 2003 December 1; 168(11): 1262-3.
  http://www.ncbi.nlm.nih.gov/entrez/query.fcgi?cmd=Retrieve&db=pubmed&dopt=Abstract&list_uids=14644917

- **Incidence and geographical distribution of sudden infant death syndrome in relation to content of nitrate in drinking water and groundwater levels.**
  Author(s): George M, Wiklund L, Aastrup M, Pousette J, Thunholm B, Saldeen T, Wernroth L, Zaren B, Holmberg L.
  Source: European Journal of Clinical Investigation. 2001 December; 31(12): 1083-94.
  http://www.ncbi.nlm.nih.gov/entrez/query.fcgi?cmd=Retrieve&db=pubmed&dopt=Abstract&list_uids=11903496

- **Increase of pulmonary density of macrophages in sudden infant death syndrome.**
  Author(s): Lorin de la Grandmaison G, Dorandeu A, Carton M, Patey A, Durigon M.
  Source: Forensic Science International. 1999 October 11; 104(2-3): 179-87.
  http://www.ncbi.nlm.nih.gov/entrez/query.fcgi?cmd=Retrieve&db=pubmed&dopt=Abstract&list_uids=10581724

- **Increased facial temperature as an early warning in Sudden Infant Death Syndrome.**
  Author(s): Russell MJ, Vink R.
  Source: Medical Hypotheses. 2001 July; 57(1): 61-3.
  http://www.ncbi.nlm.nih.gov/entrez/query.fcgi?cmd=Retrieve&db=pubmed&dopt=Abstract&list_uids=11421627

- **Infant sleeping position and the risk of sudden infant death syndrome in California, 1997-2000.**
  Author(s): Li DK, Petitti DB, Willinger M, McMahon R, Odouli R, Vu H, Hoffman HJ.
  Source: American Journal of Epidemiology. 2003 March 1; 157(5): 446-55.
  http://www.ncbi.nlm.nih.gov/entrez/query.fcgi?cmd=Retrieve&db=pubmed&dopt=Abstract&list_uids=12615609

- **Infant stress and sleep deprivation as an aetiological basis for the sudden infant death syndrome.**
  Author(s): Simpson JM.
  Source: Early Human Development. 2001 February; 61(1): 1-43. Review.
  http://www.ncbi.nlm.nih.gov/entrez/query.fcgi?cmd=Retrieve&db=pubmed&dopt=Abstract&list_uids=11172974

- **Inflammatory responses in sudden infant death syndrome -- past and present views.**
  Author(s): Vege A, Rognum TO.
  Source: Fems Immunology and Medical Microbiology. 1999 August 1; 25(1-2): 67-78. Review.
  http://www.ncbi.nlm.nih.gov/entrez/query.fcgi?cmd=Retrieve&db=pubmed&dopt=Abstract&list_uids=10443493

- **Inspired CO(2) and O(2) in sleeping infants rebreathing from bedding: relevance for sudden infant death syndrome.**
  Author(s): Patel AL, Harris K, Thach BT.
  Source: Journal of Applied Physiology (Bethesda, Md. : 1985). 2001 December; 91(6): 2537-45.
  http://www.ncbi.nlm.nih.gov/entrez/query.fcgi?cmd=Retrieve&db=pubmed&dopt=Abstract&list_uids=11717216

- **Intra-alveolar haemorrhage in sudden infant death syndrome: a cause for concern?**
  Author(s): Yukawa N, Carter N, Rutty G, Green MA.
  Source: Journal of Clinical Pathology. 1999 August; 52(8): 581-7.
  http://www.ncbi.nlm.nih.gov/entrez/query.fcgi?cmd=Retrieve&db=pubmed&dopt=Abstract&list_uids=10645227

- **Intra-alveolar haemorrhage in sudden infant death syndrome: a cause for concern?**
  Author(s): Berry PJ.
  Source: Journal of Clinical Pathology. 1999 August; 52(8): 553-4.
  http://www.ncbi.nlm.nih.gov/entrez/query.fcgi?cmd=Retrieve&db=pubmed&dopt=Abstract&list_uids=10645223

- **Intrathoracic petechiae in sudden infant death syndrome: relationship to face position when found.**
  Author(s): Krous HF, Nadeau JM, Silva PD, Blackbourne BD.
  Source: Pediatric and Developmental Pathology : the Official Journal of the Society for Pediatric Pathology and the Paediatric Pathology Society. 2001 March-April; 4(2): 160-6.
  http://www.ncbi.nlm.nih.gov/entrez/query.fcgi?cmd=Retrieve&db=pubmed&dopt=Abstract&list_uids=11178632

- **Is sudden infant death syndrome a problem in Zimbabwe?.**
  Author(s): Wolf BH, Ikeogu MO.
  Source: Annals of Tropical Paediatrics. 1996 June; 16(2): 149-53.
  http://www.ncbi.nlm.nih.gov/entrez/query.fcgi?cmd=Retrieve&db=pubmed&dopt=Abstract&list_uids=8790679

- **Is sudden infant death syndrome associated with Helicobacter pylori infection in children?**
  Author(s): Elitsur Y, Btriest W, Sabet Z, Neace C, Jiang C, Thomas E.
  Source: Helicobacter. 2000 December; 5(4): 227-31.
  http://www.ncbi.nlm.nih.gov/entrez/query.fcgi?cmd=Retrieve&db=pubmed&dopt=Abstract&list_uids=11179988

- **Is sudden infant death syndrome still more common in very low birthweight infants in the 1990s?**
  Author(s): Sowter B, Doyle LW, Morley CJ, Altmann A, Halliday J.
  Source: The Medical Journal of Australia. 1999 October 18; 171(8): 411-3.
  http://www.ncbi.nlm.nih.gov/entrez/query.fcgi?cmd=Retrieve&db=pubmed&dopt=Abstract&list_uids=10590743

- **Is the G985A allelic variant of medium-chain acyl-CoA dehydrogenase a risk factor for sudden infant death syndrome? A pooled analysis.**
  Author(s): Wang SS, Fernhoff PM, Khoury MJ.
  Source: Pediatrics. 2000 May; 105(5): 1175-6.
  http://www.ncbi.nlm.nih.gov/entrez/query.fcgi?cmd=Retrieve&db=pubmed&dopt=Abstract&list_uids=10836898

- **Is there a familial association between obstructive sleep apnoea/hypopnoea and the sudden infant death syndrome?**
  Author(s): Vennelle M, Brander PE, Kingshott RN, Rees K, Warren PM, Keeling JW, Douglas NJ.
  Source: Thorax. 2004 April; 59(4): 337-41.
  http://www.ncbi.nlm.nih.gov/entrez/query.fcgi?cmd=Retrieve&db=pubmed&dopt=Abstract&list_uids=15047958

- **JAMA patient page. Sudden infant death syndrome.**
  Author(s): Parmet S, Lynm C, Glass RM.
  Source: Jama : the Journal of the American Medical Association. 2002 December 4; 288(21): 2772.
  http://www.ncbi.nlm.nih.gov/entrez/query.fcgi?cmd=Retrieve&db=pubmed&dopt=Abstract&list_uids=12460105

- **Labor and delivery events and risk of sudden infant death syndrome (SIDS)**
  Author(s): Buck GM, Michalek AM, Kramer AA, Batt RE.
  Source: American Journal of Epidemiology. 1991 May 1; 133(9): 900-6.
  http://www.ncbi.nlm.nih.gov/entrez/query.fcgi?cmd=Retrieve&db=pubmed&dopt=Abstract&list_uids=2028979

- **Laryngospasm and diaphragmatic arrest in immature dogs after laryngeal acid exposure: a possible model for sudden infant death syndrome.**
  Author(s): Duke SG, Postma GN, McGuirt WF Jr, Ririe D, Averill DB, Koufman JA.
  Source: The Annals of Otology, Rhinology, and Laryngology. 2001 August; 110(8): 729-33.
  http://www.ncbi.nlm.nih.gov/entrez/query.fcgi?cmd=Retrieve&db=pubmed&dopt=Abstract&list_uids=11510729

- **Lessons from sudden infant death syndrome.**
  Author(s): Kearney PJ.
  Source: Ir J Med Sci. 2000 January-March; 169(1): 17-8. No Abstract Available.
  http://www.ncbi.nlm.nih.gov/entrez/query.fcgi?cmd=Retrieve&db=pubmed&dopt=Abstract&list_uids=10846850

- **Lethal challenge of gnotobiotic weanling rats with bacterial isolates from cases of sudden infant death syndrome (SIDS).**
  Author(s): Lee S, Barson AJ, Drucker DB, Morris JA, Telford DR.
  Source: Journal of Clinical Pathology. 1987 December; 40(12): 1393-6.
  http://www.ncbi.nlm.nih.gov/entrez/query.fcgi?cmd=Retrieve&db=pubmed&dopt=Abstract&list_uids=3323245

- **Lethal synergistic action of toxins of bacteria isolated from sudden infant death syndrome.**
  Author(s): Drucker DB, Aluyi HS, Morris JA, Telford DR, Gibbs A.
  Source: Journal of Clinical Pathology. 1992 September; 45(9): 799-801.
  http://www.ncbi.nlm.nih.gov/entrez/query.fcgi?cmd=Retrieve&db=pubmed&dopt=Abstract&list_uids=1401211

- **Lethal synergy between toxins of staphylococci and enterobacteria: implications for sudden infant death syndrome.**
  Author(s): Sayers NM, Drucker DB, Morris JA, Telford DR.
  Source: Journal of Clinical Pathology. 1995 October; 48(10): 929-32.
  http://www.ncbi.nlm.nih.gov/entrez/query.fcgi?cmd=Retrieve&db=pubmed&dopt=Abstract&list_uids=8537492

- **Life events, social support and the risk of sudden infant death syndrome.**
  Author(s): Ford RP, Hassall IB, Mitchell EA, Scragg R, Taylor BJ, Allen EM, Stewart AW.
  Source: Journal of Child Psychology and Psychiatry, and Allied Disciplines. 1996 October; 37(7): 835-40.
  http://www.ncbi.nlm.nih.gov/entrez/query.fcgi?cmd=Retrieve&db=pubmed&dopt=Abstract&list_uids=8923226

- **Light is recognized best through darkness: mast cells and Sudden Infant Death Syndrome.**
  Author(s): Schwartz LB.
  Source: Clinical and Experimental Allergy : Journal of the British Society for Allergy and Clinical Immunology. 2001 November; 31(11): 1657-9.
  http://www.ncbi.nlm.nih.gov/entrez/query.fcgi?cmd=Retrieve&db=pubmed&dopt=Abstract&list_uids=11696039

- **Lipid-containing cells in the brain in sudden infant death syndrome.**
  Author(s): Esiri MM, Urry P, Keeling J.
  Source: Developmental Medicine and Child Neurology. 1990 April; 32(4): 319-24.
  http://www.ncbi.nlm.nih.gov/entrez/query.fcgi?cmd=Retrieve&db=pubmed&dopt=Abstract&list_uids=2332122

- **Liver fatty acids and the sudden infant death syndrome.**
  Author(s): Fogerty AC, Ford GL, Willcox ME, Clancy SL.
  Source: The American Journal of Clinical Nutrition. 1984 February; 39(2): 201-8.
  http://www.ncbi.nlm.nih.gov/entrez/query.fcgi?cmd=Retrieve&db=pubmed&dopt=Abstract&list_uids=6230001

- **Liver iron concentrations in sudden infant death syndrome.**
  Author(s): Moore CA, Raha-Chowdhury R, Fagan DG, Worwood M.
  Source: Archives of Disease in Childhood. 1994 April; 70(4): 295-8.
  http://www.ncbi.nlm.nih.gov/entrez/query.fcgi?cmd=Retrieve&db=pubmed&dopt=Abstract&list_uids=8185362

- **Living at high altitude and risk of sudden infant death syndrome.**
  Author(s): Kohlendorfer U, Kiechl S, Sperl W.
  Source: Archives of Disease in Childhood. 1998 December; 79(6): 506-9.
  http://www.ncbi.nlm.nih.gov/entrez/query.fcgi?cmd=Retrieve&db=pubmed&dopt=Abstract&list_uids=10210996

- **Location of smoking and the sudden infant death syndrome (SIDS).**
  Author(s): Mitchell EA, Scragg L, Clements M.
  Source: Aust N Z J Med. 1995 April; 25(2): 155-6. No Abstract Available.
  http://www.ncbi.nlm.nih.gov/entrez/query.fcgi?cmd=Retrieve&db=pubmed&dopt=Abstract&list_uids=7605299

- **Loss of neonatal hypoxia tolerance after prenatal nicotine exposure: implications for sudden infant death syndrome.**
  Author(s): Slotkin TA, Lappi SE, McCook EC, Lorber BA, Seidler FJ.
  Source: Brain Research Bulletin. 1995; 38(1): 69-75.
  http://www.ncbi.nlm.nih.gov/entrez/query.fcgi?cmd=Retrieve&db=pubmed&dopt=Abstract&list_uids=7552377

- **Lung development: number of terminal bronchiolar duct endings and gas exchange surface area in victims of sudden infant death syndrome.**
  Author(s): Beech DJ, Sibbons PD, Howard CV, van Velzen D.
  Source: Pediatric Pulmonology. 2001 May; 31(5): 339-43.
  http://www.ncbi.nlm.nih.gov/entrez/query.fcgi?cmd=Retrieve&db=pubmed&dopt=Abstract&list_uids=11340679

- **Lung immunoglobulins in the sudden infant death syndrome.**
  Author(s): Matthews TG, Fox GP.
  Source: Bmj (Clinical Research Ed.). 1989 February 25; 298(6672): 522.
  http://www.ncbi.nlm.nih.gov/entrez/query.fcgi?cmd=Retrieve&db=pubmed&dopt=Abstract&list_uids=2495093

- **Lung immunoglobulins in the sudden infant death syndrome.**
  Author(s): Forsyth KD, Weeks SC, Koh L, Skinner J, Bradley J.
  Source: Bmj (Clinical Research Ed.). 1989 January 7; 298(6665): 23-6.
  http://www.ncbi.nlm.nih.gov/entrez/query.fcgi?cmd=Retrieve&db=pubmed&dopt=Abstract&list_uids=2492843

- **Lung surfactant and sudden infant death syndrome.**
  Author(s): Morley C, Hill C, Brown B.
  Source: Annals of the New York Academy of Sciences. 1988; 533: 289-95.
  http://www.ncbi.nlm.nih.gov/entrez/query.fcgi?cmd=Retrieve&db=pubmed&dopt=Abstract&list_uids=3421631

- **Lung tissue concentrations of nicotine in sudden infant death syndrome (SIDS).**
  Author(s): McMartin KI, Platt MS, Hackman R, Klein J, Smialek JE, Vigorito R, Koren G.
  Source: The Journal of Pediatrics. 2002 February; 140(2): 205-9.
  http://www.ncbi.nlm.nih.gov/entrez/query.fcgi?cmd=Retrieve&db=pubmed&dopt=Abstract&list_uids=11865272

- **Lympho-monocytic enteroviral myocarditis: traditional, immunohistological and molecularpathological methods for diagnosis in a case of suspected sudden infant death syndrome (SIDS).**
  Author(s): Dettmeyer R, Kandolf R, Schmidt P, Schlamann M, Madea B.
  Source: Forensic Science International. 2001 June 1; 119(1): 141-4.
  http://www.ncbi.nlm.nih.gov/entrez/query.fcgi?cmd=Retrieve&db=pubmed&dopt=Abstract&list_uids=11348811

- **Magnesium deficit and sudden infant death syndrome (SIDS): SIDS due to magnesium deficiency and SIDS due to various forms of magnesium depletion: possible importance of the chronopathological form.**
  Author(s): Durlach J, Pages N, Bac P, Bara M, Guiet-Bara A.
  Source: Magnes Res. 2002 December; 15(3-4): 269-78. Review.
  http://www.ncbi.nlm.nih.gov/entrez/query.fcgi?cmd=Retrieve&db=pubmed&dopt=Abstract&list_uids=12635883

- **Maternal and paternal recreational drug use and sudden infant death syndrome.**
  Author(s): Klonoff-Cohen H, Lam-Kruglick P.
  Source: Archives of Pediatrics & Adolescent Medicine. 2001 July; 155(7): 765-70.
  http://www.ncbi.nlm.nih.gov/entrez/query.fcgi?cmd=Retrieve&db=pubmed&dopt=Abstract&list_uids=11434841

- **Maternal awareness of sudden infant death syndrome in North Queensland, Australia: an analysis of infant care practices.**
  Author(s): Douglas TA, Buettner PG, Whitehall J.
  Source: Journal of Paediatrics and Child Health. 2001 October; 37(5): 441-5.
  http://www.ncbi.nlm.nih.gov/entrez/query.fcgi?cmd=Retrieve&db=pubmed&dopt=Abstract&list_uids=11885706

- **Maternal pre-eclampsia/eclampsia and the risk of sudden infant death syndrome in offspring.**
  Author(s): Li DK, Wi S.
  Source: Paediatric and Perinatal Epidemiology. 2000 April; 14(2): 141-4.
  http://www.ncbi.nlm.nih.gov/entrez/query.fcgi?cmd=Retrieve&db=pubmed&dopt=Abstract&list_uids=10791657

- **Maternal selenium levels and sudden infant death syndrome (SIDS).**
  Author(s): McGlashan ND, Cook SJ, Melrose W, Martin PL, Chelkowska E, von Witt RJ.
  Source: Aust N Z J Med. 1996 October; 26(5): 677-82.
  http://www.ncbi.nlm.nih.gov/entrez/query.fcgi?cmd=Retrieve&db=pubmed&dopt=Abstract&list_uids=8958364

- **Maternal smoking and pulmonary neuroendocrine cells in sudden infant death syndrome.**
  Author(s): Cutz E, Perrin DG, Hackman R, Czegledy-Nagy EN.
  Source: Pediatrics. 1996 October; 98(4 Pt 1): 668-72.
  http://www.ncbi.nlm.nih.gov/entrez/query.fcgi?cmd=Retrieve&db=pubmed&dopt=Abstract&list_uids=8885943

- **Medial smooth muscle thickness in small pulmonary arteries in sudden infant death syndrome revisited.**
  Author(s): Krous HF, Floyd CW, Nadeau JM, Silva PD, Blackbourne BD, Langston C.
  Source: Pediatric and Developmental Pathology : the Official Journal of the Society for Pediatric Pathology and the Paediatric Pathology Society. 2002 July-August; 5(4): 375-85. Epub 2002 May 21.
  http://www.ncbi.nlm.nih.gov/entrez/query.fcgi?cmd=Retrieve&db=pubmed&dopt=Abstract&list_uids=12016526

- **Medullary serotonergic network deficiency in the sudden infant death syndrome: review of a 15-year study of a single dataset.**
  Author(s): Kinney HC, Filiano JJ, White WF.
  Source: Journal of Neuropathology and Experimental Neurology. 2001 March; 60(3): 228-47. Review.
  http://www.ncbi.nlm.nih.gov/entrez/query.fcgi?cmd=Retrieve&db=pubmed&dopt=Abstract&list_uids=11245208

- **Mitochondrial DNA point mutations detected in four cases of sudden infant death syndrome.**
  Author(s): Opdal SH, Rognum TO, Torgersen H, Vege A.
  Source: Acta Paediatrica (Oslo, Norway : 1992). 1999 September; 88(9): 957-60.
  http://www.ncbi.nlm.nih.gov/entrez/query.fcgi?cmd=Retrieve&db=pubmed&dopt=Abstract&list_uids=10519336

- **Molecular biology in cerebral cortex of sudden infant death syndrome.**
  Author(s): Sawaguchi T, Takashima S, Ito M, Sawaguchi A.
  Source: Forensic Science International. 2002 September 14; 130 Suppl: S60-2.
  http://www.ncbi.nlm.nih.gov/entrez/query.fcgi?cmd=Retrieve&db=pubmed&dopt=Abstract&list_uids=12350302

- **Molecular diagnosis in a child with sudden infant death syndrome.**
  Author(s): Schwartz PJ, Priori SG, Bloise R, Napolitano C, Ronchetti E, Piccinini A, Goj C, Breithardt G, Schulze-Bahr E, Wedekind H, Nastoli J.
  Source: Lancet. 2001 October 20; 358(9290): 1342-3.
  http://www.ncbi.nlm.nih.gov/entrez/query.fcgi?cmd=Retrieve&db=pubmed&dopt=Abstract&list_uids=11684219

- **Molecular link between Sudden Infant Death Syndrome and long-QT syndrome is "proof of concept".**
  Author(s): SoRelle R.
  Source: Circulation. 2000 August 22; 102(8): E9014-5.
  http://www.ncbi.nlm.nih.gov/entrez/query.fcgi?cmd=Retrieve&db=pubmed&dopt=Abstract&list_uids=10952968

- **Monolateral hypoplasia of the motor vagal nuclei in a case of sudden infant death syndrome.**
  Author(s): Macchi V, Snenghi R, De Caro R, Parenti A.
  Source: Journal of Anatomy. 2002 February; 200(Pt 2): 195-8.
  http://www.ncbi.nlm.nih.gov/entrez/query.fcgi?cmd=Retrieve&db=pubmed&dopt=Abstract&list_uids=11895117

- **Myocarditis and sudden infant death syndrome.**
  Author(s): Rasten-Almqvist P, Eksborg S, Rajs J.
  Source: Apmis : Acta Pathologica, Microbiologica, Et Immunologica Scandinavica. 2002 June; 110(6): 469-80.
  http://www.ncbi.nlm.nih.gov/entrez/query.fcgi?cmd=Retrieve&db=pubmed&dopt=Abstract&list_uids=12193208

- **Nasal and intrapulmonary haemorrhage in sudden infant death syndrome.**
  Author(s): Becroft DM, Thompson JM, Mitchell EA.
  Source: Archives of Disease in Childhood. 2001 August; 85(2): 116-20.
  http://www.ncbi.nlm.nih.gov/entrez/query.fcgi?cmd=Retrieve&db=pubmed&dopt=Abstract&list_uids=11466185

- **Near miss sudden infant death syndrome episodes? A clinical and electrocardiographic correlation.**
  Author(s): Krongrad E, O'Neill L.
  Source: Pediatrics. 1986 June; 77(6): 811-5.
  http://www.ncbi.nlm.nih.gov/entrez/query.fcgi?cmd=Retrieve&db=pubmed&dopt=Abstract&list_uids=3714372

- **Neck extension and rotation in sudden infant death syndrome and other natural infant deaths.**
  Author(s): Krous HF, Nadeau JM, Silva PD, Blackbourne BD.
  Source: Pediatric and Developmental Pathology : the Official Journal of the Society for Pediatric Pathology and the Paediatric Pathology Society. 2001 March-April; 4(2): 154-9.
  http://www.ncbi.nlm.nih.gov/entrez/query.fcgi?cmd=Retrieve&db=pubmed&dopt=Abstract&list_uids=11178631

- **Negative effect of a short interpregnancy interval on birth weight following loss of an infant to sudden infant death syndrome.**
  Author(s): Spiers PS, Onstad L, Guntheroth WG.
  Source: American Journal of Epidemiology. 1996 June 1; 143(11): 1137-41.
  http://www.ncbi.nlm.nih.gov/entrez/query.fcgi?cmd=Retrieve&db=pubmed&dopt=Abstract&list_uids=8633603

- **Neuronal apoptosis in sudden infant death syndrome.**
  Author(s): Waters KA, Meehan B, Huang JQ, Gravel RA, Michaud J, Cote A.
  Source: Pediatric Research. 1999 February; 45(2): 166-72.
  http://www.ncbi.nlm.nih.gov/entrez/query.fcgi?cmd=Retrieve&db=pubmed&dopt=Abstract&list_uids=10022585

- **Newborn acoustic cry characteristics of infants subsequently dying of sudden infant death syndrome.**
  Author(s): Corwin MJ, Lester BM, Sepkoski C, Peucker M, Kayne H, Golub HL.
  Source: Pediatrics. 1995 July; 96(1 Pt 1): 73-7.
  http://www.ncbi.nlm.nih.gov/entrez/query.fcgi?cmd=Retrieve&db=pubmed&dopt=Abstract&list_uids=7596727

- **Nicotine, serotonin, and sudden infant death syndrome.**
  Author(s): Nattie E, Kinney H.
  Source: American Journal of Respiratory and Critical Care Medicine. 2002 December 15; 166(12 Pt 1): 1530-1.
  http://www.ncbi.nlm.nih.gov/entrez/query.fcgi?cmd=Retrieve&db=pubmed&dopt=Abstract&list_uids=12471066

- **Nighttime child care: inadequate sudden infant death syndrome risk factor knowledge, practice, and policies.**
  Author(s): Moon RY, Weese-Mayer DE, Silvestri JM.
  Source: Pediatrics. 2003 April; 111(4 Pt 1): 795-9.
  http://www.ncbi.nlm.nih.gov/entrez/query.fcgi?cmd=Retrieve&db=pubmed&dopt=Abstract&list_uids=12671114

- **NMDA receptor 1 expression in the brainstem of human infants and its relevance to the sudden infant death syndrome (SIDS).**
  Author(s): Machaalani R, Waters KA.
  Source: Journal of Neuropathology and Experimental Neurology. 2003 October; 62(10): 1076-85.
  http://www.ncbi.nlm.nih.gov/entrez/query.fcgi?cmd=Retrieve&db=pubmed&dopt=Abstract&list_uids=14575242

- **Numbers of infant deaths in Scotland, with special reference to sudden infant death syndrome.**
  Author(s): Arrundale J.
  Source: Health Bull (Edinb). 1993 March; 51(2): 106-17.
  http://www.ncbi.nlm.nih.gov/entrez/query.fcgi?cmd=Retrieve&db=pubmed&dopt=Abstract&list_uids=8514487

- **Objective measurements of nicotine exposure in victims of sudden infant death syndrome and in other unexpected child deaths.**
  Author(s): Milerad J, Vege A, Opdal SH, Rognum TO.
  Source: The Journal of Pediatrics. 1998 August; 133(2): 232-6.
  http://www.ncbi.nlm.nih.gov/entrez/query.fcgi?cmd=Retrieve&db=pubmed&dopt=Abstract&list_uids=9709711

- **Obstructive sleep apnea in infants: relation to family history of sudden infant death syndrome, apparent life-threatening events, and obstructive sleep apnea.**
  Author(s): McNamara F, Sullivan CE.
  Source: The Journal of Pediatrics. 2000 March; 136(3): 318-23.
  http://www.ncbi.nlm.nih.gov/entrez/query.fcgi?cmd=Retrieve&db=pubmed&dopt=Abstract&list_uids=10700687

- **On listening to parents: the sudden infant death syndrome over 25 years.**
  Author(s): Tonkin S.
  Source: Pediatrics. 1996 June; 97(6 Pt 1): 896-7.
  http://www.ncbi.nlm.nih.gov/entrez/query.fcgi?cmd=Retrieve&db=pubmed&dopt=Abstract&list_uids=8657533

- **Ondine's curse and sudden infant death syndrome.**
  Author(s): Long KJ.
  Source: Pediatric Emergency Care. 1992 February; 8(1): 61-2.
  http://www.ncbi.nlm.nih.gov/entrez/query.fcgi?cmd=Retrieve&db=pubmed&dopt=Abstract&list_uids=1603697

- **One more thought on sudden infant death syndrome.**
  Author(s): Albers S, Levy HL.
  Source: Pediatrics. 2001 April; 107(4): 809.
  http://www.ncbi.nlm.nih.gov/entrez/query.fcgi?cmd=Retrieve&db=pubmed&dopt=Abstract&list_uids=11380009

- **Ontogenesis of CYP2C-dependent arachidonic acid metabolism in the human liver: relationship with sudden infant death syndrome.**
  Author(s): Treluyer JM, Benech H, Colin I, Pruvost A, Cheron G, Cresteil T.
  Source: Pediatric Research. 2000 May; 47(5): 677-83.
  http://www.ncbi.nlm.nih.gov/entrez/query.fcgi?cmd=Retrieve&db=pubmed&dopt=Abstract&list_uids=10813596

- **Ontogeny of peptides in human hypothalamus in relation to sudden infant death syndrome (SIDS).**
  Author(s): Kopp N, Najimi M, Champier J, Chigr F, Charnay Y, Epelbaum J, Jordan D.
  Source: Prog Brain Res. 1992; 93: 167-87; Discussion 187-8. Review.
  http://www.ncbi.nlm.nih.gov/entrez/query.fcgi?cmd=Retrieve&db=pubmed&dopt=Abstract&list_uids=1336202

- **Organ weights in sudden infant death syndrome.**
  Author(s): Siebert JR, Haas JE.
  Source: Pediatr Pathol. 1994 November-December; 14(6): 973-85.
  http://www.ncbi.nlm.nih.gov/entrez/query.fcgi?cmd=Retrieve&db=pubmed&dopt=Abstract&list_uids=7855017

- **Overview of sudden infant death syndrome in Japan.**
  Author(s): Nishida H.
  Source: Acta Paediatr Jpn. 1994 June; 36(3): 301-3. Review.
  http://www.ncbi.nlm.nih.gov/entrez/query.fcgi?cmd=Retrieve&db=pubmed&dopt=Abstract&list_uids=8091984

- **Oxidative stress in sudden infant death syndrome.**
  Author(s): Huggle S, Hunsaker JC 3rd, Coyne CM, Sparks DL.
  Source: Journal of Child Neurology. 1996 November; 11(6): 433-8.
  http://www.ncbi.nlm.nih.gov/entrez/query.fcgi?cmd=Retrieve&db=pubmed&dopt=Abstract&list_uids=9120219

- **Pacifier use and sudden infant death syndrome: should health professionals recommend pacifier use based on present knowledge?**
  Author(s): Zotter H, Kerbl R, Kurz R, Muller W.
  Source: Wiener Klinische Wochenschrift. 2002 September 30; 114(17-18): 791-4. Review.
  http://www.ncbi.nlm.nih.gov/entrez/query.fcgi?cmd=Retrieve&db=pubmed&dopt=Abstract&list_uids=12416286

- **Patterns of symptoms in siblings of sudden infant death syndrome infants.**
  Author(s): Wailoo M, Thompson JR, Waite AJ, Coombs RC, Jackson JA.
  Source: Child: Care, Health and Development. 2002 September; 28 Suppl 1: 19-21.
  http://www.ncbi.nlm.nih.gov/entrez/query.fcgi?cmd=Retrieve&db=pubmed&dopt=Abstract&list_uids=12515433

- PCR-based diagnosis of enterovirus and parvovirus B19 in paraffin-embedded heart tissue of children with suspected sudden infant death syndrome.
  Author(s): Baasner A, Dettmeyer R, Graebe M, Rissland J, Madea B.
  Source: Laboratory Investigation; a Journal of Technical Methods and Pathology. 2003 October; 83(10): 1451-5.
  http://www.ncbi.nlm.nih.gov/entrez/query.fcgi?cmd=Retrieve&db=pubmed&dopt=Abstract&list_uids=14563946

- Polymorphisms in genes involved in glucose metabolism in cases of sudden infant death syndrome.
  Author(s): Burchell A, Forsyth L, Hume R.
  Source: Child: Care, Health and Development. 2002 September; 28 Suppl 1: 37-9.
  http://www.ncbi.nlm.nih.gov/entrez/query.fcgi?cmd=Retrieve&db=pubmed&dopt=Abstract&list_uids=12515438

- Population trends in sudden infant death syndrome.
  Author(s): Ponsonby AL, Dwyer T, Cochrane J.
  Source: Semin Perinatol. 2002 August; 26(4): 296-305. Review.
  http://www.ncbi.nlm.nih.gov/entrez/query.fcgi?cmd=Retrieve&db=pubmed&dopt=Abstract&list_uids=12211620

- Population-based recurrence risk of sudden infant death syndrome compared with other infant and fetal deaths.
  Author(s): Oyen N, Skjaerven R, Irgens LM.
  Source: American Journal of Epidemiology. 1996 August 1; 144(3): 300-5.
  http://www.ncbi.nlm.nih.gov/entrez/query.fcgi?cmd=Retrieve&db=pubmed&dopt=Abstract&list_uids=8686699

- Prepregnancy body mass index and sudden infant death syndrome.
  Author(s): Wisborg K, Vesterggard M, Kristensen J, Kesmodel U.
  Source: Epidemiology (Cambridge, Mass.). 2003 September; 14(5): 630.
  http://www.ncbi.nlm.nih.gov/entrez/query.fcgi?cmd=Retrieve&db=pubmed&dopt=Abstract&list_uids=14501281

- Prevalence of modifiable risk factors for sudden infant death syndrome in British Forces Germany.
  Author(s): Miller SA, Morrison MM.
  Source: J R Army Med Corps. 1996 June; 142(2): 72-8.
  http://www.ncbi.nlm.nih.gov/entrez/query.fcgi?cmd=Retrieve&db=pubmed&dopt=Abstract&list_uids=8819036

- **Prevention of sudden infant death syndrome.**
  Author(s): Wennergren G.
  Source: Pediatr Pulmonol Suppl. 2004; 26: 110-1. No Abstract Available.
  http://www.ncbi.nlm.nih.gov/entrez/query.fcgi?cmd=Retrieve&db=pubmed&dopt=Abstract&list_uids=15029618

- **PrP Sc-like prion protein conformer in sudden infant death syndrome brain.**
  Author(s): Bergmann J, Bergmann R, Janetzky B, Singh S, Preddie E.
  Source: Acta Neuropathologica. 2004 January; 107(1): 66-8. Epub 2003 November 06.
  http://www.ncbi.nlm.nih.gov/entrez/query.fcgi?cmd=Retrieve&db=pubmed&dopt=Abstract&list_uids=14605831

- **QT interval measurements before sudden infant death syndrome.**
  Author(s): Southall DP, Arrowsmith WA, Stebbens V, Alexander JR.
  Source: Archives of Disease in Childhood. 1986 April; 61(4): 327-33.
  http://www.ncbi.nlm.nih.gov/entrez/query.fcgi?cmd=Retrieve&db=pubmed&dopt=Abstract&list_uids=3707181

- **QTc and R-R intervals in victims of the sudden infant death syndrome.**
  Author(s): Weinstein SL, Steinschneider A.
  Source: Am J Dis Child. 1985 October; 139(10): 987-90.
  http://www.ncbi.nlm.nih.gov/entrez/query.fcgi?cmd=Retrieve&db=pubmed&dopt=Abstract&list_uids=4036903

- **Quantitation of medullary astrogliosis in sudden infant death syndrome.**
  Author(s): Bruce K, Becker LE.
  Source: Pediatric Neurosurgery. 1991-92; 17(2): 74-9.
  http://www.ncbi.nlm.nih.gov/entrez/query.fcgi?cmd=Retrieve&db=pubmed&dopt=Abstract&list_uids=1815732

- **Quantitative neuropathological analysis of sudden infant death syndrome.**
  Author(s): Ansari T, Sibbons PD, Parsons A, Rossi ML.
  Source: Child: Care, Health and Development. 2002 September; 28 Suppl 1: 3-6.
  http://www.ncbi.nlm.nih.gov/entrez/query.fcgi?cmd=Retrieve&db=pubmed&dopt=Abstract&list_uids=12515429

- **Recent trend of the incidence of sudden infant death syndrome in Japan.**
  Author(s): Sawaguchi T, Namiki M.
  Source: Early Human Development. 2003 December; 75 Suppl: S175-9.
  http://www.ncbi.nlm.nih.gov/entrez/query.fcgi?cmd=Retrieve&db=pubmed&dopt=Abstract&list_uids=14693403

- **Reducing the incidence of sudden infant death syndrome in the Delta region of Mississippi: a three-pronged approach.**
  Author(s): Kum-Nji P, Mangrem CL, Wells PJ.
  Source: Southern Medical Journal. 2001 July; 94(7): 704-10. Review.
  http://www.ncbi.nlm.nih.gov/entrez/query.fcgi?cmd=Retrieve&db=pubmed&dopt=Abstract&list_uids=11531178

- **Reduction in sudden infant death syndrome may be due to parents checking their babies more often.**
  Author(s): Davies DP, Ansari BM, Evans IE.
  Source: Bmj (Clinical Research Ed.). 1996 September 21; 313(7059): 752-3.
  http://www.ncbi.nlm.nih.gov/entrez/query.fcgi?cmd=Retrieve&db=pubmed&dopt=Abstract&list_uids=8819460

- **Relationship between arousal reaction and autonomic nervous system in the sudden infant death syndrome.**
  Author(s): Sawaguchi T, Franco P, Groswasser J, Kahn A.
  Source: The American Journal of Forensic Medicine and Pathology : Official Publication of the National Association of Medical Examiners. 2001 June; 22(2): 213-4.
  http://www.ncbi.nlm.nih.gov/entrez/query.fcgi?cmd=Retrieve&db=pubmed&dopt=Abstract&list_uids=11394765

- **Relationship of substance P and gliosis in medulla oblongata in neonatal sudden infant death syndrome.**
  Author(s): Obonai T, Takashima S, Becker LE, Asanuma M, Mizuta R, Horie H, Tanaka J.
  Source: Pediatric Neurology. 1996 October; 15(3): 189-92.
  http://www.ncbi.nlm.nih.gov/entrez/query.fcgi?cmd=Retrieve&db=pubmed&dopt=Abstract&list_uids=8916154

- **Review of risk factors for sudden infant death syndrome.**
  Author(s): Sullivan FM, Barlow SM.
  Source: Paediatric and Perinatal Epidemiology. 2001 April; 15(2): 144-200.
  Review. Erratum In: Paediatr Perinat Epidemiol 2002 January; 16(1): 96.
  http://www.ncbi.nlm.nih.gov/entrez/query.fcgi?cmd=Retrieve&db=pu
  bmed&dopt=Abstract&list_uids=11383580

- **Risk factors for sudden infant death syndrome among northern plains Indians.**
  Author(s): Iyasu S, Randall LL, Welty TK, Hsia J, Kinney HC, Mandell F, McClain M, Randall B, Habbe D, Wilson H, Willinger M.
  Source: Jama : the Journal of the American Medical Association. 2002 December 4; 288(21): 2717-23. Erratum In: Jama. 2003 January 15; 289(3): 303.
  http://www.ncbi.nlm.nih.gov/entrez/query.fcgi?cmd=Retrieve&db=pu
  bmed&dopt=Abstract&list_uids=12460095

- **Risk factors for sudden infant death syndrome: changes associated with sleep position recommendations.**
  Author(s): Paris CA, Remler R, Daling JR.
  Source: The Journal of Pediatrics. 2001 December; 139(6): 771-7.
  http://www.ncbi.nlm.nih.gov/entrez/query.fcgi?cmd=Retrieve&db=pu
  bmed&dopt=Abstract&list_uids=11743500

- **Risk factors for sudden infant death syndrome: further change in 1992-3.**
  Author(s): Hiley CM, Morley CJ.
  Source: Bmj (Clinical Research Ed.). 1996 June 1; 312(7043): 1397-8.
  http://www.ncbi.nlm.nih.gov/entrez/query.fcgi?cmd=Retrieve&db=pu
  bmed&dopt=Abstract&list_uids=8646098

- **Risk of sudden infant death syndrome and week of gestation of term birth.**
  Author(s): Smith GC, Pell JP, Dobbie R.
  Source: Pediatrics. 2003 June; 111(6 Pt 1): 1367-71.
  http://www.ncbi.nlm.nih.gov/entrez/query.fcgi?cmd=Retrieve&db=pu
  bmed&dopt=Abstract&list_uids=12777554

- **Seasonal variation in sudden infant death syndrome and bronchiolitis-- a common mechanism?**
  Author(s): Gupta R, Helms PJ, Jolliffe IT, Douglas AS.
  Source: American Journal of Respiratory and Critical Care Medicine. 1996 August; 154(2 Pt 1): 431-5.
  http://www.ncbi.nlm.nih.gov/entrez/query.fcgi?cmd=Retrieve&db=pubmed&dopt=Abstract&list_uids=8756818

- **Smoking during pregnancy and poor antenatal care: two major preventable risk factors for sudden infant death syndrome.**
  Author(s): Schlaud M, Kleemann WJ, Poets CF, Sens B.
  Source: International Journal of Epidemiology. 1996 October; 25(5): 959-65.
  http://www.ncbi.nlm.nih.gov/entrez/query.fcgi?cmd=Retrieve&db=pubmed&dopt=Abstract&list_uids=8921481

- **Sudden infant death syndrome and baby care practices.**
  Author(s): Coyne I.
  Source: Paediatric Nursing. 1996 December; 8(10): 16-8. Review.
  http://www.ncbi.nlm.nih.gov/entrez/query.fcgi?cmd=Retrieve&db=pubmed&dopt=Abstract&list_uids=9052212

- **Sudden infant death syndrome in Pacific Islands infants in Auckland.**
  Author(s): Tukuitonga C.
  Source: N Z Med J. 1996 October 11; 109(1031): 388. No Abstract Available.
  http://www.ncbi.nlm.nih.gov/entrez/query.fcgi?cmd=Retrieve&db=pubmed&dopt=Abstract&list_uids=8890883

- **Sudden infant death syndrome.**
  Author(s): Koehler SA.
  Source: Acta Paediatrica (Oslo, Norway : 1992). 1996 December; 85(12): 1514-5.
  http://www.ncbi.nlm.nih.gov/entrez/query.fcgi?cmd=Retrieve&db=pubmed&dopt=Abstract&list_uids=9001672

- **Sudden infant death syndrome.**
  Author(s): Beal SM.
  Source: The Medical Journal of Australia. 1996 August 19; 165(4): 179-80.
  http://www.ncbi.nlm.nih.gov/entrez/query.fcgi?cmd=Retrieve&db=pubmed&dopt=Abstract&list_uids=8773641

- **Sudden infant death syndrome. Many infants move from position in which they are put to sleep.**
  Author(s): De Jonge GA, Engelberts AC.
  Source: Bmj (Clinical Research Ed.). 1996 November 23; 313(7068): 1333; Author Reply 1333-4.
  http://www.ncbi.nlm.nih.gov/entrez/query.fcgi?cmd=Retrieve&db=pubmed&dopt=Abstract&list_uids=8942710

- **Sudden infant death syndrome. More attention should have been paid to socioeconomic factors.**
  Author(s): Macfarlane A.
  Source: Bmj (Clinical Research Ed.). 1996 November 23; 313(7068): 1332.
  http://www.ncbi.nlm.nih.gov/entrez/query.fcgi?cmd=Retrieve&db=pubmed&dopt=Abstract&list_uids=8942708

- **Sudden infant death syndrome. Smoking is part of a causal chain.**
  Author(s): Logan S, Spencer N, Blackburn C.
  Source: Bmj (Clinical Research Ed.). 1996 November 23; 313(7068): 1332-3; Author Reply 1333-4.
  http://www.ncbi.nlm.nih.gov/entrez/query.fcgi?cmd=Retrieve&db=pubmed&dopt=Abstract&list_uids=8942709

- **Sudden infant death syndrome: the role of bedding revisited.**
  Author(s): Kemp JS.
  Source: The Journal of Pediatrics. 1996 December; 129(6): 946-7.
  http://www.ncbi.nlm.nih.gov/entrez/query.fcgi?cmd=Retrieve&db=pubmed&dopt=Abstract&list_uids=8969748

- **Temperament ratings do not predict arousability in normal infants and infants at increased risk of sudden infant death syndrome.**
  Author(s): Parslow PM, Horne RS, Ferens D, Bandopadhayay P, Mitchell K, Watts AM, Adamson TM.
  Source: Journal of Developmental and Behavioral Pediatrics : Jdbp. 2002 October; 23(5): 365-70.
  http://www.ncbi.nlm.nih.gov/entrez/query.fcgi?cmd=Retrieve&db=pubmed&dopt=Abstract&list_uids=12394525

- **The brainstem and vulnerability to sudden infant death syndrome.**
  Author(s): Thach BT.
  Source: Neurology. 2003 November 11; 61(9): 1170-1.
  http://www.ncbi.nlm.nih.gov/entrez/query.fcgi?cmd=Retrieve&db=pubmed&dopt=Abstract&list_uids=14610114

- **The contribution of prone sleeping position to the racial disparity in sudden infant death syndrome: the Chicago Infant Mortality Study.**
  Author(s): Hauck FR, Moore CM, Herman SM, Donovan M, Kalelkar M, Christoffel KK, Hoffman HJ, Rowley D.
  Source: Pediatrics. 2002 October; 110(4): 772-80.
  http://www.ncbi.nlm.nih.gov/entrez/query.fcgi?cmd=Retrieve&db=pubmed&dopt=Abstract&list_uids=12359794

- **The epidemiology of sudden infant death syndrome.**
  Author(s): Platt MJ, Pharoah PO.
  Source: Archives of Disease in Childhood. 2003 January; 88(1): 27-9.
  http://www.ncbi.nlm.nih.gov/entrez/query.fcgi?cmd=Retrieve&db=pubmed&dopt=Abstract&list_uids=12495955

- **The role of bacterial toxins in sudden infant death syndrome (SIDS).**
  Author(s): Blackwell CC, Gordon AE, James VS, MacKenzie DA, Mogensen-Buchanan M, El Ahmer OR, Al Madani OM, Toro K, Csukas Z, Sotonyi P, Weir DM, Busuttil A.
  Source: International Journal of Medical Microbiology : Ijmm. 2002 February; 291(6-7): 561-70. Review.
  http://www.ncbi.nlm.nih.gov/entrez/query.fcgi?cmd=Retrieve&db=pubmed&dopt=Abstract&list_uids=11892683

- **The significance of ante- and perinatal periods for formation of risk of sudden infant death syndrome.**
  Author(s): Aryayev N, Kukushkin V, Nepomyashcha V.
  Source: Ginekol Pol. 2001 December; 72(12): 931-9.
  http://www.ncbi.nlm.nih.gov/entrez/query.fcgi?cmd=Retrieve&db=pubmed&dopt=Abstract&list_uids=11883247

- **The triple risk hypotheses in sudden infant death syndrome.**
  Author(s): Guntheroth WG, Spiers PS.
  Source: Pediatrics. 2002 November; 110(5): E64. Review.
  http://www.ncbi.nlm.nih.gov/entrez/query.fcgi?cmd=Retrieve&db=pubmed&dopt=Abstract&list_uids=12415070

- **Toxicologic analysis in cases of possible sudden infant death syndrome: a worthwhile exercise?**
  Author(s): Langlois NE, Ellis PS, Little D, Hulewicz B.
  Source: The American Journal of Forensic Medicine and Pathology : Official Publication of the National Association of Medical Examiners. 2002 June; 23(2): 162-6.
  http://www.ncbi.nlm.nih.gov/entrez/query.fcgi?cmd=Retrieve&db=pubmed&dopt=Abstract&list_uids=12040261

- **Tracking strategies involving fourteen sources for locating a transient study sample: parents of sudden infant death syndrome infants and control infants.**
  Author(s): Klonoff-Cohen H.
  Source: American Journal of Epidemiology. 1996 July 1; 144(1): 98-101.
  http://www.ncbi.nlm.nih.gov/entrez/query.fcgi?cmd=Retrieve&db=pubmed&dopt=Abstract&list_uids=8659490

- **Trends in postneonatal aspiration deaths and reclassification of sudden infant death syndrome: impact of the "Back to Sleep" program.**
  Author(s): Malloy MH.
  Source: Pediatrics. 2002 April; 109(4): 661-5.
  http://www.ncbi.nlm.nih.gov/entrez/query.fcgi?cmd=Retrieve&db=pubmed&dopt=Abstract&list_uids=11927712

- **Understanding and preventing sudden infant death syndrome.**
  Author(s): Fleming PJ.
  Source: Current Opinion in Pediatrics. 1994 April; 6(2): 158-62. Review.
  http://www.ncbi.nlm.nih.gov/entrez/query.fcgi?cmd=Retrieve&db=pubmed&dopt=Abstract&list_uids=8032395

- **Unexpected infant death: occult cardiac disease and sudden infant death syndrome-how much of an overlap is there?**
  Author(s): Byard RW.
  Source: The Journal of Pediatrics. 2002 September; 141(3): 303-5.
  http://www.ncbi.nlm.nih.gov/entrez/query.fcgi?cmd=Retrieve&db=pubmed&dopt=Abstract&list_uids=12219047

- **Unexplained stillbirths and sudden infant death syndrome.**
  Author(s): Walsh S, Mortimer G.
  Source: Medical Hypotheses. 1995 July; 45(1): 73-5.
  http://www.ncbi.nlm.nih.gov/entrez/query.fcgi?cmd=Retrieve&db=pubmed&dopt=Abstract&list_uids=8524185

- **Unraveling the mysteries of sudden infant death syndrome.**
  Author(s): Brooks JG.
  Source: Current Opinion in Pediatrics. 1993 June; 5(3): 266-72. Review.
  http://www.ncbi.nlm.nih.gov/entrez/query.fcgi?cmd=Retrieve&db=pubmed&dopt=Abstract&list_uids=8374644

- **Unsafe sleep practices and an analysis of bedsharing among infants dying suddenly and unexpectedly: results of a four-year, population-based, death-scene investigation study of sudden infant death syndrome and related deaths.**
  Author(s): Kemp JS, Unger B, Wilkins D, Psara RM, Ledbetter TL, Graham MA, Case M, Thach BT.
  Source: Pediatrics. 2000 September; 106(3): E41.
  http://www.ncbi.nlm.nih.gov/entrez/query.fcgi?cmd=Retrieve&db=pubmed&dopt=Abstract&list_uids=10969125

- **Updates on attention deficit hyperactivity disorder, child abuse and neglect, and sudden infant death syndrome.**
  Author(s): Daley KC.
  Source: Current Opinion in Pediatrics. 2003 April; 15(2): 216-25.
  http://www.ncbi.nlm.nih.gov/entrez/query.fcgi?cmd=Retrieve&db=pubmed&dopt=Abstract&list_uids=12640282

- **Upper airway resistance in infants at risk for sudden infant death syndrome.**
  Author(s): Guilleminault C, Stoohs R, Skrobal A, Labanowski M, Simmons J.
  Source: The Journal of Pediatrics. 1993 June; 122(6): 881-6.
  http://www.ncbi.nlm.nih.gov/entrez/query.fcgi?cmd=Retrieve&db=pubmed&dopt=Abstract&list_uids=8501563

- **Up-regulated epithelial expression of HLA-DR and secretory component in salivary glands: reflection of mucosal immunostimulation in sudden infant death syndrome.**
  Author(s): Thrane PS, Rognum TO, Brandtzaeg P.
  Source: Pediatric Research. 1994 May; 35(5): 625-8.
  http://www.ncbi.nlm.nih.gov/entrez/query.fcgi?cmd=Retrieve&db=pubmed&dopt=Abstract&list_uids=8065849

- **Use of duvets and the risk of sudden infant death syndrome.**
  Author(s): Mitchell EA, Williams SM, Taylor BJ.
  Source: Archives of Disease in Childhood. 1999 August; 81(2): 117-9.
  http://www.ncbi.nlm.nih.gov/entrez/query.fcgi?cmd=Retrieve&db=pubmed&dopt=Abstract&list_uids=10490515

- **Used infant mattresses and sudden infant death syndrome in Scotland: case-control study.**
  Author(s): Tappin D, Brooke H, Ecob R, Gibson A.
  Source: Bmj (Clinical Research Ed.). 2002 November 2; 325(7371): 1007.
  http://www.ncbi.nlm.nih.gov/entrez/query.fcgi?cmd=Retrieve&db=pubmed&dopt=Abstract&list_uids=12411359

- **Vagal nerve complex in normal development and sudden infant death syndrome.**
  Author(s): Becker LE, Zhang W.
  Source: The Canadian Journal of Neurological Sciences. Le Journal Canadien Des Sciences Neurologiques. 1996 February; 23(1): 24-33. Review.
  http://www.ncbi.nlm.nih.gov/entrez/query.fcgi?cmd=Retrieve&db=pubmed&dopt=Abstract&list_uids=8673958

- **Vagal overactivity: a risk factor of sudden infant death syndrome?**
  Author(s): Shojaei-Brosseau T, Bonaiti-Pellie C, Lyonnet S, Feingold J, Lucet V.
  Source: Archives of Disease in Childhood. 2003 January; 88(1): 88.
  http://www.ncbi.nlm.nih.gov/entrez/query.fcgi?cmd=Retrieve&db=pubmed&dopt=Abstract&list_uids=12495979

- **Variations in acromial ossification simulating infant abuse in victims of sudden infant death syndrome.**
  Author(s): Curto TL.
  Source: The Journal of Emergency Medicine. 1992 March-April; 10(2): 206.
  http://www.ncbi.nlm.nih.gov/entrez/query.fcgi?cmd=Retrieve&db=pubmed&dopt=Abstract&list_uids=1607628

- **Variations in acromial ossification simulating infant abuse in victims of sudden infant death syndrome.**
  Author(s): Kleinman PK, Spevak MR.
  Source: Radiology. 1991 July; 180(1): 185-7.
  http://www.ncbi.nlm.nih.gov/entrez/query.fcgi?cmd=Retrieve&db=pubmed&dopt=Abstract&list_uids=2052690

- **Vascular endothelial growth factor in the cerebrospinal fluid of infants who died of sudden infant death syndrome: evidence for antecedent hypoxia.**
  Author(s): Jones KL, Krous HF, Nadeau J, Blackbourne B, Zielke HR, Gozal D.
  Source: Pediatrics. 2003 February; 111(2): 358-63.
  http://www.ncbi.nlm.nih.gov/entrez/query.fcgi?cmd=Retrieve&db=pubmed&dopt=Abstract&list_uids=12563064

- **Ventilatory responses to carbon dioxide in infants at risk for sudden infant death syndrome.**
  Author(s): Graff MA, Novo RP, Smith C, Zapanta V, Diaz M, Hiatt IM, Hegyi T.
  Source: Critical Care Medicine. 1986 October; 14(10): 873-7.
  http://www.ncbi.nlm.nih.gov/entrez/query.fcgi?cmd=Retrieve&db=pubmed&dopt=Abstract&list_uids=3093148

- **Vertebral artery compression resulting from head movement: a possible cause of the sudden infant death syndrome.**
  Author(s): Pamphlett R, Raisanen J, Kum-Jew S.
  Source: Pediatrics. 1999 February; 103(2): 460-8.
  http://www.ncbi.nlm.nih.gov/entrez/query.fcgi?cmd=Retrieve&db=pubmed&dopt=Abstract&list_uids=9925842

- **Virulence factors associated with strains of Escherichia coli from cases of sudden infant death syndrome (SIDS).**
  Author(s): Bettelheim KA, Chang BJ, Elliott SJ, Gunzburg ST, Pearce JL.
  Source: Comparative Immunology, Microbiology and Infectious Diseases. 1995 June; 18(3): 179-88.
  http://www.ncbi.nlm.nih.gov/entrez/query.fcgi?cmd=Retrieve&db=pubmed&dopt=Abstract&list_uids=7554819

- **Vitamin A and sudden infant death syndrome in Scandinavia 1992-1995.**
  Author(s): Alm B, Wennergren G, Norvenius SG, Skjaerven R, Lagercrantz H, Helweg-Larsen K, Irgens LM; Nordic Epidemiological SIDS Study.
  Source: Acta Paediatrica (Oslo, Norway : 1992). 2003; 92(2): 162-4.
  http://www.ncbi.nlm.nih.gov/entrez/query.fcgi?cmd=Retrieve&db=pubmed&dopt=Abstract&list_uids=12710640

- **Vulnerability of the infant brain stem to ischemia: a possible cause of sudden infant death syndrome.**
  Author(s): Pamphlett R, Murray N.
  Source: Journal of Child Neurology. 1996 May; 11(3): 181-4.
  http://www.ncbi.nlm.nih.gov/entrez/query.fcgi?cmd=Retrieve&db=pubmed&dopt=Abstract&list_uids=8734017

- **Water fluoridation and the sudden infant death syndrome.**
  Author(s): Dick AE, Ford RP, Schluter PJ, Mitchell EA, Taylor BJ, Williams SM, Stewart AW, Becroft DM, Thompson JM, Scragg R, Hassall IB, Barry DM, Allen EM.
  Source: N Z Med J. 1999 August 13; 112(1093): 286-9.
  http://www.ncbi.nlm.nih.gov/entrez/query.fcgi?cmd=Retrieve&db=pubmed&dopt=Abstract&list_uids=10493424

- **Weather and the risk of sudden infant death syndrome: the effect of wind.**
  Author(s): Macey PM, Schluter PJ, Ford RP.
  Source: Journal of Epidemiology and Community Health. 2000 May; 54(5): 333-9.
  http://www.ncbi.nlm.nih.gov/entrez/query.fcgi?cmd=Retrieve&db=pubmed&dopt=Abstract&list_uids=10814652

- **Weather temperatures and sudden infant death syndrome: a regional study over 22 years in New Zealand.**
  Author(s): Schluter PJ, Ford RP, Brown J, Ryan AP.
  Source: Journal of Epidemiology and Community Health. 1998 January; 52(1): 27-33.
  http://www.ncbi.nlm.nih.gov/entrez/query.fcgi?cmd=Retrieve&db=pubmed&dopt=Abstract&list_uids=9604038

- **Weight gain and sudden infant death syndrome: changes in weight z scores may identify infants at increased risk.**
  Author(s): Blair PS, Nadin P, Cole TJ, Fleming PJ, Smith IJ, Platt MW, Berry PJ, Golding J.
  Source: Archives of Disease in Childhood. 2000 June; 82(6): 462-9.
  http://www.ncbi.nlm.nih.gov/entrez/query.fcgi?cmd=Retrieve&db=pubmed&dopt=Abstract&list_uids=10833177

- What are the national rates for sudden infant death syndrome for Aboriginal and Torres Strait Islander infants?
  Author(s): Read AW.
  Source: Journal of Paediatrics and Child Health. 2002 April; 38(2): 122-3.
  http://www.ncbi.nlm.nih.gov/entrez/query.fcgi?cmd=Retrieve&db=pubmed&dopt=Abstract&list_uids=12030990

- WHO to revamp statistics to include sudden infant death syndrome.
  Author(s): Watson R.
  Source: Bmj (Clinical Research Ed.). 2004 January 17; 328(7432): 128.
  http://www.ncbi.nlm.nih.gov/entrez/query.fcgi?cmd=Retrieve&db=pubmed&dopt=Abstract&list_uids=14726335

- Why does maternal smoke exposure increase the risk of sudden infant death syndrome?
  Author(s): Sundell H.
  Source: Acta Paediatrica (Oslo, Norway : 1992). 2001 July; 90(7): 718-20.
  http://www.ncbi.nlm.nih.gov/entrez/query.fcgi?cmd=Retrieve&db=pubmed&dopt=Abstract&list_uids=11519971

- Why is smoking a risk factor for sudden infant death syndrome?
  Author(s): Gordon AE, El Ahmer OR, Chan R, Al Madani OM, Braun JM, Weir DM, Busuttil A, Blackwell CC.
  Source: Child: Care, Health and Development. 2002 September; 28 Suppl 1: 23-5.
  http://www.ncbi.nlm.nih.gov/entrez/query.fcgi?cmd=Retrieve&db=pubmed&dopt=Abstract&list_uids=12515434

- Why is sudden infant death syndrome more common at weekends? The New Zealand National Cot Death Study Group.
  Author(s): Williams SM, Mitchell EA, Scragg R.
  Source: Archives of Disease in Childhood. 1997 November; 77(5): 415-9.
  http://www.ncbi.nlm.nih.gov/entrez/query.fcgi?cmd=Retrieve&db=pubmed&dopt=Abstract&list_uids=9487964

Vocabulary Builder

Ablation: The removal of an organ by surgery. [NIH]

Antagonism: Interference with, or inhibition of, the growth of a living organism by another living organism, due either to creation of unfavorable conditions (e. g. exhaustion of food supplies) or to production of a specific antibiotic substance (e. g. penicillin). [NIH]

Applicability: A list of the commodities to which the candidate method can be applied as presented or with minor modifications. [NIH]

Attenuated: Strain with weakened or reduced virulence. [NIH]

Autoradiography: A process in which radioactive material within an object produces an image when it is in close proximity to a radiation sensitive emulsion. [NIH]

Bacterium: Microscopic organism which may have a spherical, rod-like, or spiral unicellular or non-cellular body. Bacteria usually reproduce through asexual processes. [NIH]

Berger: A binocular loupe with the lenses mounted at the anterior end of a light-excluding chamber fitting over the eyes and held in place by an elastic headband. [NIH]

Biophysics: The science of physical phenomena and processes in living organisms. [NIH]

Bowen: Intraepithelial epithelioma affecting the skin and sometimes the mucous membranes. [NIH]

CDNA: Synthetic DNA reverse transcribed from a specific RNA through the action of the enzyme reverse transcriptase. DNA synthesized by reverse transcriptase using RNA as a template. [NIH]

Clamp: A u-shaped steel rod used with a pin or wire for skeletal traction in the treatment of certain fractures. [NIH]

Clone: The term "clone" has acquired a new meaning. It is applied specifically to the bits of inserted foreign DNA in the hybrid molecules of the population. Each inserted segment originally resided in the DNA of a complex genome amid millions of other DNA segment. [NIH]

Confounder: A factor of confusion which blurs a specific connection between a disease and a probable causal factor which is being studied. [NIH]

Consumption: Pulmonary tuberculosis. [NIH]

Cyanide: An extremely toxic class of compounds that can be lethal on inhaling of ingesting in minute quantities. [NIH]

Density: The logarithm to the base 10 of the opacity of an exposed and processed film. [NIH]

Diaphragm: Contraceptive intra-uterine device. [NIH]

Disparity: Failure of the two retinal images of an object to fall on corresponding retinal points. [NIH]

EEG: A graphic recording of the changes in electrical potential associated with the activity of the cerebral cortex made with the electroencephalogram. [NIH]

Effector: It is often an enzyme that converts an inactive precursor molecule into an active second messenger. [NIH]

Electrode: Component of the pacing system which is at the distal end of the lead. It is the interface with living cardiac tissue across which the stimulus is transmitted. [NIH]

EMG: Recording of electrical activity or currents in a muscle. [NIH]

Evoke: The electric response recorded from the cerebral cortex after stimulation of a peripheral sense organ. [NIH]

Excitatory: When cortical neurons are excited, their output increases and each new input they receive while they are still excited raises their output markedly. [NIH]

Fluoridation: The addition of fluorine usually as a fluoride to something, as the adding of a fluoride to drinking water or public water supplies for prevention of tooth decay in children. [NIH]

Generator: Any system incorporating a fixed parent radionuclide from which is produced a daughter radionuclide which is to be removed by elution or by any other method and used in a radiopharmaceutical. [NIH]

Genetics: The biological science that deals with the phenomena and mechanisms of heredity. [NIH]

Gestational: Psychosis attributable to or occurring during pregnancy. [NIH]

Glutamate: Excitatory neurotransmitter of the brain. [NIH]

Growth: The progressive development of a living being or part of an organism from its earliest stage to maturity. [NIH]

Habitat: An area considered in terms of its environment, particularly as this determines the type and quality of the vegetation the area can carry. [NIH]

Hemosiderin: Molecule which can bind large numbers of iron atoms. [NIH]

Heterogeneity: The property of one or more samples or populations which implies that they are not identical in respect of some or all of their parameters, e. g. heterogeneity of variance. [NIH]

Hospice: Institution dedicated to caring for the terminally ill. [NIH]

Hyperpnea: Increased ventilation in proportion to increased metabolism. [NIH]

Impairment: In the context of health experience, an impairment is any loss or abnormality of psychological, physiological, or anatomical structure or function. [NIH]

Initiation: Mutation induced by a chemical reactive substance causing cell changes; being a step in a carcinogenic process. [NIH]

Insight: The capacity to understand one's own motives, to be aware of one's own psychodynamics, to appreciate the meaning of symbolic behavior. [NIH]

Involuntary: Reaction occurring without intention or volition. [NIH]

Kainate: Glutamate receptor. [NIH]

Ligands: A RNA simulation method developed by the MIT. [NIH]

Linkage: The tendency of two or more genes in the same chromosome to remain together from one generation to the next more frequently than expected according to the law of independent assortment. [NIH]

Loop: A wire usually of platinum bent at one end into a small loop (usually 4 mm inside diameter) and used in transferring microorganisms. [NIH]

Mesencephalic: Ipsilateral oculomotor paralysis and contralateral tremor, spasm. or choreic movements of the face and limbs. [NIH]

Modeling: A treatment procedure whereby the therapist presents the target behavior which the learner is to imitate and make part of his repertoire. [NIH]

Monogenic: A human disease caused by a mutation in a single gene. [NIH]

MRNA: The RNA molecule that conveys from the DNA the information that is to be translated into the structure of a particular polypeptide molecule. [NIH]

Mycotoxins: Toxins derived from bacteria or fungi. [NIH]

Nerve: A cordlike structure of nervous tissue that connects parts of the nervous system with other tissues of the body and conveys nervous impulses to, or away from, these tissues. [NIH]

Networks: Pertaining to a nerve or to the nerves, a meshlike structure of interlocking fibers or strands. [NIH]

Neurotrophins: A nerve growth factor. [NIH]

Nuclei: A body of specialized protoplasm found in nearly all cells and containing the chromosomes. [NIH]

Otology: The branch of medicine which deals with the diagnosis and treatment of the disorders and diseases of the ear. [NIH]

Pacemakers: A center or a substance that controls the rhythm of a body process; the term usually refers to the cardiac pacemaker. [NIH]

Paralysis: Loss or impairment of muscle function or sensation. [NIH]

Patch: A piece of material used to cover or protect a wound, an injured part, etc.: a patch over the eye. [NIH]

Pathologies: The study of abnormality, especially the study of diseases. [NIH]

Phenotypes: An organism as observed, i. e. as judged by its visually perceptible characters resulting from the interaction of its genotype with the environment. [NIH]

Physiology: The science that deals with the life processes and functions of organismus, their cells, tissues, and organs. [NIH]

Plasticity: In an individual or a population, the capacity for adaptation: a) through gene changes (genetic plasticity) or b) through internal physiological modifications in response to changes of environment (physiological plasticity). [NIH]

Polymorphism: The occurrence together of two or more distinct forms in the same population. [NIH]

Pontine: A brain region involved in the detection and processing of taste. [NIH]

Potassium: It is essential to the ability of muscle cells to contract. [NIH]

Potentiating: A degree of synergism which causes the exposure of the organism to a harmful substance to worsen a disease already contracted. [NIH]

Potentiation: An overall effect of two drugs taken together which is greater than the sum of the effects of each drug taken alone. [NIH]

Prion: Small proteinaceous infectious particles that resist inactivation by procedures modifying nucleic acids and contain an abnormal isoform of a cellular protein which is a major and necessary component. [NIH]

Probe: An instrument used in exploring cavities, or in the detection and dilatation of strictures, or in demonstrating the potency of channels; an elongated instrument for exploring or sounding body cavities. [NIH]

Protocol: The detailed plan for a clinical trial that states the trial's rationale, purpose, drug or vaccine dosages, length of study, routes of administration, who may participate, and other aspects of trial design. [NIH]

Restoration: Broad term applied to any inlay, crown, bridge or complete denture which restores or replaces loss of teeth or oral tissues. [NIH]

Salivary: The duct that convey saliva to the mouth. [NIH]

Secretory: Secreting; relating to or influencing secretion or the secretions. [NIH]

Sensor: A device designed to respond to physical stimuli such as temperature, light, magnetism or movement and transmit resulting impulses for interpretation, recording, movement, or operating control. [NIH]

Serotypes: A cause of haemorrhagic septicaemia (in cattle, sheep and pigs), fowl cholera of birds, pasteurellosis of rabbits, and gangrenous mastitis of ewes. It is also commonly found in atrophic rhinitis of pigs. [NIH]

Spike: The activation of synapses causes changes in the permeability of the dendritic membrane leading to changes in the membrane potential. This difference of the potential travels along the axon of the neuron and is called spike. [NIH]

Stillbirth: The birth of a dead fetus or baby. [NIH]

Stimulus: That which can elicit or evoke action (response) in a muscle, nerve, gland or other excitable issue, or cause an augmenting action upon any function or metabolic process. [NIH]

Synapse: The region where the processes of two neurons come into close contiguity, and the nervous impulse passes from one to the other; the fibers of the two are intermeshed, but, according to the general view, there is no direct contiguity. [NIH]

Temporal: One of the two irregular bones forming part of the lateral surfaces and base of the skull, and containing the organs of hearing. [NIH]

Therapeutics: The branch of medicine which is concerned with the treatment of diseases, palliative or curative. [NIH]

Thorax: A part of the trunk between the neck and the abdomen; the chest. [NIH]

Tractus: A part of some structure, usually that part along which something passes. [NIH]

Transduction: The transfer of genes from one cell to another by means of a viral (in the case of bacteria, a bacteriophage) vector or a vector which is similar to a virus particle (pseudovirion). [NIH]

Trauma: Any injury, wound, or shock, must frequently physical or structural shock, producing a disturbance. [NIH]

Trigeminal: Cranial nerve V. It is sensory for the eyeball, the conjunctiva, the eyebrow, the skin of face and scalp, the teeth, the mucous membranes in the mouth and nose, and is motor to the muscles of mastication. [NIH]

Tropism: Directed movements and orientations found in plants, such as the turning of the sunflower to face the sun. [NIH]

Vector: Plasmid or other self-replicating DNA molecule that transfers DNA between cells in nature or in recombinant DNA technology. [NIH]

Venom: That produced by the poison glands of the mouth and injected by the fangs of poisonous snakes. [NIH]

Vertebrae: A bony unit of the segmented spinal column. [NIH]

Vitro: Descriptive of an event or enzyme reaction under experimental investigation occurring outside a living organism. Parts of an organism or microorganism are used together with artificial substrates and/or conditions. [NIH]

Vivo: Outside of or removed from the body of a living organism. [NIH]

Chapter 4. Patents on Sudden Infant Death Syndrome

Overview

You can learn about innovations relating to sudden infant death syndrome by reading recent patents and patent applications. Patents can be physical innovations (e.g. chemicals, pharmaceuticals, medical equipment) or processes (e.g. treatments or diagnostic procedures). The United States Patent and Trademark Office defines a patent as a grant of a property right to the inventor, issued by the Patent and Trademark Office.[20] Patents, therefore, are intellectual property. For the United States, the term of a new patent is 20 years from the date when the patent application was filed. If the inventor wishes to receive economic benefits, it is likely that the invention will become commercially available within 20 years of the initial filing. It is important to understand, therefore, that an inventor's patent does not indicate that a product or service is or will be commercially available. The patent implies only that the inventor has "the right to exclude others from making, using, offering for sale, or selling" the invention in the United States. While this relates to U.S. patents, similar rules govern foreign patents.

In this chapter, we show you how to locate information on patents and their inventors. If you find a patent that is particularly interesting to you, contact the inventor or the assignee for further information.

[20]Adapted from The U. S. Patent and Trademark Office:
http://www.uspto.gov/web/offices/pac/doc/general/whatis.htm.

Patents on Sudden Infant Death Syndrome

By performing a patent search focusing on sudden infant death syndrome, you can obtain information such as the title of the invention, the names of the inventor(s), the assignee(s) or the company that owns or controls the patent, a short abstract that summarizes the patent, and a few excerpts from the description of the patent. The abstract of a patent tends to be more technical in nature, while the description is often written for the public. Full patent descriptions contain much more information than is presented here (e.g. claims, references, figures, diagrams, etc.). We will tell you how to obtain this information later in the chapter. The following is an example of the type of information that you can expect to obtain from a patent search on sudden infant death syndrome:

- **Apnoea monitor**

  Inventor(s): Thatcher; John B. (3860 Pendiente Cir., Bldg. CD-105, San Diego, CA 92124)

  Assignee(s): None Reported

  Patent Number: 4,738,266

  Date filed: May 9, 1983

  Abstract: An apnoea monitor for preventing **sudden infant death syndrome** (SIDS). The exhaled breath of the infant is collected in a hood. A source of infrared energy emits infrared energy into the hood. So long as the infant is breathing, the carbon dioxide in its breath absorbs a portion of the infrared energy in the hood. Should the infant stop breathing, an infrared detector responds to the resulting increase in infrared energy to activate an alarm so as to enable the attendant personnel to take appropriate life saving action.

  Excerpt(s): There are an estimated 10,000-15,000 deaths in the United States each year due to **sudden infant death syndrome** (SIDS), making it the most frequent cause of death in the first year of life. Many hypotheses have been formulated to explain its etiology. Most of the easily recognized post-mortem abnormalities in the victims are in the lungs and they have usually been interpreted as evidence of a sudden catastrophic event in an otherwise normal infant. Years of speculation about the nature of the catastrophic event have been unfruitful because the easily recognized post-mortem abnormalities give few clues to the dynamic events surrounding the deaths.... The term "apnoea" is often used in conjunction with SIDS as a symptom as well as a cause. Apnoea may be defined as a pause in the infant's breathing equal to or exceeding six seconds. Short periods of apnoea during sleep are normal during infancy while prolonged periods are abnormal. In 1972 Steinschneider (Pediatrics 50:646-654, 1972) reported that several SIDS victims had prolonged periods of apnoea during sleep before death.... In an attempt to combat SIDS, monitoring systems have been proposed in the past which react to any period of apnoea in the sleeping infant. Although some of the indications may be false alarms due to normal periods of apnoea by the infant, in any event, the parents or attending nurses are alerted by the monitors whenever the infant stops breathing, even for a short period.

Web site: http://www.delphion.com/details?pn=US04738266__

- **Apparatus and method for preventing sudden infant death syndrome**

  Inventor(s): von der Heyde; Christian P. (182 Great Hill Rd. Extension, East Sandwich, MA 02537)

  Assignee(s): None Reported

  Patent Number: 5,887,304

  Date filed: July 10, 1997

  Abstract: An apparatus and method for preventing asphyxiation of an infant due to breathing of exhaled carbon dioxide. A mattress with optional mattress pad provides an even air flow that removes exhaled carbon dioxide that accumulates at or near the surface of the mattress or mattress pad. The infant may be located anywhere on the surface of the mattress or mattress pad as the even air flow disperses carbon dioxide across the entire surface. In a preferred embodiment, the even air flow is accomplished by forcing air into a cavity, or plenum chamber, in the body of the mattress which air distributes equally to air flow holes on the top surfaces of the mattress and mattress pad. Optional temperature regulating or medicine dispensing devices respectively heat or cool the air flow, or introduce medicine into the air flow. In another embodiment, the mattress is itself a mattress pad. That is, the mattress pad provides an even air flow as described and may be placed on the sleeping surface of a conventional mattress.

  Excerpt(s): This invention generally relates to apparatuses and methods for preventing **sudden infant death syndrome,** and more particularly to mattresses and pads that remove exhaled carbon dioxide from the vicinity of a sleeping infant's mouth to prevent asphyxiation.... Sudden Infant Death Syndrome (SIDS) claims the lives of thousands of infants in the United States each year. These infants generally appear to be normal and healthy, but succumb without warning in their cribs. The cause of SIDS is not known, and thus there is no certain means of preventing these tragedies. Medical specialists have, however, advanced several theories to explain the onset of SIDS. U.S. Pat. No. 5,483,711 issued to Hargest et al. reviews these theories, provides statistics regarding the impact of SIDS in the United States, and explains the advantage of placing an infant on its stomach for rest or sleep to prevent choking on regurgitated fluids. This advantage may be accentuated in the case of a premature or newborn infant with relatively undeveloped lungs. However, placing the infant on its stomach has certain drawbacks. As noted in Hargest, one theory regarding the cause of SIDS is that an infant sleeping or resting on its stomach, and thus with its mouth near the mattress or mattress pad of its crib, inhales the carbon dioxide products of breathing that have accumulated near the top surface of the mattress or mattress pad resulting in "carbon dioxide poisoning." This result may alternatively be described as suffocation due to an insufficient amount of oxygen in the carbon-dioxide rich air near the infant's mouth. The presence of bedding may contribute to such accumulation and thus contribute to the possibility of suffocation by the infant.... As a result, there are reasons to conclude that SIDS may be prevented by avoiding the accumulation of carbon dioxide near the top surface of the mattress or mattress pad of an infant's crib. Known apparatuses for attempting to prevent such accumulation, and in some cases for attempting to provide a fresh flow of air or oxygen, include that of Hargest and also the mattresses disclosed in U.S. Pat. No. 5,546,618 issued to Beedy et al., U.S. Pat. No. 4,536,906 issued to Varndell et al., and U.S. Pat. No. 3,339,216 issued to Ormerod.

Web site: http://www.delphion.com/details?pn=US05887304__

- **Assay and method for determining newborn risk for sudden infant death syndrome**

  Inventor(s): Beach; Peter G. (6780 SW. 205th Ct., Portland, OR 97007)

  Assignee(s): None Reported

  Patent Number: 5,556,759

  Date filed: August 2, 1993

  Abstract: An assay and method for screening newborns to determine risk of Sudden Infant Syndrome is described. The assay and method is based on the detection of elevated IgM-anti-IgG (MAG) levels in newborns' serum within the first year of birth. In particular, it has been discovered that elevated MAG levels indicate an increased risk of **Sudden Infant Death Syndrome** (SIDS).In a preferred embodiment of the invention, an ELISA is utilized in which a first binding agent having specific affinity for IgM is used to capture and separate IgM antibodies from the newborn's blood sample. A second binding agent having specific affinity for IgG which has been separated from the sample eluant by complexing with MAG, is then used in conjunction with an enzyme conjugate to indirectly determine the amount of MAG in the newborn's blood. The MAG level is then compared to a cut-off which is selected to separate out approximately 4% of the newborns which have the highest MAG levels. These newborns are designated "high risk" and are recommended for more testing and/or monitoring.

Excerpt(s): The invention relates to newborn diagnostic screening. In particular, the invention involves an assay and method for determining the level of IgM-anti-IgG ("MAG") in a newborn's blood, and correlating the MAG level with an empirically determined cut-off to determine whether the newborn has an elevated risk of premature death.... Approximately five thousand infants under the age of one die in the United States each year for unexplained reasons, their death ultimately being classified as being caused by "Sudden Infant Death Syndrome" ("SIDS"). The cause of SIDS is not known and no methods for identifying those babies that either have SIDS or are at high risk of developing SIDS, have been previously disclosed.... Prior investigators have suggested that Sudden Infant Death may be related to elevated immunoglobulin concentrations. Urquhart et al., Sudden Unexplained Death in Infancy and Hyperimmunization, J. Clin. Path.; 24:736-739 (Feb. 24, 1971). Urquhart et al. determined postmortem antibody levels in SIDS cases. Urquhart et al.'s studies showed that antiglobulin antibodies were detected in Sudden Infant Death cases more frequently (56%) than in living control cases (5%). Urquhart et al. suggest that anti-antibodies might participate in fatal anaphylaxis in SIDS cases. However, Urquhart et al. did not suggest any technique for identifying newborns who are at elevated risk for SIDS, where the identification can be made at a time early enough to implement measures to prevent premature death.

Web site: http://www.delphion.com/details?pn=US05556759__

- **Breathing monitor articles of wearing apparel**

  Inventor(s): Stephens; David L. (6221 La Tijera Blvd., Los Angeles, CA 90056)

  Assignee(s): None Reported

  Patent Number: 5,454,376

  Date filed: August 16, 1993

  Abstract: A breathing monitor article of wearing apparel, adapted for child users in order to monitor breathing conditions of a child user. The apparatus and the method of the invention are particularly adaptable for infant child users in order to prevent conditions such as **Sudden Infant Death Syndrome** and similar conditions arising from apnea. The article of wearing apparel comprises a shirt or like garment adapted to extend around the chest and/or abdomen portion of the child user and which contains a pocket having a monitor therein. An elastic belt extends about the chest and/or abdomen of the user and particularly, in the region of the user's lungs. A strain gauge is secured to the elastic belt and detects breathing movement through the expansion and contraction of the chest wall. The monitor is electronically operated and constructed so as to generate an alarm signal if there is a cessation of breathing for a minimum predetermined time period. The shirt, or like garment, is also constructed so that when it is secured to the child user, it automatically energizes the monitor, thereby eliminating the necessity of an attendant to the child from turning the monitor on or off.

Excerpt(s): This invention relates in general to certain new and useful improvements in breathing monitor articles of wearing apparel and more particularly, to an article of wearing apparel which is constructed so as to detect and generate an alarm signal when there is a cessation of breathing of the child user for a minimum predetermined time period.... Detection of breathing patterns of children, and particularly infant children, has proved to be a more difficult task than one would initially envision. There has been a long-felt need for an apparatus and a method to monitor infant child breathing conditions in order to ensure that the child does not lapse into a non-breathing state.... The syndrome of sudden infant death ("SIDS"), is one which is moderately rare, although not uncommon. In the **sudden infant death syndrome,** oftentimes for some inexplicable reason, the child stops breathing and since there is usually utter silence, a parent, or other attendant to the child, does not recognize the cessation of breathing until long after the death of the infant child. The same situation exists when an infant child becomes entangled in clothing, blankets or the like and is unable to extricate himself or herself. Here, again, suffocation usually occurs, silently resulting in the death of the infant child.

Web site: http://www.delphion.com/details?pn=US05454376__

- **Cervical appliance to ameliorate sleep apneas**

Inventor(s): Bennett; C. Richard (15 Forest Glen Dr., Pittsburgh, PA 15228), Mundell; Robert D. (542 Lucia Dr., Pittsburgh, PA 15221)

Assignee(s): None Reported

Patent Number: 4,700,697

Date filed: May 9, 1985

Abstract: A cervical appliance for preventing ventral flexion of the head to reduce the possibility of **sudden infant death syndrome** and/or adult sleep apnea, both of which have common characteristics which are at least partially obviated with the use of the invention.

Excerpt(s): A variety of theories have been proposed to explain **sudden infant death syndrome** (SIDS). SIDS is defined as "the sudden death of an infant or young child which is unexpectd by history, and in which a thorough post-mortem examination fails to reveal an adequate cause for death". While SIDS may occur for different reasons, one attribute of this phenomenon, included in the great majority of the cases described in the literature, is apnea (or respiratoray pause or periodic breathing) which occurs during sleep and is fatal. The autopsy reports describe conditions that are consistent with a condition of hypoxia and/or hypoxemia having existed for some time prior to the fatal apneic episode. It is the apneic character of SIDS which is addressed when "SIDS-risks" infants are placed on a cardiopulmonary monitor or treated with respiratory stimulants.... Some adult humans also suffer severe apnea during sleep (adult sleep apnea, or hypersomnia with periodic apnea [HPA]). SIDS and HPA share the fact that they occur during sleep, and that at least part of the apnea occurs without the subject's making any attempt to breathe. This latter condition is called "central apnea" because it appears to be ordered by the central nervous system. HPA oocurs most frequently in overweight males, over 40 years of age, who are given to strident or stentorian snoring. Typically, their obesity causes such individuals to sleep in a supine position. Careful observations have shown that they possess redundancy of tissue in the soft palate and the walls of the oropharynx. Part of this may be due to fatty deposit; part may be due to anatomical variation.... During sleep, especially "quiet sleep" or "REM (rapid eye-movement) sleep", facial muscles become hypotonic. During the inspiratory phase of the respiratory cycle the walls of the oropharynx and the base of the tongue tend to collapse onto the oropharynx. This is partly due to muscular hypotonia, partly due to negative pressure. The latter may be caused by negative intrathoracic pressure as air is breathed in, or by the Bernoulli effect (in which rapid airflow through a restricted space decreases the pressure).

Web site: http://www.delphion.com/details?pn=US04700697__

- **Crib death (SIDS) warning device**

Inventor(s): Macias; Helene (5333 Russell Ave., Ste. 301, Hollywood, CA 90027-3513), Winke; Angos (5333 Russell Ave., Ste. 301, Hollywood, CA 90027-3513)

Assignee(s): None Reported

Patent Number: 4,851,816

Date filed: February 24, 1987

Abstract: An apparatus for specific fluid detection in prophylactic prognosis of a medical condition known as **Sudden Infant Death Syndrome,** that in one embodiment features a casing which is removably affixable to a sensor configured for receiving and transmitting the information of manifestation of micturition to an embodied acquisitioning accommodation embracing a variable frequency oscillator, the output of which interconnects with a signal converter conceptualized to transition a switching provision into energizing a built-in alarm system consequential to the signal converter's having sampled and found the oscillator's frequency to be representative of a manifestation of micturition in precursor to a CNS agonal episode derived laryngospasm attack, while in another embodiment, a switching structure provides for the energizing of an alarm configuration that injects its modulation into the signal circuitry of a baby listening device, and in yet another embodiment, provides for the switching on of a code modulator and thereto connected propagation device in a manner for propagating the information of manifestation of micturition to an independent capture accommodation connected to a compatible signal converter that is conceptualized upon such code's acquisition to consequently cause the transition of a switching faculty, the configuration of which, results in a bi-directionally spliced signal flow of which one is directed to initiate the tasking of a multi-ported microprocessor that controls an ACLS arrangement operationally architectured to induce increased negative intrathoracic pressure relief when not cancelled by supervising personnel or the microprocessor itself accessing the receipt of data that is comprised of co-processed signals.

Excerpt(s): This invention relates to a system for detecting the moment of micturition in babies.... More particularly, this invention relates to a system which will interdict enuresis alarm circuitry incorporated in it or attached to it from being tricked into switching itself on when in fact the sensor striping, screens, clips or stripes used in and with swaddles or latest embodiment the plastic layered disposable diaper is not wet with urine but condensation permeated.... An inspection of the numerous art precursive to this invention amply demonstrates that enuresis monitors continue to present a challenge to practitioners in the art.

Web site: http://www.delphion.com/details?pn=US04851816__

- **Infant blood oxygen monitor and SIDS warning device**

Inventor(s): Jackson, III; William H. (P.O. Box 4795, Wilmington, NC 28406)

Assignee(s): None Reported

Patent Number: 6,047,201

Date filed: April 2, 1998

Abstract: A device to help a caregiver monitor an infant to discover the onset of a **Sudden Infant Death Syndrome** event and to intervene to prevent the **Sudden Infant Death Syndrome** event. A foot and ankle wrap containing rechargeable batteries and a radio transmitter is connected to a toe cap containing a pulse oximeter by adjustable cords. Blood oxygen and pulse readouts from the pulse oximeter are transmitted to a monitor kept by the caregiver. Visible readouts of the blood oxygen and pulse are shown on the monitor for continuous view by the caregiver. The monitor sounds an alarm if the infant's blood oxygen drops to a dangerous level for predetermined period. The time delay prevents false alarms, therefore, provides a greater degree of alertness to the caregiver using the device. When not in use the device is recharged on a stand.

Excerpt(s): This invention is a monitoring device to detect warning signs indicative in **Sudden Infant Death Syndrome** (SIDS) and other respiratory or cardiac conditions threatening to infants. It is designed to minimize false alarms, to be easily used by parents or other caregivers who have no special training, to be portable, affordable, and practical.... Sudden Infant Death Syndrome is the term used to designate the death of seemingly healthy infants commonly between the ages of two weeks and one year. **Sudden Infant Death Syndrome** [usually abbreviated SIDS, sometimes called crib death] is the leading cause of infant deaths up to the age of one year.... The exact cause of SIDS has not been determined. It has been suggested that SIDS occurs in healthy infants as the result of the occurrence of a series of unrelated events. Infants who have periods of apnea, changes in skin color, changes in muscle tone, or who sometimes require help in breathing are more likely to die of SIDS. It is sometimes thought that the infant's position in the crib is a factor in SIDS, and various arrangements of pillows around the infant have been proposed to reduce the risk of SIDS.

Web site: http://www.delphion.com/details?pn=US06047201__

- **Mattress for cribs and basinets for sudden infant death prevention**

   Inventor(s): Mahdavi; Habib (11504 Canton Dr., Studio City, CA 91604)

   Assignee(s): None Reported

   Patent Number: 5,857,232

   Date filed: December 4, 1995

   Abstract: The present invention provides a safety device and a method to counter a potential cause of **Sudden infant death syndrome.** A frame, fit to the dimensions of a crib or bassinet is equipped with an air permeable material that allows for the free flow of fresh air to an infant's mouth and offsets any exhaled carbon dioxide that lingers by the infant's air passages. The material is of a particular elasticity that an infant's weight does not cause the material to collapse on itself, thereby keeping the supply of fresh air retained in the material in place.

   Excerpt(s): The present invention relates generally to an apparatus for the prevention of **sudden infant death syndrome,** and more particularly to a mattress for bassinets or cribs which provides for a supply of fresh air to an infant's mouth and prevents the infant's asphyxiation from carbon dioxide poisoning.... Each year, thousands of infants (aged 2 weeks to 1 year) die from **Sudden Infant Death Syndrome** (SIDS), a mysterious disorder in which otherwise healthy infants seemingly stop breathing. Although scientific and medical research has uncovered factors which indicate a predisposition to the disorder (i.e., low birth weight, age of mothers) no specific cause has been uncovered. Moreover, there are varied theories put forth by the medical community as to the cause of SIDS. Some theories suggest a neurological disorder in the infants which intercepts the breathing functions while sleeping and leads to the infant's death by asphyxiation.... Applicant believes a contributing cause of SIDS is that infants fall victim to asphyxiation from carbon dioxide poisoning. More specifically, infants sleeping face down rebreathe the carbon dioxide in the exhaled air trapped in the air pocket of their bedding near their air passages. Doctors, nurses and medical journals have for years recommended placing an infant on its back for sleeping to avoid this concern. However, many parents and caregivers are reluctant to follow this advice. Some infants prefer sleeping on their stomachs, and do not adjust to the changed position well. Moreover after 5-6 months, most infants can roll themselves over to their preferred sleeping position.

Further, many infants have a tendency to regurgitate and parents are concerned their infant may choke on the regurgitated matter.

Web site: http://www.delphion.com/details?pn=US05857232__

- **Means of aiding in the prevention of sudden infant death syndrome**

Inventor(s): Moore; Luana (Miami Beach, FL)

Assignee(s): Key Pharmaceuticals, Inc. (miami, Fl)

Patent Number: 4,639,455

Date filed: October 2, 1984

Abstract: A means of aiding in the prevention of **Sudden Infant Death Syndrome** (SIDS) is disclosed. The means comprises administering a pharmaceutically effective amount of the drug 6-methylene-6-desoxy-N-cylopryplymethyl-14-hydroxydihydronormorphone to an infant determined to be susceptible to SIDS. The drug is preferably administered bi-daily via the GI tract. The drug attaches to the nerve receptor sites responsible for the actuation of respiration thus blocking the attachment of endogenous endorphins which, if present in high levels, prevents such actuation resulting in apnea and SIDS. A suppository containing the drug for use in carrying out the method is also disclosed.

Excerpt(s): The present invention relates to the field of means for aiding in the prevention of **Sudden Infant Death Syndrome** (hereinafter SIDS). More specifically, the invention relates to administering the drug 6-methylene-6-desoxy-N-cyclopropylmethyl-14-hydroxydihydronormorphone to an infant determined to be susceptible to SIDS and to an anal suppository containing such a drug.... Sudden Infant Death Syndrome (SIDS), also called "Crib Death", can be defined as the sudden death of any infant which is unexpected according to history and in which a post-mortem fails to demonstrate an adequate cause of death. Although the death might be unexpected according to the infant's history as examined in a conventional manner a SIDS death might have been predictable or at least determined to be more probable with that specific infant due to its history. For example, premature infants, low birth weight infants and those with respiratory distress syndrome are more likely to suffer a SIDS death than other infants. Another group of infants more likely to be susceptible to a SIDS death would be the "Near-Miss" infants, i.e. those who have been successfully revived after respiration ceased. A number of other factors are known to be associated with an increased likelihood of suffering a SIDS death.... In an attempt to reduce the number of SIDS deaths, attempts have been made to identify those infants who would be more likely to suffer a SIDS death. After identifying such infants, the parents are notified and mechanical devices can be attached to the infant. These mechanical devices monitor the respiration and/or heartbeat of the infant and actuate an alarm when respiration and/or heartbeat ceases. The parents can respond to the alarm and revive the infant. Such devices are advantageous in that they do not require the administration of any drugs to the infant. However, they are undesirable in that they may fail due to mechanical malfunction or an interruption of their power supply. Further, individuals might fail to respond to the alarm or fail to respond fast enough in order to revive the infant. Perhaps most importantly, such devices do nothing to prevent respiratory arrest and respiratory arrest for even a short period of time can of course cause brain damage.

Web site: http://www.delphion.com/details?pn=US04639455__

- **Method and apparatus for correlating respiration and heartbeat variability**

Inventor(s): Nishimura; Toshihiro (Ooita, JP)

Assignee(s): Nippon Kayaku Kabushiki Kaisha (tokyo, Jp)

Patent Number: 5,105,354

Date filed: January 23, 1989

Abstract: An evaluation method of respiration and heart beat and its apparatus which permits one to forecast **sudden infant death syndrome** by investigating correlation between respiration and heart beat in the normal state and sleep-apnea of a newborn.

Excerpt(s): This invention relates to a method of evaluating data pertaining to respiration and heart beat and an apparatus for evaluating them, especially for forecasting **sudden infant death syndrome** (SIDS) by investigating the correlation between respiration and heart beat in a normal state and respiratory standstill in sleep.... Generally, the data from organisms includes EEG, cardiac electricity, respiration, ocular movement, and EMG. Signal forms of this data are relatively more useful than from EEG etc. It is therefore easier to analyze an R--R interval as a change of peak interval of an ECG wave, chronologically.... Considering that respiratory arrhythmia depends upon an efferent impulse from an extension receptor, standstill of the efferent impulse from an extension receptor in respiratory arrest in sleep will have an effect on heart beat. It has been already reported that in Cheyne Stokes respiration during hyperrespiration the increase of heart beat and decrease of blood pressure are observed; during its apnea the decrease of heart beat and increase of blood pressure occur.

Web site: http://www.delphion.com/details?pn=US05105354__

- **Method and apparatus for improving the respiratory efficiency of an infant**

Inventor(s): Hale; Theodore M. (39 Celano La., West Islip, NY 11795)

Assignee(s): None Reported

Patent Number: 5,389,037

Date filed: July 15, 1993

Abstract: A method and apparatus for reducing respiratory abnormalities in infants and the incidence of **crib death** by providing a flow of room air to a sleeping infant's environment to stimulate breathing. In a preferred embodiment of the invention, room air is delivered into a crib through an air plenum that is removably attached to the vertical bars of a crib and positioned within 1 cm to 20 cm of the infant's mouth, nose, larynx and trachea. The flow of room air from the air plenum safely assists the respiration of an infant with inadequate shallow end tidal volume, decreases rebreathing of expired carbon dioxide from the nose, mouth, oral cavity and trachea, prevents pockets of increasing carbon dioxide from developing within the cushions and beddings surrounding the infant, and decreases the likelihood of overheating and other conditions associated with **sudden infant death syndrome,** apnea syndromes and hypoventilation.

Excerpt(s): The present invention relates to a method and apparatus for providing room oxygen to an infant and removing expired carbon dioxide from the infant's environment by directing a flow of room oxygen to the infant's mouth and nose in a non-intrusive manner. More particularly, the present invention relates to an air plenum assembly that may be permanently or removably mounted to a crib or playpen such that the air flow from the plenum is directed toward the mouth and nose of the child.... The present invention is directed toward preventing infant deaths due to prolonged periodic breathing and **sudden infant death syndrome.**... Periodic breathing is a normal phenomenon where an infant's breathing pattern is interrupted by recurrent apneas or absences of breathing. It has been shown in independent studies that an increase in ambient oxygen concentration correlates with a reduction in the incidence of apnea in infants. Kattwinkel, J., Neonatal/Apnea: Pathogenesis and Therapy, 90 J. Pediatric 342 (1977); Hoppen-Brouwers, T., Hodgman, J. E., Harper, R. M., et al., Polygraphic Studies of Normal Infants During the

First Six Months of Life: I. V. Incidence of Apnea and Periodic Breathing, 60 Pediatrics 418 (1977). Pharmacological therapies have been used to treat prolonged periodic breathing, but the effect of these therapies remains uncertain. Neil N. Finer, M.D., Keith J. Barrington, M.D., and Barbara Hayes, R.N., Prolonged Periodic Breathing: Significance in Sleep Studies, Pediatrics, Vol. 89, No. 3, pp. 450-52 (March 1992).

Web site: http://www.delphion.com/details?pn=US05389037__

- **Method and apparatus for monitoring and treating sudden infant death syndrome**

Inventor(s): Gliner; Bradford F. (Issaquah, WA), Jorgenson; Dawn Billie (Seattle, WA)

Assignee(s): Agilent Technologies, Inc. (palo Alto, Ca)

Patent Number: 6,208,897

Date filed: April 27, 1999

Abstract: This invention relates generally to a device for monitoring an infant for the onset of **sudden infant death syndrome** (SIDS), detecting the onset of SIDS and providing immediate treatment. In the broadest sense, the invention includes an apparatus for detecting and treating SIDS. The apparatus comprises a data gatherer for monitoring an infant parameter, a controller for communicating with the data gatherer, an energy source operable to power the data gatherer for monitoring the infant parameter and further operable to provide energy to an energy delivery system which is operable to deliver an electric shock from an energy source to an electrode interface, and an alarm which is activated by the controller for alerting a remote caregiver to the onset of symptoms associated with SIDS. The invention also relates to a method of operating a SIDS monitor. The method comprises the steps of monitoring an infant parameter, determining whether the monitored parameter is an acceptable value. If the monitored parameter is an acceptable value, then an alarm is activated to alert a caretaker of the onset of SIDS symptoms, if the monitored parameter is within an acceptable value, then continuing to monitor the infant parameter.

Excerpt(s): This invention relates generally to a device for monitoring an infant for the onset of **sudden infant death syndrome** (SIDS), detecting the onset of SIDS and providing immediate treatment. Treatment could include instructions for administering cardiopulmonary resuscitation (CPR) as well as delivery of a defibrillation pulse from an automatic or semi-automatic external defibrillator (AED). The device may be a SIDS monitor as well as a SIDS trainer, or a SIDS monitor which has the ability to function as a trainer.... Because SIDS is identified in situations where no explanation for the death can be found, the potential causes of SIDS has been largely speculative. Potential causes include cardiac disorders, respiratory abnormalities, gastrointestinal diseases, metabolic disorders, injury and child abuse.... Many devices have been developed that provide a way to monitor an infant for the onset of SIDS by detecting cessation of movement, cessation of respiration or detection of urination that may accompany agonal movement. Other devices have been developed to prevent SIDS from occuring, such as by providing an oxygenated mattress. The following summarizes a selection of previously patented approaches to SIDS detection and/or prevention.

Web site: http://www.delphion.com/details?pn=US06208897__

- **Method and apparatus to prevent positional plagiocephaly in infants**

  Inventor(s): Dixon; Donald L. (Anchorage, KY), Havens; Robert L. (Marysville, IN)

  Assignee(s): Center for Orthotic & Prosthetic Care, L.l.c. (louisville, Ky)

  Patent Number: 6,052,849

  Date filed: March 18, 1998

  Abstract: A cranial suspension apparatus to prevent positional plagiocephaly in an infant by distributing loads on the head of the infant lying in the supine position on a horizontal surface. The infant is placed in the apparatus such that the head of the infant is supported on a flexible porous support material with the tension of the material adjusted to support the head just above or just touching the sleep surface. The flexible porous support material may be a net with an open weave. The apparatus prevents localized pressure on the infant's head in an area contacting a sleep surface when infants are routinely placed in the supine position, which is recommended to avoid **sudden infant death syndrome.**

  Excerpt(s): The invention relates to an apparatus and the use of the apparatus to prevent positional plagiocephaly by more evenly distributing loads on the head of an infant lying on a sleep surface in the supine position.... Cranial asymmetry (plagiocephaly) and deformations are common in the neonatal period. They may occur from various causes including premature closure of the cranial vault and/or skull base sutures (craniosynostosis), syndromal craniofacial dysostosis, intracranial volume disorders such as hydrocephalus, microcephaly or tumor, metabolic bone disorders such as rickets, and birth trauma such as depressed skull fractures. A subset of patients with plagiocephaly are recognized that do not exhibit pathology of the sutures and do not fall into any of the above categories. These patients are referred to as having plagiocephaly without synostosis (PWS), also known as "positional" or "gestational" plagiocephaly.... The etiology of cranial asymmetry in PWS has been suggested to result from two possible mechanisms. One proposed mechanism is intrauterine constraint that develops from early descent of the fetal head into the pelvis, effectively placing uneven pressure on one area of the cranium within a confined space. This leads to constraint of one side of the occiput (back of the head) with a compensatory change to the contralateral skull. Another mechanism that can perpetuate the fetal constraint or even lead to the misshapen head is supine positioning of the infant. Once the occiput develops even a mildly flattened area, placing the infant on the back or supine position will perpetuate the deformity. The head will roll to the flattened area by the forces of gravity and, because motor control is lacking in the neonate, the deformity will remain or worsen. This effect is especially illustrated in infants with neuromuscular disorders and hypotonia where deformation of the cranium can be quite profound. This phenomena has been recognized for many years and recommendations for changing the infant's environment with relationship to the crib and placement within the sleeping area are well established.

Web site: http://www.delphion.com/details?pn=US06052849__

- **Method for correcting plasma melatonin levels and pharmaceutical formulation comprising melatonin**

Inventor(s): Zisapel; Nava (Tel Aviv, IL)

Assignee(s): Neurim Pharmaceuticals (1991) Ltd. (il)

Patent Number: 5,498,423

Date filed: February 14, 1994

Abstract: In order to correct a melatonin deficiency or distortion in the plasma melatonin level and profile in a human subject, there is administered to a human in which such a deficiency or distortion had been diagnosed, over a predetermined time period including at least part of the nocturnal period, an amount of melatonin in controlled-release form, such that the melatonin is released according to a profile which, taking into account the existing profile, simulates the profile in plasma of a human having a normal endogenous melatonin plasma profile. The invention also relates to a pharmaceutical controlled-release formulation, which comprises melatonin in combination with at least one pharmaceutical carrier, diluent or coating, the formulation being adapted to release melatonin over a predetermined time period, according to a profile which, taking into account the existing profile, simulates the profile in plasma of a human having a normal endogenous melatonin profile. The method of the invention may be e.g. applied to the prevention of **sudden infant death syndrome** in infants, and then comprises a preliminary screening step in order to determine the plasma melatonin levels, in order to select infants having a deficient plasma melatonin level.

Excerpt(s): The present invention relates to a method for correcting a deficiency or distortion in the plasma melatonin level and profile in a human subject and to a pharmaceutical controlled-release formulation which comprises melatonin.... Melatonin is the principal hormone secreted by the pineal gland in all vertebrates. In all mammals studied to date, including humans, a nocturnal rise in the production of melatonin by the pineal gland is evident, regardless of whether the mammals are nocturnal or diurnal, and conversely, melatonin production by the body is acutely suppressed by light. Melatonin is involved in the coordination of photoperiod and physiological processes, e.g. in animals which use changes in the photoperiod to time their thermoregulation, temporal signals to the thermoregulatory system are controlled by the daily rhythm in the duration of melatonin during the dark phase. Numerous studies have shown that melatonin has a potent influence on gonadal activity.... The timing of melatonin administration has been shown to be crucial for its biological activities. E.g., while in the case of rats whose circadian rhythms are disrupted or arrhythmic in constant light, as well as in the case of rats free running in constant darkness, their rhythms are synchronized by daily melatonin injections, by contrast it has been found that continuous availability of melatonin in circulation, of injection of melatonin in the morning, sometimes prevents gonodal responses to melatonin in the afternoon. The inventor has shown, e.g. in Zisapel et al, Neuroendocrinology 40: 102 (1985), that the inhibition by melatonin of the stimulated release of dopamine from rat hypothalamus, was highest in the early photophase and lowest in the early afternoon.

Web site: http://www.delphion.com/details?pn=US05498423__

- **Method for determination of urine components and for preventing sudden infant death syndrome**

Inventor(s): Laudon; Moshe (Kfar Saba, IL), Zisapel; Nava (Tel Aviv, IL)

Assignee(s): Neurim Pharmaceuticals (1991) Ltd. (tel Aviv, Il)

Patent Number: 5,500,225

Date filed: October 19, 1993

Abstract: Non-volatile organic components of interest in the urine of humans using diapers are assayed by carrying out the following sequence of steps at least once and up to as many times as the diapers are changed in a given 24-hour period, namely: removing the outer cover and any extraneous material from a used diaper so as to leave only diaper pulp with absorbed urine, estimating the amount of water in the used diaper, extracting a weighed portion of the diaper pulp with a water-miscible organic solvent, in which the diaper pulp is insoluble, to give an extract containing a component of interest, and determining the amount of the component of interest per unit volume of urine absorbed on the diaper pulp by analyzing an aliquot of the extract. The method may be applied e.g. to the prevention of **sudden infant death syndrome** in infants, by selecting infants for medication with melatonin where diaper urine indicates a deficiency of its metabolite 6-sulfatoxymelatonin in a 24-hour period. The melatonin may be administered in the form of a pharmaceutical formulation, or in an infant food which is included within the invention.

Excerpt(s): The present invention relates to a method for determination of components of urine in diapers, as well as to a method for preventing **sudden infant death syndrome** (i.e. cot death), which makes use of the results of such determination.... In another aspect, the prior patent application (U.S. Ser. No. 07/697,714) relates to a method for correcting a melatonin deficiency or distortion in the plasma melatonin level and profile in a human subject, which comprises administering to a human in which such a deficiency or distortion had been diagnosed, over a time period including at least part of the nocturnal period, an effective plasma melatonin deficiency or distortion correcting amount of melatonin in the form of a pharmaceutical controlled-release formulation defined in the preceding paragraph.... (c) administering an effective plasma melatonin deficiency correcting amount of melatonin to the at least one selected infant from step (b), the melatonin being in the form of a pharmaceutical controlled-release formulation defined above.

Web site: http://www.delphion.com/details?pn=US05500225__

- **Motion monitor useful for sleeping humans**

Inventor(s): Miller; William (1735 Caminito Ardiente, La Jolla, CA 92037)

Assignee(s): None Reported

Patent Number: 5,796,340

Date filed: August 12, 1996

Abstract: A motion monitor which detects respiration and/or cardiac activity of a human, particularly a sleeping human, has a mattress, for example, an air mattress, for supporting a sleeping human. The mattress has an interior cavity isolated from and at a pressure equal to or greater than ambient atmospheric pressure. A pressure transducer is connected with the interior cavity of the mattress and generates a signal representative of the pressure in the interior cavity. An indication unit is connected to the pressure transducer and presents a signal based on the output of the pressure transducer. This sleep monitor is useful for infants, particularly infants at risk for **sudden infant death syndrome** (SIDS).

Excerpt(s): The present invention relates to motion monitors, particularly sleep monitors useful with children suspected of being at risk for **sudden infant death syndrome** ("SIDS").... Sleep monitors are used to detect occurrences of apnea (transient cessation of respiration), bradycardia (relatively slow heart action), and tachycardia (relatively rapid heart action) when there is some medical reason to believe that infants (or adults) are at risk for these events. A sleep monitor can also be used with infants who are suspected of being at risk for SIDS. SIDS, which affects one out of every 500 to 600 live births, is the largest single cause of death among infants less than one year of age, and accounts for 6,000 to 10,000 deaths per year in the United States.... Conventional sleep monitors measure respiration and heart action by measuring transthoracic impedance and the electrocardiogram (TTI/ECG) and are designed to sound an alarm when apnea, bradycardia or tachycardia is detected and found to persist for more than a predetermined amount of time. The measurements taken by conventional sleep monitors are electrical in nature, and require attaching electrodes to the subject's skin, usually on the chest. Wires from a control box are attached to the electrodes, and a band is wrapped around the chest to keep the wires in place during sleep. The electrodes must be attached each time the subject goes to sleep, and the band, the electrodes and the wires must be removed at the end of each sleep session. Special care must be taken to assure good electrical contact between the electrodes and the skin. Foreign matter on the skin, such as talc, can cause a faulty contact. Motion of the subject during sleep can cause electrical noise at the contacts, can cause the wires to come loose, or can cause the wires to break. In a recent study in which 182 patients were monitored in their sleep, of 30,059 recorded events (i.e., machine-indicated occurrences of apnea and/or bradycardia and/or tachycardia) 91.9% were false alarms. 68.5% of the recorded events were false alarms caused by body motion and/or loose leads, and 23.4% were other machine errors such as interpretation of a low-amplitude respiratory signal as apnea. In addition to the functional problems of using a sleep monitor, there is also the matter of cost. The rental fee for such a machine is several hundred dollars per month. Weese-Mayer DE, Morrow AS, Conway LP et al., Assessing clinical significance of apnea exceeding 15 seconds with event recording. J. Pediatrics 117:568, 1990. Also see Nathanson I, O'Donnell J, Commins MF Am Dis Child 143:476.

Web site: http://www.delphion.com/details?pn=US05796340

- **Optical monitor for sudden infant death syndrome**

  Inventor(s): Flock; Stephen T. (Mt. Eliza, AU), Marchitto; Kevin S. (Mt. Eliza, AU)

  Assignee(s): Rocky Mountain Biosystems, Inc. (golden, Co)

  Patent Number: 6,492,634

  Date filed: May 2, 2001

  Abstract: The present invention provides devices and/or methods of monitoring extremely small movements associated with infant breathing and heart rate, therefore monitoring **sudden infant death syndrome** (SIDS). Provided is a system for monitoring movement of an infant, comprising: a light source which produces radiant energy; an optical device; and an imaging device. Further provided is a method of monitoring movement of an infant, comprising the steps of: producing radiant energy by a light source; coupling said radiant energy into an optical device so as to create a matrix of images; projecting said images into a field of interest; and detecting movement of said infant using an imaging device.

  Excerpt(s): The present invention relates generally to the field of medical devices. More specifically, the present invention relates to an optical monitor for **sudden infant death syndrome.**... Sudden Infant Death Syndrome (SIDS) is the sudden and unexpected death of an apparently healthy infant, whose death remains unexplained after further medical investigation such as an autopsy. **Sudden Infant Death Syndrome** is neither a disease, nor can it be a diagnosis for a living baby [1]. SIDS occurs at a rate of approximately 2 per 1,000 live births in the United States and occurs most often (90%) in under six months of age; of these, 18% were preterm infants [2].... One of the events that occurs during

Sudden Infant Death Syndrome is a period of apnea (stoppage of breathing) during which it may be possible that the infant may be resuscitated. However, most **Sudden Infant Death Syndrome** events occur at night when the infant's caregiver is asleep. Since **Sudden Infant Death Syndrome** is not normally associated with verbal distress, few infants get a chance to be resuscitated.

Web site: http://www.delphion.com/details?pn=US06492634__

- **Passive apnea monitor**

  Inventor(s): Sullivan; Patrick K. (Honolulu, HI)

  Assignee(s): Ocean Laboratories, Inc. (honolulu, Hi)

  Patent Number: 6,375,621

  Date filed: December 27, 1994

  Abstract: The instrument monitors the acoustic and electromechanical signals of the patient and calculates an energy spectrum periodogram or histogram using time series analysis techniques. The patient lies down on a large piezoelectric film (few microns thick) that has the capability of measuring signals from very high to very low frequencies. The heart and respiration rates as well as obstructive apnea can be observed, detected and measured from the spectral peaks in the resulting energy spectrum. A microcomputing machine provides calculations to determine the energy spectrum and provides for discrimination between noise and a true apnea episode. An alarm calls for assistance in the event of an apnea, including obstructive apnea, or a **Sudden Infant Death Syndrome** (SIDS) episode.

  Excerpt(s): An interesting application of the proposed technology, to which the invention relates preferably, but not exclusively, is the detection of apnea, the monitoring of biological functions such as heart rate and respiration rates, as well as obstructive apnea, particularly for infants.... The invention relates to a system that uses acoustic and electromechanical transducers, such as a piezoelectric film, to measure biological respirative signals over time. Time series analysis techniques are then applied to the measured signals whereby an energy spectrum (periodogram/histogram) is calculated that identifies the rhythmic and pseudo-rhythmic biological functions such as respiration and heart rate and obstructions in the breathing passage (obstructive apnea.).... The apnea monitoring instrument offers researchers, clinicians, parents and other people who are involved in child and adult apnea monitoring an inexpensive way to monitor respiration, heart rate and obstructive apnea without the use of restrictive electrical wiring. It makes available a low cost monitoring instrument to be used as a highly reliable tool for researching and monitoring **Sudden Infant Death Syndrome** (SIDS).

Web site: http://www.delphion.com/details?pn=US06375621__

- **Position monitor and alarm apparatus for reducing the possibility of sudden infant death syndrome (SIDS)**

Inventor(s): Clark, Jr.; Leonard R. (Oreland, PA), Mesibov; Barbara (Mill Neck, NY)

Assignee(s): Waterview Llc (east Norwich, Ny)

Patent Number: 5,914,660

Date filed: March 26, 1998

Abstract: A device for reducing the possibility of **sudden infant death syndrome** (SIDS) comprises a position-indicating device effectively coupled to a signal-producing circuit and attached to the clothing of the infant. The position-indicating device provides signals varying in response to prone and other positions assumed by the infant during sleep, allowing an associated alarm device to be activated in response to the infant's assuming a SIDS-dangerous prone or side-lying position. In one embodiment, the position of the infant can be determined by an optical sensor interacting with a reflective or other marker adhered to the infant. Gravity or pressure switches may also be used to provide position-responsive signals. A signal generated upon assumption of the SIDS-dangerous prone or side-lying positions is transmitted to a remote receiver located proximate the infant's care-giver whereupon an alarm is generated to indicate the need to reposition the infant. A constant low-level or intermittent maintenance signal can be produced to assure the continued and proper operation of the apparatus. An additional awakening alarm can be produced near the sleeping infant to further reduce the likelihood of a SIDS event.

Excerpt(s): The present invention relates to an apparatus for continuously monitoring the position assumed by a sleeping infant. More particularly, the invention relates to the provision of an alarm to indicate when the infant has taken a position considered to be conducive to the onset of **Sudden Infant Death Syndrome** (SIDS).... Sudden Infant Death Syndrome (SIDS) has been defined as the "sudden death of an infant under one year of age which remains unexplained after a thorough case investigation, including performance of a complete autopsy, examination of the death scene, and a review of the clinical history." SIDS occurs in all types of families and is generally independent of race and socioeconomic level. It is unexpected and usually occurs in apparently healthy infants from one month to one year of age. Death occurs without warning and is accompanied by no signs of suffering. Five to six thousand infant deaths per year were attributed to SIDS during the late eighties and early nineties.... The horror of SIDS, also commonly known as "crib death", lies in the thus far unsolved mystery of why a seemingly healthy baby dies suddenly, without warning and without apparent reason. A form of undiagnosed apnea has been suspected; various maternal risk factors, including cigarette smoking during pregnancy, maternal age less than 20 years, poor prenatal care, low weight gain, anemia, drug abuse and a history of sexually transmitted disease and/or urinary tract infection have all been suspected of heightening the likelihood of occurrence; and the presence of soft bedding materials and the breathing of second-hand smoke have also been cited as possible contributing factors. Recent studies at the National Institute of Child Health and Human Development (NICHD) have identified defects in the regions of the brains of SIDS-susceptible infants that control breathing. However, whatever the root cause of SIDS is eventually determined to be, it appears that pro-active parenting can substantially reduce the risk to the newborn.

Web site: http://www.delphion.com/details?pn=US05914660__

- **Prevention of sudden infant death**

  Inventor(s): Hedner; Jan (Gothenburg, SE), Pettersson; Anders (Kode, SE)

  Assignee(s): Diabact AB (se)

  Patent Number: 6,083,756

  Date filed: May 7, 1998

  Abstract: A method for identification of an infant being particularly susceptible to **sudden infant death syndrome** (SIDS) comprises the determination of an Helicobacter pylori infection in the infant's mother, particularly by detection of antibodies to H. pylori of the IgG type, in a blood sample drawn from the infant's mother or by determination of carbon dioxide formed from urea in the air exhaled from the infant's mother upon oral administration of a challenge dose of urea. Also disclosed is the use of an antibiotic effective against H. pylori for the manufacture of a medicament for administration to mothers and other persons infected by H. pylori and coming into close bodily contact with infants below two years of age, and a method of prevention of SIDS by administration of that antibiotic.

  Excerpt(s): The present invention relates to the identification of infants with increased risk of sudden death (sudden death syndrome; SIDS), and to methods and means for SIDS prevention.... Sudden infant death syndrome (SIDS) occurs in young infants during a narrow time range that peaks at 3 months and extends over about two years from birth. It is relatively common (7,000 deaths in the United States per year). Usually it is defined in the negative: "The sudden death of any infant or young child which is unexpected in history and in which a thorough post-mortem examination fails to demonstrate an adequate cause for death".... Several factors identified in epidemiological studies of SIDS are associated with increased susceptibility of infants to infectious diseases, particularly upper respiratory tract infections. The period in which infants are at highest risk roughly corresponds to the period when maternal antibodies in the infant are decreasing while its immature immune system is not able to provide full compensation. The vast majority of SIDS-related deaths occur below the age of two years. Not only are breast-fed infants less vulnerable to infections but also less susceptible to SIDS. Many babies who died from SIDS had mild gastrointestinal tract infection shortly before death; IgA response of their duodenal mucosa was found to be significantly increased (Stoltenberg L et al., Pediatr. Res. 32 (1992) 372-375).

Web site: http://www.delphion.com/details?pn=US06083756__

- **Respiratory stimulator bed**

    Inventor(s): Totten; Bertram F. (912 Yosemite La., El Dorado Hills, CA 95630)

    Assignee(s): None Reported

    Patent Number: 4,969,451

    Date filed: April 23, 1987

    Abstract: Unique crib or bed structure designed and constructed to combat and overcome **sudden infant death syndrome** by effecting an external and intermittent jarring stimulus to weak, slow and undeveloped body functions in accordance with the age and respiratory rate of an infant or other body reclining upon the crib or bed. In its preferred form in order to effect this intermittent jarring stimulus to a body reclining upon the crib or bed, an electronically controlled cam is positioned beneath the mattress supporting structure of the crib or bed intermittently when rotated to strike the underside of the mattress supporting structure, thereby jarring it in a manner effecting intermittent cycles of upward and downward motions of the mattress supporting structure and a mattress supported thereon, with a momentary pause or rest period between each cycle of cam rotation at which time the cam is completely out of contact with the mattress supporting structure.

Excerpt(s): The present invention relates to bio-engineered beds but more particularly to such crib structures wherein its unique construction and best mode of operation is designed to stimulate the respiratory rate of infants while sleeping upon its mattress and thereby overcome the mysterious infant sudden death syndrome.... While the known prior art discloses crib structures for moving crib mattresses in a number of ways and directions, none has specifically dwelt with this infant death syndrome, and none discloses a construction and mode of operation which would be effective to overcome it, as has the present invention.... The primary object of the present invention is to provide a unique bio-engineered bed or crib structure which, in its best mode of operation is effective to overcome the mysterious infant death syndrome.

Web site: http://www.delphion.com/details?pn=US04969451__

- **Sleeping pad, beddings and bumpers to improve respiratory efficiency and environmental temperature of an infant and reduce the risks of sudden infant death syndrome (SIDS) and asphyxiation**

Inventor(s): Koenig; J. Frank (407 Kramer Dr. SE., Vienna, VA 22180)

Assignee(s): None Reported

Patent Number: 6,055,690

Date filed: November 1, 1995

Abstract: Rebreathing carbon dioxide and overheating of the infant are contributing causes of **Sudden Infant Death Syndrome** (SIDS) and asphyxiation. The characteristics of conventional crib mattresses, beddings and bumper pads contribute to rebreathing of carbon dioxide and overheating of the infant and may be contributing environmental causes of SIDS, asphyxiation, apnea syndromes and hypoventilation. The present invention consists of improved sleeping pads, beddings and bumper pads which reduce rebreathing of carbon dioxide and overheating and provide increased crib ventilation to stimulate breathing.

Excerpt(s): The present invention relates to apparatus for reducing the risk of **sudden infant death syndrome,** asphyxiation, apnea syndrome and hypoventilation through the use of improved sleeping pads, beddings and bumper pads within a crib or the like to improve the respiratory efficiency and environmental temperature of an infant.... Sudden infant death syndrome (SIDS) is the leading cause of postneonatal infant death in the United States. About 7,000 deaths occur each year from SIDS. In addition, many infants die each year of asphyxiation while in a crib.... Prone sleeping is associated with spontaneous face-down sleeping in infants. The face-down position is associated with rebreathing expired gases, including carbon dioxide, and increased carbon dioxide lung pressure in normal infants. In some cases the amount of rebreathed carbon dioxide is sufficient to cause death in normal infants. B. A. Chiodini and B. T. Thach, Impaired ventilation in infants sleeping facedown: Potential significance for **sudden infant death syndrome,** J. Pediatrics, Vol. 123, 686 (1993); J. S. Kemp and B. T. Thach, Sudden Death in Infants Sleeping on Polystyrene-Filled Cushions, New England Journal of Medicine, Vol. 324, 1858 (1991). In that case the cause of death is asphyxiation, not SIDS. However in SIDS's cases the rebreathing of carbon dioxide, short of asphyxiation, may be a contributing cause of death of the infant.

Web site: http://www.delphion.com/details?pn=US06055690__

- **Sudden Infant Death Syndrome (SIDS) monitor and stimulator**

  Inventor(s): Scanlon; Michael (Silver Spring, MD)

  Assignee(s): The United States of America AS Represented by the Secretary of the Army (washington, Dc)

  Patent Number: 5,515,865

  Date filed: April 22, 1994

  Abstract: A movement and sound monitor and stimulator which is particularly useful for preventing death in human infants from **sudden infant death syndrome** is disclosed. The movement and sound monitor and stimulator has a base member which may be a fluid-filled sensing pad for supporting the infant or other animate object which is being monitored and a transducer positioned for detecting movement or acoustic activity (e.g., heartbeat, breathing) of the object on the base member to provide an output signal in response to forces applied thereto which are generated by such movement. A circuit is connected to monitor the output signal from the transducer and activates a stimulator which is operable to provide movement to the base member to stimulate movement in the object when output from the transducer to the circuit corresponds to no movement from the object. The transducer may be a pressure transducer in fluid communication with the fluid interior of the sensing pad. In the alternative, a piezo-electric sheet operatively connected to a surface of the sensing pad to detect such movement as well as movement cessation. The circuit may also be connected to an alarm which can provide an audible or visual indication to third parties when there is no movement from the object.

Excerpt(s): The present invention relates to a movement monitor suitable for detecting movement and, more particularly, to a movement monitor suitable for monitoring and stimulating/resuscitating a human or other living organism's breathing movement.... Sudden Infant Death Syndrome (SIDS) is a medical condition whereby an infant suddenly stops breathing, leading to the eventual death of the infant. Although the cause and initial symptoms of SIDS is not completely understood, it is felt that a child can be awakened from the SIDS condition.... Unfortunately, many currently available baby monitors are usually only provided with a microphone/transmitter and a receiver/speaker, enabling the parents to monitor baby noises such as crying, coughing, sneezing and sniffling. If the parents do not hear anything, they assume the baby is sleeping, and therefore do not need to check in on the child. Unfortunately, in some tragic situations, the absence of baby noises can be deadly to the child.

Web site: http://www.delphion.com/details?pn=US05515865__

- **Sudden infant death syndrome monitor**

  Inventor(s): Kim; Bill H. (702 Doubletree La., Long Beach, CA 90815)

  Assignee(s): None Reported

  Patent Number: 5,505,199

  Date filed: December 1, 1994

  Abstract: A **sudden infant death syndrome,** SIDS, monitor which monitors the infant to determine oxygen desaturation and movement. No alarm indication is produced if movement is detected, a low alarm condition is produced if desaturation occurs while movement is detected and a high condition is produced if desaturation is occurs and no movement is detected. A video monitor is provided to bring the image of the infant into the presence of the caregiver when either alarm is produced. The substantially reduced number of false alarms, due for example to motion artifacts, improves the level of alarm response over the long term that can reasonably be provided by parents and caregivers.

  Excerpt(s): Sudden infant death syndrome is the medical terminology used to designate the almost inexplicable deaths of seemingly healthy infants. Commonly known as **crib death,** SIDS is the leading category of infant deaths between the ages of two weeks and one year and account for one-third of all deaths after the new born period.... Despite limited information, a scientific consensus suggests that SIDS occurred in healthy infants as a result of the simultaneous occurrence of a series of seemingly unrelated biological events. Infants who have periods of apnea, or difficulty in breathing, sudden skin color change to blue or pale, changes in muscle tone either to limpness or rigidity and who appear to require help in breathing are more likely to die of SIDS. These episodes can occur during sleep, feeding or while awake and are now known as apparent life-threatening events or ALTEs.... Specially designed apnea/bradycardia alarm systems became available for home use in the late 1970s to monitor infant breathing in an attempt to reduce SIDS. Conventional apnea/bradycardia monitors use electrodes attached to the infant's skin. The monitors provide an audible alarm if the baby stops breathing for a pre-determined period of time, or when the heart rate drops below a designated level, to indicate to the parent or guardian that the baby may need assistance in breathing. Conventional home monitors may now also include means for recording the electrocardiogram and respiratory wave form before, during or after the alarm event.

Web site: http://www.delphion.com/details?pn=US05505199__

- **Sudden infant death syndrome prevention apparatus and method**

  Inventor(s): Hargest; Thomas S. (14 Lockwood Blvd., Apt. 10J., Charleston, SC 29401), Hargest; William M. (8470 Doar Rd., Awendaw, SC 29429)

  Assignee(s): None Reported

  Patent Number: 5,317,767

  Date filed: June 16, 1992

  Abstract: A safety pad or mattress such as for use in a crib prevents **sudden infant death syndrome** by ensuring an oxygenated breathing space beneath the infant. Reticulated foam or other air permeable material is made into the shape of a pad or even a mattress and covered with a fitted open weave fabric covering. An air tube is embedded in the pad or mattress and interconnected with an air pump which circulates fresh, i.e., oxygenated, air in a breathing space formed beneath an infant by the air permeable mattress. The forced air circulation flushes any exhaled carbon dioxide from the breathing space, even when the infant is face down or otherwise in a prone position on the mattress, to prevent carbon dioxide poisoning. The materials of the fabric covering and air permeable mattress permit any fluids regurgitated from the infant to drain away from the infant's face. A relatively tight fit for the fitted covering obviates loose fitting sheets to further prevent potential entanglement and suffocation of a recumbent infant.

Excerpt(s): The present invention relates in general to apparatus and method for the prevention of **sudden infant death syndrome** and in particular to an infant safety pad or mattress and corresponding method for the prevention of infant asphyxiation from carbon dioxide poisoning.... Several thousand apparently healthy infants (children under the age of 1 year) die each year in the United States from **Sudden Infant Death Syndrome** (SIDS). Deaths from SIDS have been estimated at 7,000 to 10,000 per year. See for example Womens Day, volume 55, issue 3, Jan. 7, 1992, pages 38 through 43; and USA Today, volume 117, issue 2626, February 1989, page 11. The occurrence of SIDS in a given family can be particularly devastating emotionally because, in general, there is no warning that the infant is at risk and the parent or care giver has no knowledge of any problem until he or she discovers an unconscious or deceased infant thought to be safely sleeping in its crib.... The specific cause of SIDS is generally unknown, which unfortunately leads to the result that heretofore there has generally been no known treatment and generally no means of prevention.

Web site: http://www.delphion.com/details?pn=US05317767__

- **Vital signs monitor**

  Inventor(s): Cestaro; Victor L. (Farmingville, NY), Sciarra; Michael J. (Southampton, NY)

  Assignee(s): F. William Carr (houston, Tx)

  Patent Number: 4,494,553

  Date filed: April 1, 1981

  Abstract: Provision is made to monitor for vital signs, such as respiratory activity and cardiac activity. The monitoring equipment is mounted by a belt to a person being monitored. Multiple Inductance coils carried by the belt move relative to each other in response to breathing, and the associated mutual inductance changes provide sensory signals to reflect the breathing. Electrical signals indicative of such vital signs are transmitted by radio wave to a central monitor which can monitor the activity of numerous persons. A plurality of such patient units including vital signs sensors and transmitters in combination with a single central monitor may be used to monitor multiple patients. The present invention is useful in monitoring to attempt to prevent **sudden infant death syndrome,** or **crib death,** and in intensive care units or cardiac units of hospitals and the like.

  Excerpt(s): The present invention relates to electronic systems for monitoring vital signs, such as respiration and cardiac activity.... There have been several types of vital sign monitors to detect interrupted respiration. However, each of these types has suffered from several shortcomings. A first type of monitor was based on detecting the temperature differential between inhaled and exhaled air. Usually, a temperature sensor was mounted near a patient's nose to detect changes in temperature in the air between inhaling and exhaling. However, since a person normally breathes once every five or more seconds, a substantial time delay in seconds lapsed, usually twenty or more, before an abnormal condition was sensed.... Another type of monitor utilized a strain gage sensor whose resistance changed as the patient's chest cavity expanded and contracted during breathing. However, for reference reading purposes, the strain gage was required to be applied to the patient's body in a set or fixed state of tension. Usually the strain gage was contained in a bandage or wrap in some manner about the patient's thorax. If the wrap loosened in any way, however, the readings obtained by the strain gage were no longer accurate.

Web site: http://www.delphion.com/details?pn=US04494553__

Patent Applications on Sudden Infant Death Syndrome

As of December 2000, U.S. patent applications are open to public viewing.[21] Applications are patent requests which have yet to be granted (the process to achieve a patent can take several years). The following patent applications have been filed since December 2000 relating to sudden infant death syndrome:

- **Alkylaryl polyether alcohol polymers for treatment and prophylaxis of snoring, sleep apnea, sudden infant death syndrome and for improvement of nasal breathing**

  Inventor(s): Hofmann, Thomas; (Seattle, WA)

  Correspondence: Hana Verny; Peters, Verny, Jones & Schmitt, Llp; Suite 6; 385 Sherman Avenue; Palo Alto; CA; 94306; US

  Patent Application Number: 20030053956

  Date filed: January 23, 2002

  Abstract: A method and composition for treatment and prophylaxis of snoring, sleep apnea or **sudden infant death syndrome** and for improvement of nasal breathing in mammals by nasal and/or pharyngeal administration of tyloxapol or a related alkylaryl polyether alcohol

---

[21] This has been a common practice outside the United States prior to December 2000.

polymer. A spray, liquid or solid composition comprising from about 0.01 to about 20% (w/v), equivalent to about 100.mu.g/ml to about 200 mg/ml, of tyloxapol or another alkylaryl polyether alcohol polymer alone or in admixture with pharmaceutically acceptable excipients and additives. The composition is administered as a spray, liquid, liquid drops, lozenges or powder suitable for nasal and/or pharyngeal application.

Excerpt(s): This application is based on and claims priority of the provisional application Ser. No. 60/264,166 filed on Jan. 24, 2001.... The current invention concerns a method and composition for treatment and prophylaxis of snoring, sleep apnea or **sudden infant death syndrome** and for improvement of nasal breathing in mammals by nasal and/or pharyngeal administration of tyloxapol or a related alkylaryl polyether alcohol polymer. In particular, the present invention provides a spray, liquid or solid composition comprising from about 0.01 to about 20% (w/v), equivalent to about 100.mu.g/ml to about 200 mg/ml, of tyloxapol or another selected alkylaryl polyether alcohol polymer alone, in combination, or in admixture with pharmaceutically acceptable excipients and additives. The composition is administered as a spray, liquid, liquid drops, lozenges or powder suitable for nasal and/or pharyngeal application.... Snoring and related sleep apnea are amongst the most troublesome sleeping impairments. Snoring is not only a nuisance for other people, but it has been shown, similarly to sleep apnea, to correlate with increased daytime sleepiness and decreased alertness and work performance.

Web site: http://appft1.uspto.gov/netahtml/PTO/search-bool.html

- **Computer powered wire(less) ultra-intelligent real-time monitor**

  Inventor(s): Ridley, Alfred Dennis; (Tallahassee, FL)

  Correspondence: Dr. Alfred Dennis Ridley; P.o. Box 12518; Tallahassee; FL; 32317-2518; US

  Patent Application Number: 20030164762

  Date filed: December 2, 2002

  Abstract: A device (1)(2) and method to monitor, in real time, one or more variables by an at least 2500 hour water proof sensor/transmitter, not requiring recharge, placed at the source where data are automatically collected and transmitted by wire or wireless means (2A)(2B) to a battery-free computer-powered (2C) receiver connected to a computer, where software continuously analyzes and charts the data. The software auto and cross correlates the variables, continuously updates and displays the data on simple aggregate charts (4A) or decomposes the data and displays them on newly created common cause charts (4B)(4C) of internal systematically related effects and newly created special cause charts (4D)(4E) of external random unrelated effects, including summary data, and creates graduated progressive sound, color, print and world wide, fax, email and telephone alarm signals when the chart values exceed user specified limits, either in terms of actual units (4B)(4D) or standard deviations (4C)(4E), or when any particular pattern occurs. The device helps determine ahead of time, when the source of the monitored variables is functioning abnormally. Advance warning thus obtained, is used to initiate corrective action (3A)(3B)(3C)(3D) so as to prevent failure at the source that is generating the variables. Examples of failure that it helps prevent include but are not limited to, sudden infant death due to **sudden infant death syndrome** in human babies, heart or respiratory failure in any human being who is either at rest or moving around within a specified area, failure in industrial machines or measuring equipment, manufacturing defects and financial irregularities.

Excerpt(s): This application is entitled to the benefit of Provisional Patent Application Ser. No. 60/352,096 filed Jan. 25, 2002.... This invention relates to universal electronic data monitoring including their collection, wire or wireless transmission, computer analysis, detection and the classification of abnormalities in the data, where such abnormalities result in automatic alarms that are transmitted to recipients locally or world wide, thereby providing a basis for taking corrective action at the source of the data.... The prior art U.S. Pat. No. 4,583,524 to Hutchins (1986) shows a instructional system for reviving the victim of a heart attach. U.S. Pat. No. 5,199,439 to Zimmerman et al. (1993) shows the use of a quality control chart for direct and simple monitoring of data. However, the chart is used in a way that is not statistically valid. The reason is as follows. Statistical quality control charts assume that the data on which they are based are independent. That is, each measurement is completely unrelated to all previous measurements. In reality, the measurements are serially related. This is known as autocorrelation. None of these patents employs correlation as part of its analysis. Since correlation analysis is at least one of the requirements to make the charts valid, no valid conclusions can be drawn from the charts that use these patents.

Web site: http://appft1.uspto.gov/netahtml/PTO/search-bool.html

- **Identifying infants at risk for sudden infant death syndrome**

Inventor(s): Cohen, Richard J.; (Chestnut Hill, MA), Haghighi-Mood, Ali; (Andover, MA)

Correspondence: Fish & Richardson P.c.; 1425 K Street, N.w.; 11th Floor; Washington; DC; 20005-3500; US

Patent Application Number: 20030233050

Date filed: June 18, 2002

Abstract: A method for identifying infants at risk for SIDS includes applying electrodes to an infant, receiving electrical signals from the electrodes, analyzing the received electrical signals to measure alternans of a heart of the infant, and identifying whether the infant is at risk for SIDS.A system for identifying infants at risk for SIDS includes an input unit configured to receive electrical signals from electrodes applied to an infant, a processor connected to the input unit and configured to process the received electrical signals to measure alternans of a heart of the infant, and a comparator configured to compare the measured alternans with alternans in a population of infants.

Excerpt(s): This disclosure is directed to the identification of infants at risk for the **Sudden infant death syndrome**.... The **Sudden Infant Death Syndrome** (SIDS) is a disorder in which infants suddenly die, usually during sleep. For every one thousand infants, between approximately one and two die of SIDS, making SIDS the leading cause of death after the neonatal period in the first year of life. SIDS is thus an enormous human tragedy that has devastating consequences for the affected infants and their families.... Improved identification of infants at risk for SIDS is provided by measurement of alternans, for example, T-wave alternans, of an infant heart. Alternans is a subtle beat-to-beat change in the repeating pattern of an infant's or other patient's electrocardiogram (ECG) waveform. Alternans results in an ABABAB... pattern of variation of waveform shape between successive beats in an ECG waveform. The level of variation is indicative of the likelihood that an infant is at risk for SIDS.

Web site: http://appft1.uspto.gov/netahtml/PTO/search-bool.html

- **Methods for diagnosing pervasive development disorders, dysautonomia and other neurological conditions**

Inventor(s): Fallon, Joan M.; (Yonkers, NY)

Correspondence: F. Chau & Associates, Llp; Suite 501; 1900 Hempstead Turnpike; East Meadow; NY; 11554; US

Patent Application Number: 20020081628

Date filed: November 16, 2001

Abstract: Methods for aiding in the diagnosis of disorders including, but not limited to, PDDs (Pervasive Development Disorders), Dysautonomic disorders, Parkinson's disease and SIDS (Sudden Infant Death Syndrome). In one aspect, a diagnosis method comprises analyzing a stool sample of an individual for the presence of a biological marker (or marker compound) comprising one or more pathogens, which provides an indication of whether the invidual has, or can develop, a disorder including, but not limited to, a PDD, Dysautonomia, Parkinsons disease and SIDS. Preferably, the presence of one or more pathogens is determined using a stool immunoassay to determine the presence of antigens in a stool sample, wherein such antigens are associated with one or more pathogens including, but not limited to, Giardia, Cryptosporidium, E. histolytica, C. difficile, Adenovirus, Rotavirus or H.pylori.

Excerpt(s): This application is based on, and claims the benefit of, United States Provisional Application No. 60/249,239, filed on Nov. 16, 2000, which is fully incorporated herein by reference.... The present invention generally relates to methods for aiding in the diagnosis of disorders including, but not limited to, PDDs (Pervasive Development Disorders), Dysautonomic disorders, Parkinsons disease and SIDS (Sudden Infant Death Syndrome). More particularly, the invention relates to a diagnosis method comprising analyzing a stool sample of an individual for the presence of a biological marker (or marker compound) comprising one or more pathogens, which provides an indication of whether the invidual has, or can develop, a disorder including, but not limited to, a PDD, a Dysautonomic disorder, Parkinson's disease or SIDS.... Currently, extensive research is being conducted to determine associations between gastrointestinal dysfunction and a variety of human disorders that, heretofore, have been of unknown etiology. For example, an association between dysautonomic conditions and gastrointestinal dysfunction has been described in U.S. patent application Ser. No. 09/929,592, filed on Aug. 14, 2001, entitled "Methods For Diagnosing and Treating Dysautonomia and Other Dysautonomic Conditions, which is commonly owned and fully incorporated herein by reference. Further, a relationship between gastrointestinal conditions and PDDs such as Autism, ADD (Attention Deficit Disorder) and ADHD (Attention Deficit Hyperactivity Disorder) has been described in detail in U.S. patent application Ser. No. 09/466,559, filed Dec. 17, 1999, entitled "Methods For Treating Pervasive Development Disorders," and U.S. Ser. No. 09/707,395, filed on Nov. 7, 2000, entitled "Methods For Treating Pervasive Development Disorders", both of which are commonly owned and incorporated herein by reference.

Web site: http://appft1.uspto.gov/netahtml/PTO/search-bool.html

- **New use of ammonium compounds and/or urea**

Inventor(s): Wiklund, Lars; (Uppsala, SE)

Correspondence: Mcdermott, Will & Emery; 600 13th Street, N.w.; Washington; DC; 20005-3096; US

Patent Application Number: 20030021856

Date filed: November 15, 2001

Abstract: The use of a physiologically innocuous ammonium compound and/or urea as an additive to an infant formula or a pap or for the preparation of a pharmaceutical composition for the prophylaxis of **sudden infant death syndrome** (SIDS) is disclosed as is also, an infant formula or a pap which in addition to conventional ingredients contains a physiologically innocuous ammonium compound an/or urea. Furthermore, a method of preventing SIDS is disclosed, which method comprises administering to the infant an infant formula or a pap as indicated above, and a method for prophylaxis of SIDS, wherein a pharmaceutical composition containing a physiologically innocuous ammonium compound and/or urea is administered to the infant or the appropriately selected or modified non-pathogenic, urease-producing bacteria are supplied to the gastrointestinal tract of the infant. Finally, a method for the diagnosis of the risks for SIDS is disclosed according to which method the faeces of the infant are analyzed with respect to the presence of urea, urease activity and/or ammonium ions, the presence of urea, the absence of abnormally low urease activity and ammonium ion, respectively, indicating risks for SIDS.

Excerpt(s): Please replace the paragraph beginning at line 5 on page 2 with the following: In order that an animal or a human being should be able to live it is required that its body functions are regulated in such a way that there is an acid-base balance. Expressed in another way: A normal pH-value must exist in the cells, in the extracellular liquid and in the cell organelles. If this is not the case first slight functional disorders, then even increasing diseases and finally death of structures, cells and the whole organism occurs. For instance, it is known that the mortality in several diseases increases when the pH value of the extracellular liquid (normally 7.40) is above 7.55 or below 7.20.... Please replace the paragraph beginning at line 17 on page 2 with the following: Under the latest decades the opinion of the acid-base balance has not changed materially. During the 1980's, however, Atkinson and co-workers [Atkinson D E et al, Curr Top Cell Regul, 21, 261-302 (1982)] again called attention to the previously known, but among physiologists and medical physicians not accepted fact that the metabolism of mammals not only produced the main metabolites carbon dioxide, water and urea but also hydrogen carbonate. His theory also meant that the metabolism by producing hydrogen carbonate above all via amino acid metabolism in order to result in the metabolic end products carbon dioxide and water must be supplied with protons and that this process for quantitative reasons had to occur via the ornithine cycle. One of the objections against this theory has been that if such an important life process does not function the animal or the human being in question should rapidly die. However, no such lacking function of the system proposed by Atkinson has even been pointed out and even less been proven which constitutes one of the deficiencies of his theory.... Please replace the paragraph beginning at line 1 on page 5 with the following: portal area, especially at acidosis, can be utilized for synthesis of glutamine in the liver. It is also known by intensive care physicians that ammonium chloride supplied intravenously and perorally lowers base excess values and such supply is accordingly used as a matter of routine for the treatment of a metabolic alkalosis. When the patient treated is breathing by himself, the supply of ammonium will bring about a so-called compensatory hyperventilation. The present inventor has administered himself 80 mmoles ammonium chloride perorally and thereby has been able to establish that this substance obviously is resorbed very quickly from the gastrointestinal tract and causes a slight hyperventilation which in turn causes an increase in RQ ("Respiratory Quotient"=the quotient between the carbon dioxide emission and the oxygen gas uptake in a person--in both cases expressed in ml/min) from a value at rest of 0.82 to 0.87 and the elimination of carbon dioxide increases by 30 ml/min and that this seems to proceed for nearly 1h, which corresponds to about 80 mmoles of carbon dioxide. Furthermore, there is a report on the concentration of urea in the vitreous body of dead SIDS patients which is compared to autopsy material from children deceased from other causes at the same age [Blumenfeld T A, et al, Am J Clin Pathol, 71, 219-223 (1979)]. It appeared that children deceased from SIDS have lower urea values than children deceased from other causes. As a normal enterohepatic circulation of urea and ammonium ion hypothetically does not function in these cases this should have the consequence that the production of urea is less than normally and since the volume of distribution is equal this means that the concentration in various body fluids decreases. The low concentration of urea found is thus not inconsistent with the hypothesis put forward here.

Web site: http://appft1.uspto.gov/netahtml/PTO/search-bool.html

- **Orthomolecular sulpho-adenosylmethionine derivatives with antioxidant properties**

Inventor(s): Wilburn, Michael D.; (Cedar Hill, TX)

Correspondence: Nath & Associates; 1030 15th Street; 6th Floor; Washington; DC; 20005; US

Patent Application Number: 20030078231

Date filed: June 22, 2001

Abstract: Orthomolecular Sulpho-Adenosylmethionine derivative compounds, compositions, and their uses for effecting a biological activity in an animal, such as neurochemical activity; liver biology activity; heart and artery function; cartilage, bone and joint health; stomach and/or intestinal lining resistance to ulceration; immune function; cell membrane integrity; and pain and inflammation. The compounds of the present invention are further useful for preventing or treating diseases or conditions; treating viral infections, infectious diseases, leukemia, and obesity; and reducing the risk of **Sudden Infant Death Syndrome** in an animal. The compounds of the present invention are of formula I: 1A is 0 or N; andX is a reaction product as defined herein.

Excerpt(s): The present invention relates to novel compounds and pharmaceutical preparations including the same which are useful in effecting a biological activity in an animal, such as neurochemical activity; liver biology activity; heart and artery function; cartilage, bone and joint health; stomach and/or intestinal lining resistance to ulceration; immune function; cell membrane integrity; and pain and inflammation; in preventing or treating diseases or conditions; in treating viral infections, infectious diseases, leukemia, and obesity; and in reducing the risk of **Sudden infant death syndrome**.... Linus Pauling coined the term "Orthomolecular Medicine" and defined it as: "The preservation of good health and the prevention and treatment of disease by varying the concentrations in the human body of the molecules or substances that are normally present, many of them required for life, such as the vitamins, essential amino acids, essential fats, and minerals." Literally, the term is derived from the Greek "ortho", for correct or right, and "molecule", or "right molecule". When these "right molecules" are out of balance, disorders and disease can result. The Orthomolecular Concomitant Theory of Convergence suggests that the duality of stress and uncontrolled free radical proliferation are major disruptive forces in the delicate balance of life, resulting in disorders, diseases, and premature death. In particular, the free radical theory of aging and disease suggests that excess free radicals can be generated by stress, simple aging, exposure to toxic pollutants in air, water, and foods, as well as cigarette smoke, alcohol, and ionizing radiation. Free radicals may produce oxidative damage to DNA and other cell components which accumulates with age and is suggested to be a major contributor to aging and degenerative diseases. Antioxidants may be used for reducing, eliminating, preventing, and reversing oxidative damage to tissues in an animal. Treatment of disorders and disease by orthomolecular methods is aimed at bringing such natural substances into healthful balance.... In a relatively recent phenomenon, traditional primary health care practitioners have begun to embrace orthomolecular nutrition as an enhancement to their practices. There are several forces promoting this trend, including consumer demand and the increasing eligibility of alternative health care for medical insurance coverage.

Web site: http://appft1.uspto.gov/netahtml/PTO/search-bool.html

- **Orthomolecular vitamin E derivatives**

  Inventor(s): Wilburn, Michael D.; (Cedar Hill, TX)

  Correspondence: Nath & Associates; 1030 15th Street; 6th Floor; Washington; DC; 20005; US

  Patent Application Number: 20030007961

  Date filed: June 22, 2001

  Abstract: Orthomolecular Vitamin E derivative compounds, compositions, and their uses for effecting aging and longevity, nerve activity, hematopoiesis and maintenance of blood cells, hepatic activity, nephritic activity, heart and cardiovascular function, pulmonary function, muscular function, cartilage, bone, and joint health, gastrointestinal function, reproductive system function, vision, immune function, cell membrane integrity, and pain and inflammation; preventing or treating diseases or conditions; treating cancers or obesity; and reducing the risk of **Sudden Infant Death Syndrome** in an animal. The compounds of the present invention are of formula I: 1or a pharmaceutically acceptable salt, ester, or solvate, thereof, wherein:A, B, C, D, and R are as defined herein.

Excerpt(s): Linus Pauling coined the term "Orthomolecular Medicine" and defined it as: "The preservation of good health and the prevention and treatment of disease by varying the concentrations in the human body of the molecules or substances that are normally present, many of them required for life, such as the vitamins, essential amino acids, essential fats, and minerals." Literally, the term is derived from the Greek "ortho", for correct or right, and "molecule", or "right molecule". When these "right molecules" are out of balance, disorders and disease can result. The Orthomolecular Concomitant Theory of Convergence suggests that the duality of stress and uncontrolled free radical proliferation are major disruptive forces in the delicate balance of life, resulting in disorders, diseases, and premature death. In particular, the free radical theory of aging and disease suggests that excess free radicals can be generated by simple aging or exposure to toxic pollutants in air, water, and foods, as well as cigarette smoke, alcohol, and ionizing radiation. Free radicals may produce oxidative damage to DNA and other cell components which accumulates with age and is suggested to be a major contributor to aging and degenerative diseases. Antioxidants may be used for reducing, eliminating, preventing, and reversing oxidative damage to tissues in an animal. Treatment of disorders and disease by orthomolecular methods is aimed at bringing such natural substances into healthful balance.... In a relatively recent phenomenon, traditional primary health care practitioners have begun to embrace orthomolecular nutrition as an enhancement to their practices. There are several forces promoting this trend, including consumer demand and the increasing eligibility of alternative health care for medical insurance coverage.... The National Institutes of Health (NIH) has established the National Center for Complementary and Alternative Medicine (NCCAM) to assist in prioritizing applications for research grants in complementary and alternative medicine (CAM). The NCCAM classification system is divided into seven major categories and includes examples of practices or preparations in each category. The biologically-based therapies category includes natural and biologically-based practices, interventions, and products. One subcategory is orthomolecular medicine, which refers to products used as nutritional and food supplements for preventive or therapeutic purposes. The NCCAM classification system lists ascorbic acid, carotenes, tocopherols, folic acid, niacin, niacinamide, pantothenic acid, pyridoxine, riboflavin, thiamine, vitamin A, vitamin D, vitamin K, biotin, choline, s-adenosylmethionine, calcium, magnesium, selenium, potassium, taurine, lysine, tyrosine, gamma-oryzanol, iodine, iron, manganese, molybdenum, boron, silicon, vanadium, co-enzyme Q.sub.10, carnitine, probiotics, glutamine, phenylalanine, glucosamine sulfate, chondroitin sulfate, lipoic acid, amino acids, phosphatidylserine, melatonin, DHEA, inositol, glandular products, fatty acids, and medium chain triglycerides as examples of orthomolecular substances. Other examples of orthomolecular substances include omega-3 fatty acids, lycopene, soy isoflavonoids, tocotrienols, chromium, zinc, and copper.

Web site: http://appft1.uspto.gov/netahtml/PTO/search-bool.html

- **PICORNAVIRUSES, VACCINES AND DIAGNOSTIC KITS**

Inventor(s): NIKLASSON, BO; (STOCKHOLM, SE)

Correspondence: James F. Haley, Jr., Esq.; C/o Fish & Neave; 1251 Avenue of the Americas - 50th Floor; New York; NY; 10020; US

Patent Application Number: 20030044960

Date filed: March 11, 1999

Abstract: A new group of picornaviruses is disclosed. The picornaviruses of the invention comprise in the non-coding region of their viral genome a nucleotide sequence which corresponds to cDNA sequence (I) or homologous sequences having at least 75% homology to the SEQ ID NO:1, and they cause mammalian disease. Further aspects of the invention comprise a protein corresponding to a protein of the picornaviruses, antiserum or antibody directed against a protein of the picornaviruses, antigen comprising a protein of the picornaviruses, diagnostic kits, vaccines, use of the picornaviruses in medicaments, particularly for the treatment or prevention of Myocarditis, Cardiomyopathia, Guillain Barr Syndrome, and Diabetes Mellitus, Multiple Sclerosis, Chronic Fatique Syndrome, Myasthenia Gravis, Amyothrophic Lateral Sclerosis, Dermatomyositis, Polymyositis, Spontaneous Abortion, and **Sudden Infant Death Syndrome,** and methods of treatment of diseases caused by the picornaviruses. 1 SEQ ID NO: 1 (Ljungan 87-012) AGTCTAGTCT TATCTTGTAT GTGTCCTGCA CTGAACTTGT 50 TTCTGTCTCT GGAGTGCTCT ACACTTCAGT AGGGGCTGTA CCCGGGCGGT 100 CCCACTCTTC ACAGGAATCT GCACAGGTGG CTTTCACCTC TGGACAGTGC 150 (I) ATTCCACACC CGCTCCACGG TAGAAGATGA TGTGTGTCTT TGCTTGTGAA 200 AAGCTTGTGA AAATCGTGTG TAGGCGTAGC GGCTACTTGA GTGCCAGCGG 250 ATTACCCCTA GTGGTAACAC TAGC

Excerpt(s): The present invention relates to new picornaviruses, proteins expressed by the viruses, antisera and antibodies directed against said viruses, antigens comprising structural proteins of said viruses, diagnostic kits, vaccines, use of said viruses, antisera or antibodies and antigens in medicaments, and methods of treating or preventing diseases caused by said viruses, such as Myocarditis, Cardiomyopathia, Guillain Barr Syndrome, and Diabetes Mellitus, Multiple Sclerosis, Chronic Fatigue Syndrome, Myasthenia Gravis, Amyothrophic Lateral Sclerosis, Dermatomyositis, Polymyositis, Spontaneous Abortion, and **Sudden infant death syndrome**.... Recently, a sudden death syndrome among Swedish orienteers has been observed. Of approximately 200 elite orienteers six died in myocarditis during 1989-1992 (1). Orienteering, aiming to find the fastest/shortest way between several checkpoints and often in forested areas, is exceptional with respect to environmental exposure. Thus it has been speculated, that the sudden deaths syndrome among orienteers is caused by a vector borne (rodent or arthropod) infectious agent.... It has now been shown in an epidemiological study that the incidence of deaths in myocarditis in northern Sweden tracked the 3-4 year population fluctuations (cycles) of bank voles (Clethrionomys glareolus) with one year time lag. Previously, it has been shown that cardioviruses, with rodents as their natural reservoir, can cause Guillain Barr Syndrome (GBS) in man, Diabetes Mellitus (DM) in mice and myocarditis in several species including non-human primates.

Web site: http://appft1.uspto.gov/netahtml/PTO/search-bool.html

- **Sleeping pad, bedding and bumpers to improve respiratory efficiency and environmental temperature of an infant and reduce the risks of sudden infant death syndrome (SIDS) and asphyxiation**

Inventor(s): Koenig, J. Frank; (Vienna, VA)

Correspondence: Shlesinger, Arkwright & Garvey Llp; 3000 South Eads Street; Arlington; VA; 22202; US

Patent Application Number: 20020178500

Date filed: July 31, 2002

Abstract: Rebreathing carbon dioxide and overheating of the infant are contributing causes of **Sudden Infant Death Syndrome** (SIDS) and asphyxiation. The characteristics of conventional crib mattresses, bedding and bumper pads contribute to rebreathing of carbon dioxide and overheating of the infant and may be contributing environmental causes of SIDS, asphyxiation, apnea syndromes and hypoventilation. The present invention consists of improved sleeping pads, beddings and bumper pads which reduce rebreathing of carbon dioxide and overheating and provide increased crib ventilation to stimulate breathing.

Excerpt(s): This application is a continuation of U.S. application Ser. No. 09/560,139, filed Apr. 28, 2000, which is a continuation-in-part of U.S.

application Ser. No. 08/551,319, filed Nov. 1, 1995, and each of which is incorporated herein by reference.... The present invention relates to apparatus for reducing the risk of **sudden infant death syndrome,** asphyxiation, apnea syndrome and hypoventilation through the use of improved sleeping pads, bedding and bumper pads within a crib or the like to improve the respiratory efficiency and environmental temperature of an infant.... Sudden infant death syndrome (SIDS) is the leading cause of postneonatal infant death in the United States. About 7,000 deaths occur each year from SIDS. In addition, many infants die each year of asphyxiation while in a crib.

Web site: http://appft1.uspto.gov/netahtml/PTO/search-bool.html

- **Use of somatostatin receptor agonists in the treatment of human disorders of sleep hypoxia and oxygen deprivation**

Inventor(s): Young, Charles W.; (New York, NY)

Correspondence: Frommer Lawrence & Haug; 745 Fifth Avenue- 10th Fl.; New York; NY; 10151; US

Patent Application Number: 20030083241

Date filed: October 25, 2002

Abstract: The invention relates to a method of treating diverse human disorders that may arise, in part, out of sleep hypoxia and oxygen deprivation occurring in the context of sleep apnea/hypopnea disturbances. The disorders that may be treated by the invention comprise gastroesophageal reflux disease (GERD), asthma-associated gastroesophageal reflux (GER), GER-associated asthma, asthma, cardiomyopathy, cardioarrhythmia, congestive heart failure, **sudden infant death syndrome,** and diverse neurologic conditions. The mode of treatment uses somatostatin receptor ligands (SstRLs), particularly somatostatin-receptor agonists. The invention concerns the method of treatment utilizing, and compositions comprising SstRLs and somatostatin receptor agonists, including agonists of the somatostatin receptor types 2 and 5, particularly, the type 2A receptor (SsR-2A), including octreotide and lanreotide.

Excerpt(s): The invention relates to a method of using somatostatin receptor agonists to treat diverse human disorders of sleep hypoxia and oxygen deprivation, including but not limited to: 1) gastroesophageal reflux disease (GERD), asthma-associated gastroesophageal reflux (GER), GER-associated asthma, and asthma; 2) obstructive sleep apnea (OSA), and OSA-associated conditions, including GER, asthma, cardiomyopathy, cardioarrhythmia, congestive heart failure, median nerve compression neuropathy (carpal tunnel syndrome) and cognitive impairment; as well as sleep apnea-associated **sudden infant death syndrome** (SIDS), 3) central sleep apnea (CSA), as well as CSA-associated conditions, including GER, cardiomyopathy, cardioarrhythmia, congestive heart failure, and cognitive impairment; 4) mixed pattern sleep apneas, including but not limited to post-vascular occlusion sleep apnea, dementia-associated sleep apnea, amyotrophic lateral sclerosis-associated sleep apnea, myasthenia gravis-associated sleep apnea, and alcoholism-related sleep apnea; 5) excess calpain-activation disorders in tissues where the injured cell population expresses somatostatin receptors; including, but not limited to the central nervous system, peripheral nerves, heart, liver, kidney, and gastrointestinal tract.... Various documents are cited in this text. Citations in the text can be by way of a citation to a document in the reference list, e.g., by way of an author(s) and document year, whereby full citation in the text is to a document that may or may not also be listed in the reference list.... There is no admission that any of the various documents cited in this text are prior art as to the present invention. Any document having as an author or inventor person or persons named as an inventor herein is a document that is not by another as to the inventor of entity herein. All documents cited in this text ("herein cited documents") and all documents cited or referenced in herein cited documents are hereby incorporated herein by reference.

Web site: http://appft1.uspto.gov/netahtml/PTO/search-bool.html

Keeping Current

In order to stay informed about patents and patent applications dealing with sudden infant death syndrome, you can access the U.S. Patent Office archive via the Internet at the following Web address: **http://www.uspto.gov/patft/index.html**. You will see two broad options: (1) Issued Patent, and (2) Published Applications. To see a list of issued patents, perform the following steps: Under "Issued Patents," click "Quick Search." Then, type "sudden infant death syndrome" (or synonyms) into the "Term 1" box. After clicking on the search button, scroll down to see the various patents which have been granted to date on sudden infant death syndrome.

You can also use this procedure to view pending patent applications concerning sudden infant death syndrome. Simply go back to the following Web address: **http://www.uspto.gov/patft/index.html**. Select "Quick Search" under "Published Applications." Then proceed with the steps listed above.

Vocabulary Builder

Alertness: A state of readiness to detect and respond to certain specified small changes occurring at random intervals in the environment. [NIH]

Alternans: Ipsilateral abducens palsy and facial paralysis and contralateral hemiplegia of the limbs, due to a nuclear or infranuclear lesion in the pons. [NIH]

Anchorage: In dentistry, points of retention of fillings and artificial restorations and appliances. [NIH]

Antibiotic: A substance usually produced by vegetal micro-organisms capable of inhibiting the growth of or killing bacteria. [NIH]

Antiserum: The blood serum obtained from an animal after it has been immunized with a particular antigen. It will contain antibodies which are specific for that antigen as well as antibodies specific for any other antigen with which the animal has previously been immunized. [NIH]

Discrimination: The act of qualitative and/or quantitative differentiation between two or more stimuli. [NIH]

Dysostosis: Defective bone formation. [NIH]

Efferent: Nerve fibers which conduct impulses from the central nervous system to muscles and glands. [NIH]

ELISA: A sensitive analytical technique in which an enzyme is complexed to an antigen or antibody. A substrate is then added which generates a color proportional to the amount of binding. This method can be adapted to a solid-phase technique. [NIH]

Endorphin: Opioid peptides derived from beta-lipotropin. Endorphin is the most potent naturally occurring analgesic agent. It is present in pituitary, brain, and peripheral tissues. [NIH]

Fatigue: The feeling of weariness of mind and body. [NIH]

Gravis: Eruption of watery blisters on the skin among those handling animals and animal products. [NIH]

Ionizing: Radiation comprising charged particles, e. g. electrons, protons, alpha-particles, etc., having sufficient kinetic energy to produce ionization by collision. [NIH]

Joint: The point of contact between elements of an animal skeleton with the parts that surround and support it. [NIH]

Pauling: The breath is passed through a cold trap consisting of a stainless-steel tube chilled by dry ice; the condensate is then assayed by gas chromatography and mass spectroscopy. [NIH]

Stimulants: Any drug or agent which causes stimulation. [NIH]

Talc: A native magnesium silicate. [NIH]

Unconscious: Experience which was once conscious, but was subsequently rejected, as the "personal unconscious". [NIH]

CHAPTER 5. BOOKS ON SUDDEN INFANT DEATH SYNDROME

Overview

This chapter provides bibliographic book references relating to sudden infant death syndrome. You have many options to locate books on sudden infant death syndrome. The simplest method is to go to your local bookseller and inquire about titles that they have in stock or can special order for you. Some parents, however, prefer online sources (e.g. **www.amazon.com** and **www.bn.com**). In addition to online booksellers, excellent sources for book titles on sudden infant death syndrome include the Combined Health Information Database and the National Library of Medicine. Once you have found a title that interests you, visit your local public or medical library to see if it is available for loan.

Book Summaries: Federal Agencies

The Combined Health Information Database collects various book abstracts from a variety of healthcare institutions and federal agencies. To access these summaries, go directly to the following hyperlink: **http://chid.nih.gov/detail/detail.html**. You will need to use the "Detailed Search" option. To find book summaries, use the drop boxes at the bottom of the search page where "You may refine your search by." Select the dates and language you prefer. For the format option, select "Monograph/Book." Now type "sudden infant death syndrome" (or synonyms) into the "For these words:" box. You will only receive results on books. You should check back periodically with this database which is updated every 3 months. The following is a typical result when searching for books on sudden infant death syndrome:

- **Sudden Infant Death Syndrome: Trying to Understand the Mystery**

  Source: McLean, VA: National Sudden Infant Death Syndrome Resource Center. February 1994. 56 p.

  Contact: Available from National SIDS Resource Center, Suite 450, 2070 Chain Bridge Road, Vienna, VA 22182-2536. (703) 821-8955, (703) 821-2098 (Fax), sids@circsol.com (Email), http://www.circsol.com/sids (Website). Free of charge; distribution limited to one per customer. Order No. S106.

  Summary: Developed as a basic information resource for health professionals, social service personnel, support providers, and families of **sudden infant death syndrome** (SIDS) infants, this book discusses the basic characteristics of SIDS and its incidence, describes current theories of causation and the research behind them, examines the emotional impact of SIDS on families, and describes SIDS research and educational efforts at the Federal level. Chapter 1 provides the definition of SIDS, the most common characteristics of and risk factors for SIDS, the number of SIDS deaths by age for 1988 and 1989, how professionals diagnose SIDS, the importance of autopsies in SIDS cases, and the value of the death certificate. Chapter 2 reviews current theories and research on SIDS in the areas of epidemiology and biomedicine (e.g., fetal predisposition, arousal response, brainstem abnormalities) and on the topics of monitoring, sleep position, and bedding. Chapter 3 examines the impact of SIDS on parents, family, and the community. This chapter covers common grief reactions of parents to the loss of a child; the impact of a SIDS death on siblings, relatives, and child care providers; and the importance of community support for SIDS families. Chapter 4 describes Federal initiatives in SIDS research and services by the National Institute of Child Health and Human Development, the Maternal and Child Health Bureau, the Centers for Disease Control and Prevention, the Food and Drug Administration, the Consumer Product Safety Commission, and other collaborative interagency efforts. Chapter 5 reviews milestones in the history of SIDS dating from 1834 to 1992, including the publication of early medical findings on sudden infant death, the founding of parent and professional organizations, dates of the international SIDS conferences, the passage of significant legislation, and the initiation of major research programs. Appendices include a glossary of terms and a listing of 30 references.

- **A Baby Dies a Family Grieves: The Clergy's Response to Sudden Infant Death Syndrome**

  Source: Berkeley, CA: California SIDS Program/CAPHND. June 1991. 16 p.

Contact: Available from California Sudden Infant Death Syndrome Program, 5330 Primrose Drive, Suite 231, Fair Oaks, CA 95628-3542. (916) 536-0146, (800) 369-7437 (in CA), (916) 536-0167 (Fax). Free to residents of CA; $1.20 each to residents of other States.

Summary: Directed at members of the clergy, this booklet provides basic information about **sudden infant death syndrome** (SIDS) and discusses the range of emotions families are likely to experience after the sudden loss of an infant. The booklet offers helpful advice to clergy on ways of responding to the family's grief and acknowledging the importance of the baby's life. Clergy can also help the family by explaining the specific religious traditions of the family's faith, helping with funeral arrangements, and providing continuing support to the family after the funeral.

- **A Little Friend is Gone: A Book for Kids Dealing With SIDS (Sudden Infant Death Syndrome)**

  Source: Denver, CO: The Colorado SIDS Program, Inc. 1994. 18 p.

  Contact: Colorado SIDS Program, Inc., 6825 E. Tennessee Avenue, Suite 300, Denver, CO 80224-1631. (303) 320-7771, (800) 332-1018 (in CO), (888) 285-7437 (Nationwide), (303) 322-8775 (Fax). $3.00, postage included.

  Summary: The goal of this book is to provide day care playmates of **sudden infant death syndrome** (SIDS) babies with information on SIDS that is geared to their level of understanding and that will help alleviate the fear they may feel following a SIDS death. The book was written for use by day care providers with children who are dealing with a SIDS death. The book tells children how many babies die of SIDS each year; that no one can cause SIDS to happen; that there are many things that SIDS is not (e.g., it is not catching, it cannot be predicted); and that when a baby is found not breathing, it is a very frightening and confusing time. Children are encouraged to talk about the people who tried to help the baby and what they did to help, to write down what they remember most about their little friend, to tell the baby's family how they feel about the death, and to send a sympathy card. The first page of the book is a dedication page that children can fill in to dedicate the book to their little day care friend.

- **Crib death: Sudden infant death syndrome**

  Source: Rockville, MD: Health Services Administration (DHHS/PHS), Bureau of Community Health Services. 1980. 20 p.

  Contact: Available from National SIDS Resource Center, Suite 450, 2070 Chain Bridge Road, Vienna, VA 22182-2536. (703) 821-8955, (703) 821-

2098 (Fax), sids@circsol.com (E-mail), http://www.circsol.com/sids (Web site). Free of charge; distribution limited to one per requestor. Order No. S17, DHHS Publication No. (HSA) 81-5262.

Summary: This book provides a very basic description of **sudden infant death syndrome** (SIDS) in easy-to-understand language. The book presents information on what is known and not known about SIDS, emphasizes that these infants' deaths are no one's fault, explains that everyone will probably react differently to the death, provides suggestions to families for coping with the death, advises parents on how to explain the death to their other children, and reminds parents that no subsequent baby can take the place of the one who died. Printed in large type. The book also is available from the National SIDS Resource Center in Spanish. Chinese, Japanese, Korean, Tagalog, and Vietnamese versions are available from the California SIDS Program, (916) 536-0146.

- **Facts and Feelings: Sudden Infant Death Syndrome**

  Source: Sacramento, CA: California SIDS Program. 1990. 16 p.

  Contact: Available from California Sudden Infant Death Syndrome Program, 5330 Primrose Drive, Suite 231, Fair Oaks, CA 95628-3542. (916) 536- 0146, (800) 369-7437 (in CA), (916) 536-0167 (Fax). Free to residents of CA; $0.78 each for residents of other States.

  Summary: This booklet is designed especially for families and caregivers who have experienced a **sudden infant death syndrome** (SIDS) loss. The booklet provides information on what happens in a SIDS death; what causes SIDS; whether anyone is at fault in a SIDS death; whether the baby suffered; whether the baby vomited, choked, or suffocated; whether SIDS is contagious; whether older children can die of SIDS; whether SIDS is caused by DTP shots or child abuse; whether breast feeding helps to prevent SIDS; whether SIDS is hereditary; the feelings experienced by bereaved parents, which are often very different; the effects of the death on surviving siblings; and where families can go to get help and support. The booklet reminds child care providers that they, too, should seek out help and support. Contact information for the California SIDS Program and two national support groups is provided. The booklet also is available in Spanish (MCS000130).

- **Helping Children Grieve: Sudden Infant Death Syndrome**

  Source: Sacramento, CA: California SIDS Program. 1993. 8 p.

  Contact: Available from California Sudden Infant Death Syndrome Program, 5330 Primrose Drive, Suite 231, Fair Oaks, CA 95628-3542. (916)

536-0146, (800) 369-7437 (in CA), (916) 536-0167 (Fax). Free to residents of CA; $0.46 each for residents of other States.

Summary: This booklet is directed at persons who care for children who have lost a sibling to **sudden infant death syndrome** (SIDS), including parents, grandparents, childcare providers, clergy, teachers, and other friends and relatives. When a baby dies suddenly with no warning, the whole family must cope with confusing emotions. Surviving siblings need a way to express their feelings, they need help and support, and they need to feel loved and valued. The booklet discusses the types of emotions that children may feel while grieving for an infant sibling who has died, including fear, anger, guilt, and sadness. The booklet also discusses when parents or others should worry about a child's reactions to the death; the importance of everyone talking about the death; what one should and should not say about where the baby went; siblings' participation in the funeral; ways in which siblings can remember the brother or sister who died; and how the level of understanding of death differs with a child's age. The booklet also is available in Spanish (MCS000481).

- **Sudden infant death syndrome: A guide for child care providers. Revised edition**

Source: Salt Lake City, UT: Utah Department of Health. December 1997. 10 p.

Contact: Available from Utah Department of Health, Division of Community and Family Health Services, Sudden Infant Death Program, 288 North 1460 West, P.O. Box 142001, Salt Lake City, UT 84114-2001. (801) 538-9970, (800) 826-9662 (UT Baby Hotline), (801) 538-9409 (Fax), awest@doh.state.ut.us (E-mail), http://161.119.100.19/ (Web site).

Summary: This booklet is intended to help child care providers understand **sudden infant death syndrome** (SIDS), know what to do in an emergency situation, and know what to do if an infant dies of SIDS while in their care. The following topics are covered: the definition of SIDS; what SIDS is and is not; what causes SIDS; who is at risk for SIDS; what child care providers can do to reduce the risk of SIDS occurring; standards for safe cribs and bedding; the danger of letting an infant sleep on a sofa, waterbed, adult bed, or youth bed; what to do if an infant or child is found not breathing; what to expect if an infant dies and a death investigation is initiated; how to talk to the parents about what happened; emotions that parents are likely to experience after a SIDS death; how to explain the death to other children in the home; common expressions of children's grief; and the ways in which grief may manifest itself in child care workers. The booklet includes a personal narrative written by a child care provider who experienced a SIDS death and a list of emergency numbers for providers in the Salt Lake City, Utah, area.

- **Sudden Infant Death Syndrome: Some Facts You Should Know**

  Source: McLean, VA: National Sudden Infant Death Syndrome Resource Center. May 1994. 11 p.

  Contact: Available from National SIDS Resource Center, Suite 450, 2070 Chain Bridge Road, Vienna, VA 22182-2536. (703) 821-8955, (703) 821-2098 (Fax), sids@circsol.com (Email), http://www.circsol.com/sids (Website). Free of charge; distribution limited to one per customer. Order No. S110.

  Summary: This booklet provides a brief overview of the facts known to date concerning the causes, characteristics, and consequences of **sudden infant death syndrome** (SIDS). The booklet covers the following topics: what SIDS is and is not; why finding a cause for SIDS is so problematic; the importance of autopsies in SIDS cases; the infants who are at greatest risk for SIDS; the known risk factors for SIDS; the number of infants who die of SIDS each year; common parental reactions to the sudden, unexpected death of an infant; the effects of a SIDS death on siblings, relatives, and other caregivers; and where SIDS families can find peer support. Contact information is given for three organizations that provide SIDS families with information and support.

- **Sudden Infant Death Syndrome: Information, Services and Support**

  Source: Rancho Cordova, CA: California SIDS Program. 1999. 9 p.

  Contact: Available from California SIDS Program, 3164 Gold Camp, Suite 220, Rancho Cordova, CA 95670. (916) 463-0146, (800) 369-7437 (in CA), (916) 463-0167 (Fax), info@californiasids.com (E-mail), http://www.californiasids.com (Web Site). Free to CA residents; $0.50 each plus shipping and handling for residents of other states.

  Summary: This booklet provides basic information on **sudden infant death syndrome** (SIDS) and a description of the services the California SIDS Program offers to the residents of that state. The mission of the California SIDS Program is to help reduce the emotional suffering of SIDS families and caregivers, improve the knowledge and skills of people who interact with SIDS families, increase public awareness and knowledge of SIDS, collect and monitor data on SIDS, and encourage medical research. Through its toll-free information line the program provides California residents crisis intervention resources; assistance in identifying local resources for grief counseling and other support services; and referrals to local public health professionals, parent support groups, and trained peer counselors. The California SIDS Program also produces a wide array of educational materials in English and Spanish that are free to all residents and that can be purchased by out-of-state residents for a minimal amount of money. Program staff members conduct training sessions throughout the state for a wide variety of professionals, including emergency department personnel, public health nurses, coroners, medical examiners, pathologists, childcare workers, foster parents, and mortuary professionals. Training sessions also are available to SIDS parents and others who are interested in volunteering as peer counselors and support group facilitators. The program also maintains a roster of speakers for presentations on SIDS within the community, publishes a semi-annual newsletter, and coordinates a conference each October.

- **Sudden Infant Death Syndrome (SIDS): What Childcare Providers Should Know. Revised Edition**

  Source: Seattle, WA: SIDS Foundation of Washington. 1996. 4 p.

  Contact: Available from SIDS Foundation of Washington, 4649 Sunnyside Avenue N., Room 328, Seattle, WA 98103. (206) 548-9290 (Seattle), (509) 456-0505 (Spokane), (800) 533-0376 (WA, ID, OR), (206) 548-9445 (Fax), sids- wa@zipcon.net (Email).

  Summary: This booklet provides child care providers with information about **sudden infant death syndrome** (SIDS). The booklet covers the following topics: facts about the incidence of SIDS in Washington State; the investigative process that the law requires after every unexplained infant death and questions that investigators will probably ask the provider; some basic facts about SIDS that child care providers should know; causes of death that are not the cause of SIDS (e.g., a contagious illness, choking, suffocation, child abuse); emotions the child care provider may feel after experiencing a SIDS death; how parents may react to the death and to the provider; and how to explain the death to the other children in the child care group. The booklet stresses that there is currently no detection, treatment, or prevention for SIDS and that no one is to blame for a SIDS death. The booklet includes emergency procedures the provider should follow in a suspected SIDS case, a form for recording emergency telephone numbers, and contact information for State chapters of the SIDS Foundation of Washington.

- **Sudden Infant Death Syndrome: Role of the Clergy. Revised Edition**

  Source: Seattle, WA: National Sudden Infant Death Syndrome Foundation. 1989. 4 p.

  Contact: Available from SIDS Foundation of Washington, 4649 Sunnyside Avenue N., Room 328, Seattle, WA 98103. (206) 548-9290 (Seattle), (509)

456-0505 (Spokane), (800) 533-0376 (WA, ID, OR only), (206) 548-9445 (Fax), sids- wa@zipcon.net (Email), http://www.zipcon.net/sids-wa (Website). $0.21 each plus shipping and handling.

Summary: This booklet provides information to clergy to prepare them for comforting bereaved parents after an infant dies from **sudden infant death syndrome** (SIDS). The booklet includes a list of facts about SIDS; legal measures that should be taken to help the parents cope effectively with the loss (i.e., conduct a thorough autopsy, use the term 'SIDS' on the death certificate rather than terms that may imply neglect, notify parents of the autopsy findings, offer parents information and counseling about SIDS); and measures that the clergy can take to help the family cope with the loss. These measures are as follows: to be in touch with one's own feelings about death, to convince the family of the blamelessness of SIDS, to act as a family advocate, to make effective use of ritual and ceremony, to provide the family with long-term support, and to make use of available resources. Ten suggested readings are listed.

- **What every child-care provider should know about sudden infant death Syndrome**

  Source: St. Louis, MO: Sudden Infant Death Syndrome Resources, Inc. 1993. 6 p.

  Contact: Available from Sudden Infant Death Syndrome Resources, Inc., 143 Grand Avenue, St. Louis, MO 63122. (314) 822-2323, (800) 421-3511 (Nationwide), (314) 822-2098 (Fax), Ahrens@stlnet.com (E-mail), http://www.crn.org/sids (Web site). Copies up to 100 are free of charge; $10.00 shipping and handling is charged for each group of 100 copies.

  Summary: This booklet, part of the SIDS Building Blocks Program, presents information on **sudden infant death syndrome** for child care providers. The booklet lists the services that **Sudden Infant Death Syndrome** Resources, Inc., in St. Louis, Missouri, provides to families, caregivers, and professionals who have experienced a SIDS death; describes the emergency procedures that child care providers should follow if they find an infant unresponsive; provides basic facts about SIDS; discusses causes of death (i.e., contagious illness, child abuse, choking) that are not related to SIDS; describes infant care practices that child care providers should adopt to reduce the risk for SIDS (e.g., nonsmoking environment, back sleep position, use of a safe crib and bedding); describes the reactions that providers are likely to experience after a SIDS death; and outlines the ways in which **Sudden Infant Death Syndrome** Resources, Inc., can help providers survive a SIDS death.

Book Summaries: Online Booksellers

Commercial Internet-based booksellers, such as Amazon.com and Barnes&Noble.com, offer summaries which have been supplied by each title's publisher. Some summaries also include customer reviews. Your local bookseller may have access to in-house and commercial databases that index all published books (e.g. Books in Print®). The following have been recently listed with online booksellers as relating to sudden infant death syndrome (sorted alphabetically by title; follow the hyperlink to view more details at Amazon.com):

- **Babies sleep safest on their backs a resource kit for reducing the risk of Sudden Infant Death Syndrome (SIDS) in African American communities (SuDoc HE 20.9202:B 11/KIT)** by U.S. Dept of Health and Human Services; ISBN: B000114N2Y;
http://www.amazon.com/exec/obidos/ASIN/B000114N2Y/icongroupinterna

- **Back to sleep : reduce the risk of sudden infant death syndrome (SIDS) (SuDoc HE 20.2:SL 2/998)** by U.S. Dept of Health and Human Services; ISBN: B00010YVUO;
http://www.amazon.com/exec/obidos/ASIN/B00010YVUO/icongroupinterna

- **Control of Breathing During Development: Apnea of the Newborn and Sudden Infant Death Syndrome: Colloquium Nancy-Pone-A-Mousson, France September 7** by Charlotte Catz, et al; ISBN: 3805559755;
http://www.amazon.com/exec/obidos/ASIN/3805559755/icongroupinterna

- **Cot Deaths: Coping with Sudden Infant Death Syndrome (A Life Crisis Book)** by Jacquelynn Luben; ISBN: 0722512554;
http://www.amazon.com/exec/obidos/ASIN/0722512554/icongroupinterna

- **Crib Death**; ISBN: 0879931752;
http://www.amazon.com/exec/obidos/ASIN/0879931752/icongroupinterna

- **Crib Death: Scourge of Infants, Shame of Society** by Richard H. Raring; ISBN: 068248122X;
http://www.amazon.com/exec/obidos/ASIN/068248122X/icongroupinterna

- **Crib Death: The Sudden Infant Death Syndrome** by Warren G. Guntheroth; ISBN: 0879936185;

http://www.amazon.com/exec/obidos/ASIN/0879936185/icongroupin
terna

- **Histopathology for the Sudden Infant Death Syndrome** by Valdes-Daperna, Valdez-Depena; ISBN: 1881041050;
  http://www.amazon.com/exec/obidos/ASIN/1881041050/icongroupin
  terna

- **Mothers Bereaved by Stillbirth, Neonatal Death or Sudden Infant Death Syndrome** by M.Frances Boyle; ISBN: 1859721494;
  http://www.amazon.com/exec/obidos/ASIN/1859721494/icongroupin
  terna

- **Pludselig spµdbarnsd²d i Norden : resultater fra det nordiske studie 1990-1996 af pludselig og uforklarlig spµdbarnsd²d krybbed²d/vugged²d = Sudden infant death in the Nordic countries : results of the Nordic study of sudden infant death syndrome, 1990-1996**; ISBN: 9289301163;
  http://www.amazon.com/exec/obidos/ASIN/9289301163/icongroupin
  terna

- **Proceedings of the Second Sudden Infant Death Syndrome Family International Conference: Sids - What Does the Future Hold?** by C. McMillan (Editor); ISBN: 0916859525;
  http://www.amazon.com/exec/obidos/ASIN/0916859525/icongroupin
  terna

- **Sids: A Parent's Guide to Understanding and Preventing Sudden Infant Death Syndrome** by William Sears; ISBN: 0316779539;
  http://www.amazon.com/exec/obidos/ASIN/0316779539/icongroupin
  terna

- **Sudden Death in Infancy: The 'Cot Death' Syndrome** by Bernard Knight; ISBN: 0571130666;
  http://www.amazon.com/exec/obidos/ASIN/0571130666/icongroupin
  terna

- **Sudden Infant Death Syndrome** by Tyson J. Tildon, et al; ISBN: 0126910502;
  http://www.amazon.com/exec/obidos/ASIN/0126910502/icongroupin
  terna

- **Sudden Infant Death Syndrome**; ISBN: 3805548923;
  http://www.amazon.com/exec/obidos/ASIN/3805548923/icongroupin
  terna

- **Sudden Infant Death Syndrome** by Jan Culbertson, et al; ISBN: 034049381X;

http://www.amazon.com/exec/obidos/ASIN/034049381X/icongroupin
terna

- **Sudden Infant Death Syndrome** by Byard & Krous; ISBN: 0412800004;
  http://www.amazon.com/exec/obidos/ASIN/0412800004/icongroupin
  terna

- **Sudden Infant Death Syndrome - A Medical Dictionary, Bibliography, and Annotated Research Guide to I** by Icon Health Publications; ISBN: 0597840822;
  http://www.amazon.com/exec/obidos/ASIN/0597840822/icongroupin
  terna

- **Sudden Infant Death Syndrome (Clinical Series)** by Robert D. Walker; ISBN: 0850841402;
  http://www.amazon.com/exec/obidos/ASIN/0850841402/icongroupin
  terna

- **Sudden Infant Death Syndrome (SIDS) infant death programs : centers : National Sudden Infant Death Syndrome/Infant Death Program Support Center, National Center for Cultural Competence, National Sudden Infant Death Syndrome Resource Center (SuDoc HE 20.9202:IN 3/2)** by U.S. Dept of Health and Human Services; ISBN: B000113QYU;
  http://www.amazon.com/exec/obidos/ASIN/B000113QYU/icongroup
  interna

- **Sudden Infant Death Syndrome (Sids: Report of the Expert Working Group)** by Paul Turner; ISBN: 0113213905;
  http://www.amazon.com/exec/obidos/ASIN/0113213905/icongroupin
  terna

- **Sudden Infant Death Syndrome: Journal: Pediatrician** by Torleiv Rognum (Editor); ISBN: 8200224198;
  http://www.amazon.com/exec/obidos/ASIN/8200224198/icongroupin
  terna

- **Sudden Infant Death Syndrome: Medical Aspects and Psychological Management (John Hopkins Series in Contemporary Medicine and Public Health)** by Jan L. Culbertson (Editor), et al; ISBN: 0801836794;
  http://www.amazon.com/exec/obidos/ASIN/0801836794/icongroupin
  terna

- **Sudden Infant Death Syndrome: Problems, Progress and Possibilities** by Roger W., MD Byard (Editor), Henry F., MD Krous (Editor); ISBN: 0340759178;
  http://www.amazon.com/exec/obidos/ASIN/0340759178/icongroupin
  terna

- **Sudden Infant Death Syndrome: Proceedings.** by 2D, sea International Conference on Causes of Sudden Death in Infants; ISBN: 0295950870; http://www.amazon.com/exec/obidos/ASIN/0295950870/icongroupin terna

- **Sudden Infant Death Syndrome: Risk Factors and Basic Mechanisms** by Ronald M. Harper, Howard J. Hoffman (Editor); ISBN: 0893352489; http://www.amazon.com/exec/obidos/ASIN/0893352489/icongroupin terna

- **Sudden Infant Death Syndrome: The Possible Role of "the Fear Paralysis Reflex"** by Birger Kaada (Editor), et al; ISBN: 8200182045; http://www.amazon.com/exec/obidos/ASIN/8200182045/icongroupin terna

- **Sudden Infant Death Syndrome: Who Can Help and How** by Charles Corr (Editor), et al; ISBN: 0826167209; http://www.amazon.com/exec/obidos/ASIN/0826167209/icongroupin terna

- **The 2002 Official Patient's Sourcebook on Sudden Infant Death Syndrome** by James N. Parker (Editor), Philip M. Parker (Editor); ISBN: 0597832072; http://www.amazon.com/exec/obidos/ASIN/0597832072/icongroupin terna

- **The Best-Kept Secret to Raising a Healthy Child...and the Possible Prevention of Sudden Infant Death Syndrome (SIDS)** by Dr. Craig Wehrenberg, Dr. Tracey Mulhall-Wehrenberg; ISBN: 0615114857; http://www.amazon.com/exec/obidos/ASIN/0615114857/icongroupin terna

- **The Discovery of Sudden Infant Death Syndrome: Lessons in the Practice of Political Medicine** by Abraham B. Bergman; ISBN: 0295966017; http://www.amazon.com/exec/obidos/ASIN/0295966017/icongroupin terna

- **The Infant Survival Guide: Protecting Your Baby from the Dangers of Crib Death, Vaccines and Other Environmental Hazards** by Lendon H., Md. Smith, et al; ISBN: 1890572128; http://www.amazon.com/exec/obidos/ASIN/1890572128/icongroupin terna

- **The Sudden infant death syndrome : cardiac and respiratory mechanisms and interventions**; ISBN: 0897664639; http://www.amazon.com/exec/obidos/ASIN/0897664639/icongroupin terna

- **The Sudden Infant Death Syndrome: Cardiac and Respiratory Mechanisms and Interventions (Annals of the New York Academy of Sciences, Vol 533)** by Peter J. Schwartz, David P. Southall; ISBN: 0897664620;
  http://www.amazon.com/exec/obidos/ASIN/0897664620/icongroupin terna

- **Urea and Non-Protein Nitrogen Metabolism in Infants: With Special Reference to the Sudden Infant Death Syndrome (Sids** by Mary George; ISBN: 9155451411;
  http://www.amazon.com/exec/obidos/ASIN/9155451411/icongroupin terna

Chapters on Sudden Infant Death Syndrome

Frequently, sudden infant death syndrome will be discussed within a book, perhaps within a specific chapter. In order to find chapters that are specifically dealing with sudden infant death syndrome, an excellent source of abstracts is the Combined Health Information Database. You will need to limit your search to book chapters and sudden infant death syndrome using the "Detailed Search" option. Go directly to the following hyperlink: **http://chid.nih.gov/detail/detail.html**. To find book chapters, use the drop boxes at the bottom of the search page where "You may refine your search by." Select the dates and language you prefer, and the format option "Book Chapter." By making these selections and typing in "sudden infant death syndrome" (or synonyms) into the "For these words:" box, you will only receive results on chapters in books. The following is a typical result when searching for book chapters on sudden infant death syndrome:

- **Existing Resources**

  Source: in Corr, C.A., Fuller, H., Barnickol, C.A., Corr, D.M. Sudden Infant Death Syndrome: Who Can Help and How. New York: Springer Publishing Co. 1991. 218-239 p.

  Contact: Available from Springer Publishing Co., 536 Broadway, New York, NY 10012-3955. (212) 431-4370, (212) 941-7842 (Fax), springer@thorn.net (Email), http://www.libertyweb.com/springer.html (Website). $34.95 plus $4.00 shipping and handling. ISBN 0-8261-6720-9.

  Summary: This chapter identifies and describes organizations and resources that offer support to families of **sudden infant death syndrome** (SIDS) victims and training to professionals who come in contact with them. The organizations include those that are devoted to SIDS families and those that support bereaved families no matter how their children died. Print resources are divided into the following categories: SIDS-related literature for scientists and researchers; SIDS-related books for general readers; miscarriage, stillbirth, and neonatal death; parental bereavement; loss, grief, and mourning; and children, adolescents, and death. The audiovisual resources, mainly videotapes, include general introductions to SIDS; videos for training first responders; videos that show parents' reactions to a SIDS death and what they need to cope; and audiovisuals for helping professionals who work with SIDS families. The final section of the chapter summarizes 12 videos appropriate for parents and siblings who have experienced perinatal loss and for the professionals who work with them. Availability information for audiotapes and videotapes from four national conferences on SIDS and other fetal/infant death is included.

Directories

In addition to the references and resources discussed earlier in this chapter, a number of directories relating to sudden infant death syndrome have been published that consolidate information across various sources. These too might be useful in gaining access to additional guidance on sudden infant death syndrome. The Combined Health Information Database lists the following, which you may wish to consult in your local medical library:[22]

- **Pediatric resource guide**

   Source: New York, NY: Pfizer Pediatric Health. 1998. 29 pp.

   Contact: Available from Pfizer, Inc, 235 East 42nd Street, New York, NY 10017-5755.

   Summary: Produced in conjunction with Physician's Desk Reference, this booklet is designed to assist physicians in directing patients with special needs to suitable information sources and support groups. It includes contact information and descriptions for support groups in the following categories: advocacy; breastfeeding; child care; children with special

---

[22] You will need to limit your search to "Directories" and sudden infant death syndrome using the "Detailed Search" option. Go directly to the following hyperlink: **http://chid.nih.gov/detail/detail.html**. To find directories, use the drop boxes at the bottom of the search page where "You may refine your search by". For publication date, select "All Years", select language and the format option "Directory". By making these selections and typing in "sudden infant death syndrome" (or synonyms) into the "For these words:" box, you will only receive results on directories dealing with sudden infant death syndrome. You should check back periodically with this database as it is updated every three months.

needs; injury prevention and safety; maternal and child health information; mental health; multiple births; nutrition; parenting; physical activity; special issues; and **sudden infant death syndrome.**

- **Directory of Illinois bereavement support groups (for families who have experienced sudden, unexpected infant death). Revised edition**

Source: Springfield, IL: Illinois Department of Public Health. June 1996. 12 p.

Contact: Available from Illinois Department of Public Health, Division of Health Assessment and Screening, Statewide SIDS/Infant Mortality Program, 535 West Jefferson Street, Springfield, IL 62761. (217) 557-2931, (217) 524-2831 (Fax). Single copies free of charge.

Summary: The Illinois Statewide **Sudden Infant Death Syndrome** (SIDS) Program provides professional counseling services not only to SIDS families but to any family experiencing a sudden, unexpected infant death. In addition to receiving professional counseling, many families also are interested in talking with parents who have suffered a similar loss. This directory was compiled so that families experiencing a sudden, unexpected infant death or a SIDS death could locate a support group in which they might be interested. Although some counties in the state do not have a support group, this directory will help identify the support group most geographically accessible to a particular family. The support groups are organized by county. Each listing includes the name of the support group; the name of a contact person; a telephone number; and for most listings, meeting locations, days, and times. The support groups listed are sponsored by the following: the Statewide SIDS Program; various bereavement organizations, including the SIDS Alliance of Illinois, Inc., SHARE, The Compassionate Friends, Healing Our Lost Dreams, Bereaved Parents of the USA, and Bereavement Services/RTS; and numerous hospitals, medical centers, and churches.

General Home References

In addition to references for sudden infant death syndrome, you may want a general home medical guide that spans all aspects of home healthcare. The following list is a recent sample of such guides (sorted alphabetically by title; hyperlinks provide rankings, information, and reviews at Amazon.com):

- **American Academy of Pediatrics Guide to Your Child's Symptoms : The Official, Complete Home Reference, Birth Through Adolescence** by Donald Schiff (Editor), et al; Paperback - 256 pages (January 1997),

Villard Books; ISBN: 0375752579;
http://www.amazon.com/exec/obidos/ASIN/0375752579/icongroupinter
na

- **The Children's Hospital Guide to Your Child's Health and Development** by Alan D. Woolf (Editor), et al; Hardcover - 796 pages, 1st edition (January 15, 2001), Perseus Books; ISBN: 073820241X;
http://www.amazon.com/exec/obidos/ASIN/073820241X/icongroupinter
na

- **Helping Your Child in the Hospital: A Practical Guide for Parents** by Nancy Keene, Rachel Prentice; Paperback - 176 pages, 3rd edition (April 15, 2002), O'Reilly & Associates; ISBN: 0596500114;
http://www.amazon.com/exec/obidos/ASIN/0596500114/icongroupinter
na

- **Medical Emergencies & Childhood Illnesses: Includes Your Child's Personal Health Journal (Parent Smart)** by Penny A. Shore, William Sears (Contributor); Paperback - 115 pages (February 2002), Parent Kit Corporation; ISBN: 1896833187;
http://www.amazon.com/exec/obidos/ASIN/1896833187/icongroupinter
na

- **Taking Care of Your Child: A Parent's Guide to Complete Medical Care** by Robert H. Pantell, M.D., et al; Paperback - 524 pages, 6th edition (March 5, 2002), Perseus Press; ISBN: 0738206016;
http://www.amazon.com/exec/obidos/ASIN/0738206016/icongroupinter
na

Vocabulary Builder

Compassionate: A process for providing experimental drugs to very sick patients who have no treatment options. [NIH]

Hereditary: Of, relating to, or denoting factors that can be transmitted genetically from one generation to another. [NIH]

Miscarriage: Spontaneous expulsion of the products of pregnancy before the middle of the second trimester. [NIH]

CHAPTER 6. MULTIMEDIA ON SUDDEN INFANT DEATH SYNDROME

Overview

Information on sudden infant death syndrome can come in a variety of formats. Among multimedia sources, video productions, slides, audiotapes, and computer databases are often available. In this chapter, we show you how to keep current on multimedia sources of information on sudden infant death syndrome. We start with sources that have been summarized by federal agencies, and then show you how to find bibliographic information catalogued by the National Library of Medicine. If you see an interesting item, visit your local medical library to check on the availability of the title.

Video Recordings

Most medical conditions do not have a video dedicated to them. If they do, they are often rather technical in nature. An excellent source of multimedia information on sudden infant death syndrome is the Combined Health Information Database. You will need to limit your search to "video recording" and "sudden infant death syndrome" using the "Detailed Search" option. Go directly to the following hyperlink: **http://chid.nih.gov/detail/detail.html**. To find video productions, use the drop boxes at the bottom of the search page where "You may refine your search by." Select the dates and language you prefer, and the format option "Videorecording (videotape, videocassette, etc.)." By making these selections and typing "sudden infant death syndrome" (or synonyms) into the "For these words:" box, you will only receive results on video productions. The following is a typical result when searching for video recordings on sudden infant death syndrome:

- **A Critical Call: A Videotape About Sudden Infant Death Syndrome for Emergency Medical Technicians**

  Source: Minneapolis, MN: Minnesota Sudden Infant Death Center. 1989.

  Contact: Available from Minnesota Sudden Infant Death Center, Minneapolis Children's Self Care, 2525 Chicago Avenue South, Minneapolis, MN 55404. (612) 813-6285, (800) 732-3812 (in MN), (612) 813-7344 (Fax). $100.00.

  Summary: An emergency medical technician (EMT) may be the first person to receive a call that a baby has died. This 21-minute videotape outlines what EMTs should do in response to a **sudden infant death syndrome** (SIDS) death. The video addresses transporting the victim, making skilled observations while at the scene, and documenting what was observed and done at the scene. The video also illustrates the types of emotional displays the EMT may encounter at the scene and how they should be handled. For example, acute grief reactions may affect the family's or caregiver's ability to reason and act. Information also is provided on critical incident stress and how EMTs can overcome it, the roles of physician and medical examiner in a SIDS case, and the differences in responding to infant death in the home or in a child care facility. An instructor's guide accompanies the video. The guide provides basic information about SIDS, reviews the EMT's role in potential SIDS cases, and provides sample case studies to promote discussion among class participants. [Note: This video predates the 1992 announcement by the American Academy of Pediatrics regarding prone sleep position and the 'Back to Sleep' campaign and, therefore, does not discuss the importance of back or side sleep in reducing the risk for SIDS].

- **Back to Sleep. Sudden Infant Death Syndrome: A Video on Helping to Reduce the Risk**

  Source: Bethesda, MD: National Institute of Child Health and Human Development (NIH). 1994.

  Contact: Available from Back to Sleep, P.O. Box 29111, Washington, DC 20040. (800) 505-CRIB. Free of charge.

  Summary: This videorecording, a product of the national 'Back to Sleep' campaign in the United States, presents parents and child care providers with information on reducing the risk for **sudden infant death syndrome** (SIDS). The 'Back to Sleep' campaign was initiated in June 1994 to alert new parents and health professionals to sleeping position as a possible risk factor for SIDS. The video also is available in Spanish (MCS000503).

CHAPTER 7. PERIODICALS AND NEWS ON SUDDEN INFANT DEATH SYNDROME

Overview

Keeping up on the news relating to sudden infant death syndrome can be challenging. Subscribing to targeted periodicals can be an effective way to stay abreast of recent developments on sudden infant death syndrome. Periodicals include newsletters, magazines, and academic journals.

In this chapter, we suggest a number of news sources and present various periodicals that cover sudden infant death syndrome beyond and including those which are published by parent associations mentioned earlier. We will first focus on news services, and then on periodicals. News services, press releases, and newsletters generally use more accessible language, so if you do chose to subscribe to one of the more technical periodicals, make sure that it uses language you can easily follow.

News Services and Press Releases

Well before articles show up in newsletters or the popular press, they may appear in the form of a press release or a public relations announcement. One of the simplest ways of tracking press releases on sudden infant death syndrome is to search the news wires. News wires are used by professional journalists, and have existed since the invention of the telegraph. Today, there are several major "wires" that are used by companies, universities, and other organizations to announce new medical breakthroughs. In the following sample of sources, we will briefly describe how to access each service. These services only post recent news intended for public viewing.

PR Newswire

Perhaps the broadest of the wires is PR Newswire Association, Inc. To access this archive, simply go to **http://www.prnewswire.com**. Below the search box, select the option "The last 30 days." In the search box, type "sudden infant death syndrome" or synonyms. The search results are shown by order of relevance. When reading these press releases, do not forget that the sponsor of the release may be a company or organization that is trying to sell a particular product or therapy. Their views, therefore, may be biased.

Reuters Health

The Reuters' Medical News and Health eLine databases can be very useful in exploring news archives relating to sudden infant death syndrome. While some of the listed articles are free to view, others can be purchased for a nominal fee. To access this archive, go to **http://www.reutershealth.com/en/index.html** and search by "sudden infant death syndrome" (or synonyms). The following was recently listed in this archive for sudden infant death syndrome:

- **Nearly half of crib deaths tied to sleep position**
  Source: Reuters Health eLine
  Date: January 16, 2004

- **Sudden infant death syndrome linked to impaired arousal from sleep**
  Source: Reuters Medical News
  Date: December 25, 2003

- **Breastfeeding could lower risk of crib death**
  Source: Reuters Health eLine
  Date: May 22, 2002

- **Stomach bug linked to sudden infant death syndrome**
  Source: Reuters Health eLine
  Date: October 24, 2000

- **H. pylori may be implicated in sudden infant death syndrome**
  Source: Reuters Medical News
  Date: October 23, 2000

- **Pneumocystis carinii infection linked to sudden infant death syndrome**
  Source: Reuters Medical News
  Date: January 11, 2000

- **Genetic mutation linked to sudden infant death syndrome**
  Source: Reuters Medical News
  Date: July 02, 1999

The NIH

Within MEDLINEplus, the NIH has made an agreement with the New York Times Syndicate, the AP News Service, and Reuters to deliver news that can be browsed by the public. Search news releases at **http://www.nlm.nih.gov/medlineplus/alphanews_a.html.** MEDLINEplus allows you to browse across an alphabetical index. Or you can search by date at **http://www.nlm.nih.gov/medlineplus/newsbydate.html**. Often, news items are indexed by MEDLINEplus within their search engine.

Business Wire

Business Wire is similar to PR Newswire. To access this archive, simply go to **http://www.businesswire.com**. You can scan the news by industry category or company name.

Market Wire

Market Wire is more focused on technology than the other wires. To browse the latest press releases by topic, such as alternative medicine, biotechnology, fitness, healthcare, legal, nutrition, and pharmaceuticals, log on to Market Wire's Medical/Health channel at the following hyperlink **http://www.marketwire.com/mw/release_index?channel=MedicalHealth**. Market Wire's home page is **http://www.marketwire.com/mw/home**. From here, type "sudden infant death syndrome" (or synonyms) into the search box, and click on "Search News." As this service is technology oriented, you may wish to use it when searching for press releases covering diagnostic procedures or tests.

Search Engines

Free-to-view news can also be found in the news section of your favorite search engines (see the health news page at Yahoo: **http://dir.yahoo.com/Health/News_and_Media/,** or use this Web site's general news search page **http://news.yahoo.com/.** Type in "sudden infant death syndrome" (or synonyms). If you know the name of a company that is relevant to sudden infant death syndrome, you can go to any stock trading Web site (such as **www.etrade.com**) and search for the company name there. News items across various news sources are reported on indicated hyperlinks.

BBC

Covering news from a more European perspective, the British Broadcasting Corporation (BBC) allows the public free access to their news archive located at **http://www.bbc.co.uk/**. Search by "sudden infant death syndrome" (or synonyms).

Newsletters on Sudden Infant Death Syndrome

Given their focus on current and relevant developments, newsletters are often more useful to parents than academic articles. You can find newsletters using the Combined Health Information Database (CHID). You will need to use the "Detailed Search" option. To access CHID, go directly to the following hyperlink: **http://chid.nih.gov/detail/detail.html**. Your investigation must limit the search to "Newsletter" and "sudden infant death syndrome." Go to the bottom of the search page where "You may refine your search by." Select the dates and language that you prefer. For the format option, select "Newsletter." By making these selections and typing in "sudden infant death syndrome" or synonyms into the "For these words:" box, you will only receive results on newsletters. The following list was generated using the options described above:

- **Back to Sleep: A Newsletter of the Department of Human Resources Sudden Infant Death Syndrome Workgroup**

    Source: Atlanta, GA: Georgia State Dept. of Human Resources. March 1995-. 4 p.

    Contact: Available from Georgia State Department of Human Resources, Division of Public Health, Family Health Branch/Center for Family Resource Planning and Development, 2600 Skyland Drive, NE, Upper Level, Room 5, Atlanta, GA 30319. (404) 679-0531, (404) 679-0695 TTD, (404) 679-0686 (Fax), LTH1@ph.dhr.state.ga.us (Email), http://www.ph.dhr.state.ga.us (Website). Free of charge.

    Summary: This newsletter is published by the Georgia Department of Human Resources for the benefit of **sudden infant death syndrome**

(SIDS) service providers, administrators, policy makers, and families in the State of Georgia. The newsletter provides its audience with current information on SIDS research and risk factors; updates on State and national initiatives to reduce the risk for SIDS; contact information for organizations, workshops, and other sources of family bereavement support; and up-to-date resources (including the Internet) on SIDS and infant mortality.

Newsletter Articles

If you choose not to subscribe to a newsletter, you can nevertheless find references to newsletter articles. We recommend that you use the Combined Health Information Database, while limiting your search criteria to "newsletter articles." Again, you will need to use the "Detailed Search" option at **http://chid.nih.gov/detail/detail.html**. Go to the bottom of the search page where "You may refine your search by." Select the dates and language that you prefer. For the format option, select "Newsletter Article."

By making these selections, and typing in "sudden infant death syndrome" (or synonyms) into the "For these words:" box, you will only receive results on newsletter articles. You should check back periodically with this database as it is updated every 3 months. The following is a typical result when searching for newsletter articles on sudden infant death syndrome:

- **The Loss of a Multiple to SIDS**

  Source: Our Newsletter. 5(4): 10-11. December 1991.

  Contact: Available from Center for Loss in Multiple Birth, Inc. (CLIMB), c/o Jean Kollantai, P.O. Box 1064, Palmer, AK 99645. (907) 746-6123 (9 am-1 pm), (907) 274-7029 (Lisa Fleischer).

  Summary: This newsletter article consists of personal reflections excerpted from the journal of a mother who lost one of her twin daughters to **sudden infant death syndrome** (SIDS). The article covers a time period of almost 3 years, from the time the author discovered she was pregnant with twins, through the loss of one of the twins, and to the subsequent birth of another child.

CHAPTER 8. PHYSICIAN GUIDELINES AND DATABASES

Overview

Doctors and medical researchers rely on a number of information sources to help children with sudden infant death syndrome. Many will subscribe to journals or newsletters published by their professional associations or refer to specialized textbooks or clinical guides published for the medical profession. In this chapter, we focus on databases and Internet-based guidelines created or written for this professional audience.

NIH Guidelines

For the more common medical conditions, the National Institutes of Health publish guidelines that are frequently consulted by physicians. Publications are typically written by one or more of the various NIH Institutes. For physician guidelines, commonly referred to as "clinical" or "professional" guidelines, you can visit the following Institutes:

- Office of the Director (OD); guidelines consolidated across agencies available at **http://www.nih.gov/health/consumer/conkey.htm**

- National Institute of General Medical Sciences (NIGMS); fact sheets available at **http://www.nigms.nih.gov/news/facts/**

- National Library of Medicine (NLM); extensive encyclopedia (A.D.A.M., Inc.) with guidelines:
  http://www.nlm.nih.gov/medlineplus/healthtopics.html

- National Institute of Child Health and Human Development (NICHD); guidelines available at
  http://www.nichd.nih.gov/publications/pubskey.cfm

NIH Databases

In addition to the various Institutes of Health that publish professional guidelines, the NIH has designed a number of databases for professionals.[23] Physician-oriented resources provide a wide variety of information related to the biomedical and health sciences, both past and present. The format of these resources varies. Searchable databases, bibliographic citations, full text articles (when available), archival collections, and images are all available. The following are referenced by the National Library of Medicine:[24]

- **Bioethics:** Access to published literature on the ethical, legal and public policy issues surrounding healthcare and biomedical research. This information is provided in conjunction with the Kennedy Institute of Ethics located at Georgetown University, Washington, D.C.: **http://www.nlm.nih.gov/databases/databases_bioethics.html**

- **HIV/AIDS Resources:** Describes various links and databases dedicated to HIV/AIDS research: **http://www.nlm.nih.gov/pubs/factsheets/aidsinfs.html**

- **NLM Online Exhibitions:** Describes "Exhibitions in the History of Medicine": **http://www.nlm.nih.gov/exhibition/exhibition.html**. Additional resources for historical scholarship in medicine: **http://www.nlm.nih.gov/hmd/hmd.html**

- **Biotechnology Information:** Access to public databases. The National Center for Biotechnology Information conducts research in computational biology, develops software tools for analyzing genome data, and disseminates biomedical information for the better understanding of molecular processes affecting human health and disease: **http://www.ncbi.nlm.nih.gov/**

- **Population Information:** The National Library of Medicine provides access to worldwide coverage of population, family planning, and related health issues, including family planning technology and programs, fertility, and population law and policy: **http://www.nlm.nih.gov/databases/databases_population.html**

- **Cancer Information:** Access to caner-oriented databases: **http://www.nlm.nih.gov/databases/databases_cancer.html**

---

[23] Remember, for the general public, the National Library of Medicine recommends the databases referenced in MEDLINE*plus* (**http://medlineplus.gov/** or **http://www.nlm.nih.gov/medlineplus/databases.html**).
[24] See **http://www.nlm.nih.gov/databases/databases.html**.

- **Profiles in Science:** Offering the archival collections of prominent twentieth-century biomedical scientists to the public through modern digital technology: **http://www.profiles.nlm.nih.gov/**

- **Chemical Information:** Provides links to various chemical databases and references: **http://sis.nlm.nih.gov/Chem/ChemMain.html**

- **Clinical Alerts:** Reports the release of findings from the NIH-funded clinical trials where such release could significantly affect morbidity and mortality: **http://www.nlm.nih.gov/databases/alerts/clinical_alerts.html**

- **Space Life Sciences:** Provides links and information to space-based research (including NASA): **http://www.nlm.nih.gov/databases/databases_space.html**

- **MEDLINE:** Bibliographic database covering the fields of medicine, nursing, dentistry, veterinary medicine, the healthcare system, and the pre-clinical sciences: **http://www.nlm.nih.gov/databases/databases_medline.html**

- **Toxicology and Environmental Health Information (TOXNET):** Databases covering toxicology and environmental health: **http://sis.nlm.nih.gov/Tox/ToxMain.html**

- **Visible Human Interface:** Anatomically detailed, three-dimensional representations of normal male and female human bodies: **http://www.nlm.nih.gov/research/visible/visible_human.html**

While all of the above references may be of interest to physicians who study and treat sudden infant death syndrome, the following are particularly noteworthy.

The NLM Gateway[25]

The NLM (National Library of Medicine) Gateway is a Web-based system that lets users search simultaneously in multiple retrieval systems at the U.S. National Library of Medicine (NLM). It allows users of NLM services to initiate searches from one Web interface, providing "one-stop searching" for many of NLM's information resources or databases.[26] One target audience for the Gateway is the Internet user who is new to NLM's online resources and does not know what information is available or how best to search for it. This

---

[25] Adapted from NLM: http://gateway.nlm.nih.gov/gw/Cmd?Overview.x.

[26] The NLM Gateway is currently being developed by the Lister Hill National Center for Biomedical Communications (LHNCBC) at the National Library of Medicine (NLM) of the National Institutes of Health (NIH).

audience may include physicians and other healthcare providers, researchers, librarians, students, and, increasingly, parents and the public.[27] To use the NLM Gateway, simply go to the search site at **http://gateway.nlm.nih.gov/gw/Cmd**. Type "sudden infant death syndrome" (or synonyms) into the search box and click "Search." The results will be presented in a tabular form, indicating the number of references in each database category.

Results Summary

Category	Items Found
Journal Articles	6296
Books / Periodicals / Audio Visual	186
Consumer Health	941
Meeting Abstracts	11
Other Collections	77
Total	7511

HSTAT[28]

HSTAT is a free, Web-based resource that provides access to full-text documents used in healthcare decision-making.[29] HSTAT's audience includes healthcare providers, health service researchers, policy makers, insurance companies, consumers, and the information professionals who serve these groups. HSTAT provides access to a wide variety of publications, including clinical practice guidelines, quick-reference guides for clinicians, consumer health brochures, evidence reports and technology assessments from the Agency for Healthcare Research and Quality (AHRQ), as well as AHRQ's Put Prevention Into Practice.[30] Simply search by "sudden infant death syndrome" (or synonyms) at the following Web site: **http://text.nlm.nih.gov**.

---

[27] Other users may find the Gateway useful for an overall search of NLM's information resources. Some searchers may locate what they need immediately, while others will utilize the Gateway as an adjunct tool to other NLM search services such as PubMed® and MEDLINEplus®. The Gateway connects users with multiple NLM retrieval systems while also providing a search interface for its own collections. These collections include various types of information that do not logically belong in PubMed, LOCATORplus, or other established NLM retrieval systems (e.g., meeting announcements and pre-1966 journal citations). The Gateway will provide access to the information found in an increasing number of NLM retrieval systems in several phases.

[28] Adapted from HSTAT: **http://www.nlm.nih.gov/pubs/factsheets/hstat.html**.

[29] The HSTAT URL is **http://hstat.nlm.nih.gov/**.

[30] Other important documents in HSTAT include: the National Institutes of Health (NIH) Consensus Conference Reports and Technology Assessment Reports; the HIV/AIDS

Coffee Break: Tutorials for Biologists[31]

Some parents may wish to have access to a general healthcare site that takes a scientific view of the news and covers recent breakthroughs in biology that may one day assist physicians in developing treatments. To this end, we recommend "Coffee Break," a collection of short reports on recent biological discoveries. Each report incorporates interactive tutorials that demonstrate how bioinformatics tools are used as a part of the research process. Currently, all Coffee Breaks are written by NCBI staff.[32] Each report is about 400 words and is usually based on a discovery reported in one or more articles from recently published, peer-reviewed literature.[33] This site has new articles every few weeks, so it can be considered an online magazine of sorts, and intended for general background information. You can access Coffee Break at **http://www.ncbi.nlm.nih.gov/Coffeebreak/**.

Other Commercial Databases

In addition to resources maintained by official agencies, other databases exist that are commercial ventures addressing medical professionals. Here are some examples that may interest you:

- **CliniWeb International:** Index and table of contents to selected clinical information on the Internet; see **http://www.ohsu.edu/cliniweb/**.

- **Medical World Search:** Searches full text from thousands of selected medical sites on the Internet; see **http://www.mwsearch.com/**.

Treatment Information Service (ATIS) resource documents; the Substance Abuse and Mental Health Services Administration's Center for Substance Abuse Treatment (SAMHSA/CSAT) Treatment Improvement Protocols (TIP) and Center for Substance Abuse Prevention (SAMHSA/CSAP) Prevention Enhancement Protocols System (PEPS); the Public Health Service (PHS) Preventive Services Task Force's *Guide to Clinical Preventive Services*; the independent, nonfederal Task Force on Community Services *Guide to Community Preventive Services*; and the Health Technology Advisory Committee (HTAC) of the Minnesota Health Care Commission (MHCC) health technology evaluations.

[31] Adapted from **http://www.ncbi.nlm.nih.gov/Coffeebreak/Archive/FAQ.html**.

[32] The figure that accompanies each article is frequently supplied by an expert external to NCBI, in which case the source of the figure is cited. The result is an interactive tutorial that tells a biological story.

[33] After a brief introduction that sets the work described into a broader context, the report focuses on how a molecular understanding can provide explanations of observed biology and lead to therapies for diseases. Each vignette is accompanied by a figure and hypertext links that lead to a series of pages that interactively show how NCBI tools and resources are used in the research process.

The Genome Project and Sudden Infant Death Syndrome

With all the discussion in the press about the Human Genome Project, it is only natural that physicians, researchers, and parents want to know about how human genes relate to sudden infant death syndrome. In the following section, we will discuss databases and references used by physicians and scientists who work in this area.

Online Mendelian Inheritance in Man (OMIM)

The Online Mendelian Inheritance in Man (OMIM) database is a catalog of human genes and genetic disorders authored and edited by Dr. Victor A. McKusick and his colleagues at Johns Hopkins and elsewhere. OMIM was developed for the World Wide Web by the National Center for Biotechnology Information (NCBI).[34] The database contains textual information, pictures, and reference information. It also contains copious links to NCBI's Entrez database of MEDLINE articles and sequence information.

Go to **http://www.ncbi.nlm.nih.gov/Omim/searchomim.html** to search the database. Type "sudden infant death syndrome" (or synonyms) in the search box, and click "Submit Search." If too many results appear, you can narrow the search by adding the word "clinical." Each report will have additional links to related research and databases. By following these links, especially the link titled "Database Links," you will be exposed to numerous specialized databases that are largely used by the scientific community. These databases are overly technical and seldom used by the general public, but offer an abundance of information. The following is an example of the results you can obtain from the OMIM for sudden infant death syndrome:

- **Sudden Infant Death Syndrome**
  Web site:
  http://www.ncbi.nlm.nih.gov/entrez/dispomim.cgi?id=272120

---

[34] Adapted from **http://www.ncbi.nlm.nih.gov/**. Established in 1988 as a national resource for molecular biology information, NCBI creates public databases, conducts research in computational biology, develops software tools for analyzing genome data, and disseminates biomedical information--all for the better understanding of molecular processes affecting human health and disease.

Genes and Disease (NCBI - Map)

The Genes and Disease database is produced by the National Center for Biotechnology Information of the National Library of Medicine at the National Institutes of Health. This Web site categorizes each disorder by the system of the body. Go to **http://www.ncbi.nlm.nih.gov/disease/**, and browse the system pages to have a full view of important conditions linked to human genes. Since this site is regularly updated, you may wish to re-visit it from time to time. The following systems and associated disorders are addressed:

- **Immune System:** Fights invaders.
  Examples: Asthma, autoimmune polyglandular syndrome, Crohn's disease, DiGeorge syndrome, familial Mediterranean fever, immunodeficiency with Hyper-IgM, severe combined immunodeficiency.
  Web site: **http://www.ncbi.nlm.nih.gov/disease/Immune.html**

- **Metabolism:** Food and energy.
  Examples: Adreno-leukodystrophy, Atherosclerosis, Best disease, Gaucher disease, Glucose galactose malabsorption, Gyrate atrophy, Juvenile onset diabetes, Obesity, Paroxysmal nocturnal hemoglobinuria, Phenylketonuria, Refsum disease, Tangier disease, Tay-Sachs disease.
  Web site: **http://www.ncbi.nlm.nih.gov/disease/Metabolism.html**

- **Nervous System:** Mind and body.
  Examples: Alzheimer disease, Amyotrophic lateral sclerosis, Angelman syndrome, Charcot-Marie-Tooth disease, epilepsy, essential tremor, Fragile X syndrome, Friedreich's ataxia, Huntington disease, Niemann-Pick disease, Parkinson disease, Prader-Willi syndrome, Rett syndrome, Spinocerebellar atrophy, Williams syndrome.
  Web site: **http://www.ncbi.nlm.nih.gov/disease/Brain.html**

- **Signals:** Cellular messages.
  Examples: Ataxia telangiectasia, Baldness, Cockayne syndrome, Glaucoma, SRY: sex determination, Tuberous sclerosis, Waardenburg syndrome, Werner syndrome.
  Web site: **http://www.ncbi.nlm.nih.gov/disease/Signals.html**

- **Transporters:** Pumps and channels.
  Examples: Cystic Fibrosis, deafness, diastrophic dysplasia, Hemophilia A, long-QT syndrome, Menkes syndrome, Pendred syndrome, polycystic kidney disease, sickle cell anemia, Wilson's disease, Zellweger syndrome.
  Web site: **http://www.ncbi.nlm.nih.gov/disease/Transporters.html**

Entrez

Entrez is a search and retrieval system that integrates several linked databases at the National Center for Biotechnology Information (NCBI). These databases include nucleotide sequences, protein sequences, macromolecular structures, whole genomes, and MEDLINE through PubMed. Entrez provides access to the following databases:

- **3D Domains:** Domains from Entrez Structure,
  Web site: http://www.ncbi.nlm.nih.gov/entrez/query.fcgi?db=geo

- **Books:** Online books,
  Web site: http://www.ncbi.nlm.nih.gov/entrez/query.fcgi?db=books

- **Genome:** Complete genome assemblies,
  Web site: http://www.ncbi.nlm.nih.gov/entrez/query.fcgi?db=Genome

- **NCBI's Protein Sequence Information Survey Results:**
  Web site: http://www.ncbi.nlm.nih.gov/About/proteinsurvey/

- **Nucleotide Sequence Database (Genbank):**
  Web site:
  http://www.ncbi.nlm.nih.gov/entrez/query.fcgi?db=Nucleotide

- **OMIM:** Online Mendelian Inheritance in Man,
  Web site: http://www.ncbi.nlm.nih.gov/entrez/query.fcgi?db=OMIM

- **PopSet:** Population study data sets,
  Web site: http://www.ncbi.nlm.nih.gov/entrez/query.fcgi?db=Popset

- **ProbeSet:** Gene Expression Omnibus (GEO),
  Web site: http://www.ncbi.nlm.nih.gov/entrez/query.fcgi?db=geo

- **Protein Sequence Database:**
  Web site: http://www.ncbi.nlm.nih.gov/entrez/query.fcgi?db=Protein

- **PubMed:** Biomedical literature (PubMed),
  Web site: http://www.ncbi.nlm.nih.gov/entrez/query.fcgi?db=PubMed

- **Structure:** Three-dimensional macromolecular structures,
  Web site: http://www.ncbi.nlm.nih.gov/entrez/query.fcgi?db=Structure

- **Taxonomy:** Organisms in GenBank,
  Web site:
  http://www.ncbi.nlm.nih.gov/entrez/query.fcgi?db=Taxonomy

Access the Entrez system of the NCBI at the following hyperlink: **http://www.ncbi.nlm.nih.gov/entrez/query.fcgi?CMD=search&DB=genom e**, and then select the database that you would like to search. The databases available are listed in the drop box next to "Search." In the box next to "for," enter "sudden infant death syndrome" (or synonyms) and click "Go."

Jablonski's Multiple Congenital Anomaly/Mental Retardation (MCA/MR) Syndromes Database[35]

This online resource can be quite useful. It has been developed to facilitate the identification and differentiation of syndromic entities. Special attention is given to the type of information that is usually limited or completely omitted in existing reference sources due to space limitations of the printed form.

You can search across syndromes using an alphabetical index at **http://www.nlm.nih.gov/mesh/jablonski/syndrome_toc/toc_a.html.** At **http://www.nlm.nih.gov/mesh/jablonski/syndrome_db.html,** search by keyword.

The Genome Database[36]

Established at Johns Hopkins University in Baltimore, Maryland in 1990, the Genome Database (GDB) is the official central repository for genomic mapping data resulting from the Human Genome Initiative. In the spring of 1999, the Bioinformatics Supercomputing Centre (BiSC) at the Hospital for Sick Children in Toronto, Ontario assumed the management of GDB. The Human Genome Initiative is a worldwide research effort focusing on structural analysis of human DNA to determine the location and sequence of the estimated 100,000 human genes. In support of this project, GDB stores and curates data generated by researchers worldwide who are engaged in the mapping effort of the Human Genome Project (HGP). GDB's mission is to provide scientists with an encyclopedia of the human genome which is continually revised and updated to reflect the current state of scientific knowledge. Although GDB has historically focused on gene mapping, its focus will broaden as the Genome Project moves from mapping to sequence, and finally, to functional analysis.

To access the GDB, simply go to the following hyperlink: **http://www.gdb.org/.** Search "All Biological Data" by "Keyword." Type

[35] Adapted from the National Library of Medicine:
http://www.nlm.nih.gov/mesh/jablonski/about_syndrome.html.
[36] Adapted from the Genome Database:
http://gdbwww.gdb.org/gdb/aboutGDB.html#mission.

"sudden infant death syndrome" (or synonyms) into the search box, and review the results. If more than one word is used in the search box, then separate each one with the word "and" or "or" (using "or" might be useful when using synonyms). This database is extremely technical as it was created for specialists. The articles are the results which are the most accessible to non-professionals and often listed under the heading "Citations." The contact names are also accessible to non-professionals.

Specialized References

The following books are specialized references written for professionals interested in sudden infant death syndrome (sorted alphabetically by title; hyperlinks provide rankings, information, and reviews at Amazon.com):

- **Atlas of Pediatric Physical Diagnosis** by Basil J. Zitelli, Holly W. Davis (Editor); Hardcover, 3rd edition (March 1997), Mosby-Year Book; ISBN: 0815199309;
  http://www.amazon.com/exec/obidos/ASIN/0815199309/icongroupinterna

- **The 5-Minute Pediatric Consult** by M. William Schwartz (Editor); Hardcover - 1050 pages, 2nd edition (January 15, 2000), Lippincott, Williams & Wilkins; ISBN: 0683307444;
  http://www.amazon.com/exec/obidos/ASIN/0683307444/icongroupinterna

- **Nelson Textbook of Pediatrics** by Richard E. Behrman (Editor), et al; Hardcover - 2414 pages, 16th edition (January 15, 2000), W B Saunders Co; ISBN: 0721677673;
  http://www.amazon.com/exec/obidos/ASIN/0721677673/icongroupinterna

Vocabulary Builder

Essential Tremor: A rhythmic, involuntary, purposeless, oscillating movement resulting from the alternate contraction and relaxation of opposing groups of muscles. [NIH]

Rett Syndrome: A neurological disorder seen almost exclusively in females, and found in a variety of racial and ethnic groups worldwide. [NIH]

Tuberous Sclerosis: A rare congenital disease in which the essential pathology is the appearance of multiple tumors in the cerebrum and in other organs, such as the heart or kidneys. [NIH]

CHAPTER 9. DISSERTATIONS ON SUDDEN INFANT DEATH SYNDROME

Overview

University researchers are active in studying almost all known medical conditions. The result of research is often published in the form of Doctoral or Master's dissertations. You should understand, therefore, that applied diagnostic procedures and/or therapies can take many years to develop after the thesis that proposed the new technique or approach was written.

In this chapter, we will give you a bibliography on recent dissertations relating to sudden infant death syndrome. You can read about these in more detail using the Internet or your local medical library. We will also provide you with information on how to use the Internet to stay current on dissertations.

Dissertations on Sudden Infant Death Syndrome

ProQuest Digital Dissertations is the largest archive of academic dissertations available. From this archive, we have compiled the following list covering dissertations devoted to sudden infant death syndrome. You will see that the information provided includes the dissertation's title, its author, and the author's institution. To read more about the following, simply use the Internet address indicated. The following covers recent dissertations dealing with sudden infant death syndrome:

- AN EXAMINATION OF PARENT COPING IN SURVIVORS OF SUDDEN INFANT DEATH SYNDROME: IMPLICATIONS FOR THE

EDUCATION OF HEALTH AND HUMAN
SERVICES PROFESSIONALS by AADALEN, SHARON PRICE, PHD from
University of Minnesota, 1983, 354 pages
http://wwwlib.umi.com/dissertations/fullcit/8318034

- **AN INVESTIGATION OF THE SEASONALITY OF SUDDEN INFANT DEATH SYNDROME IN THE UNITED STATES** by HEREWARD, MARK COURTENAY, PHD from University of Pennsylvania, 1990, 343 pages
http://wwwlib.umi.com/dissertations/fullcit/9026573

- **Development of the neonatal rat as a model for sudden infant death syndrome: Cardiorespiratory effects of ethanol** by Stout, Rhett Whitman; PhD from Louisiana State University and Agricultural & Mechanical College, 2003, 158 pages
http://wwwlib.umi.com/dissertations/fullcit/3085700

- **REAL AND ARTIFACTUAL TRENDS IN SUDDEN INFANT DEATH SYNDROME: 1975-1986 (INFANT MORTALITY, SUDDEN INFANT DEATH SYNDROME)** by RUTROUGH, THYNE SIEBER, PHD from The University of Michigan, 1991, 273 pages
http://wwwlib.umi.com/dissertations/fullcit/9208644

- **Sudden infant death syndrome: Hospitals' dissemination, practice, support, and policies for the 'Back to Sleep Campaign'** by McCarthy, Cheryl Ann; PhD from Temple University, 2000, 263 pages
http://wwwlib.umi.com/dissertations/fullcit/9990338

- **Sudden infant death syndrome: Urban parents' perceptions of risk reduction messages and the use of a risk behavior diagnosis scale** by Esposito, Linda M.; PhD from Temple University, 2003, 274 pages
http://wwwlib.umi.com/dissertations/fullcit/3097689

- **THE DEVELOPMENT AND EVALUATION OF A SLIDE/SOUND PRESENTATION ON SUDDEN INFANT DEATH SYNDROME (SIDS)** by KAPP, MINNA ROCHELLE, EDD from Columbia University Teachers College, 1983, 205 pages
http://wwwlib.umi.com/dissertations/fullcit/8403268

- **THE DEVELOPMENT AND TESTING OF A PRACTICE MODEL WITH FAMILIES BEREAVED DUE TO SUDDEN INFANT DEATH SYNDROME** by PANZER, BARRY MARVIN, DSW from Columbia University, 1989, 221 pages
http://wwwlib.umi.com/dissertations/fullcit/9020588

- **The environmental niche of Aboriginal infants: Possible implications for sudden infant death syndrome** by Wilson, C. Elizabeth, PhD from The University of Manitoba (Canada), 1999, 229 pages
  http://wwwlib.umi.com/dissertations/fullcit/NQ35048

- **THE IMPACT OF THE DEATH OF A CHILD ON THE PARENT'S MARRIAGE: A CASE STUDY OF SUDDEN INFANT DEATH SYNDROME AND THE PARENT'S MARITAL RELATIONSHIP (SIDS)** by O'MALLEY, PATRICK W., PHD from Texas Woman's University, 1987, 144 pages
  http://wwwlib.umi.com/dissertations/fullcit/8715006

- **The role of medullary raphe serotonergic neurons in central chemoreception during sleep and wakefulness in newborn piglets: Relevance to the sudden infant death syndrome** by Messier, Michelle Louise; PhD from Dartmouth College, 2003, 178 pages
  http://wwwlib.umi.com/dissertations/fullcit/3097797

- **WHEN A YOUNG CHILD DIES: THE INTERACTIONIST APPROACH TO THE CRISIS OF SUDDEN INFANT DEATH SYNDROME AND ITS CASE MANAGEMENT.** by STEINMARC, PAUL LEANDRE, PHD from University of Minnesota, 1979, 800 pages
  http://wwwlib.umi.com/dissertations/fullcit/7918396

Keeping Current

As previously mentioned, an effective way to stay current on dissertations dedicated to sudden infant death syndrome is to use the database called *ProQuest Digital Dissertations* via the Internet, located at the following Web address: **http://wwwlib.umi.com/dissertations.** The site allows you to freely access the last two years of citations and abstracts. Ask your medical librarian if the library has full and unlimited access to this database. From the library, you should be able to do more complete searches than with the limited 2-year access available to the general public.

Vocabulary Builder

Niche: The ultimate unit of the habitat, i. e. the specific spot occupied by an individual organism; by extension, the more or less specialized relationships existing between an organism, individual or synusia(e), and its environment. [NIH]

PART III. APPENDICES

ABOUT PART III

Part III is a collection of appendices on general medical topics relating to sudden infant death syndrome and related conditions.

APPENDIX A. RESEARCHING YOUR CHILD'S MEDICATIONS

Overview

There are a number of sources available on new or existing medications which could be prescribed to treat sudden infant death syndrome. While a number of hard copy or CD-Rom resources are available to parents and physicians for research purposes, a more flexible method is to use Internet-based databases. In this chapter, we will begin with a general overview of medications. We will then proceed to outline official recommendations on how you should view your child's medications. You may also want to research medications that your child is currently taking for other conditions as they may interact with medications for sudden infant death syndrome. Research can give you information on the side effects, interactions, and limitations of prescription drugs used in the treatment of sudden infant death syndrome. Broadly speaking, there are two sources of information on approved medications: public sources and private sources. We will emphasize free-to-use public sources.

Your Child's Medications: The Basics[37]

The Agency for Health Care Research and Quality has published extremely useful guidelines on the medication aspects of sudden infant death syndrome. Giving your child medication can involve many steps and decisions each day. The AHCRQ recommends that parents take part in treatment decisions. Do not be afraid to ask questions and talk about your concerns. By taking a moment to ask questions, your child may be spared

---

[37] This section is adapted from AHCRQ: **http://www.ahcpr.gov/consumer/ncpiebro.htm**.

from possible problems. Here are some points to cover each time a new medicine is prescribed:

- Ask about all parts of your child's treatment, including diet changes, exercise, and medicines.

- Ask about the risks and benefits of each medicine or other treatment your child might receive.

- Ask how often you or your child's doctor will check for side effects from a given medication.

Do not hesitate to tell the doctor about preferences you have for your child's medicines. You may want your child to have a medicine with the fewest side effects, or the fewest doses to take each day. You may care most about cost. Or, you may want the medicine the doctor believes will work the best. Sharing your concerns will help the doctor select the best treatment for your child.

Do not be afraid to "bother" the doctor with your questions about medications for sudden infant death syndrome. You can also talk to a nurse or a pharmacist. They can help you better understand your child's treatment plan. Talking over your child's options with someone you trust can help you make better choices. Specifically, ask the doctor the following:

- The name of the medicine and what it is supposed to do.

- How and when to give your child the medicine, how much, and for how long.

- What food, drinks, other medicines, or activities your child should avoid while taking the medicine.

- What side effects your child may experience, and what to do if they occur.

- If there are any refills, and how often.

- About any terms or directions you do not understand.

- What to do if your child misses a dose.

- If there is written information you can take home (most pharmacies have information sheets on prescription medicines; some even offer large-print or Spanish versions).

Do not forget to tell the doctor about all the medicines your child is currently taking (not just those for sudden infant death syndrome). This includes prescription medicines and the medicines that you buy over the counter. When talking to the doctor, you may wish to prepare a list of medicines your child is currently taking including why and in what forms. Be sure to include the following information for each:

- Name of medicine
- Reason taken
- Dosage
- Time(s) of day

Also include any over-the-counter medicines, such as:

- Laxatives
- Diet pills
- Vitamins
- Cold medicine
- Aspirin or other pain, headache, or fever medicine
- Cough medicine
- Allergy relief medicine
- Antacids
- Sleeping pills
- Others (include names)

Learning More about Your Child's Medications

Because of historical investments by various organizations and the emergence of the Internet, it has become rather simple to learn about the medications the doctor has recommended for sudden infant death syndrome. One such source is the United States Pharmacopeia. In 1820, eleven physicians met in Washington, D.C. to establish the first compendium of standard drugs for the United States. They called this compendium the "U.S. Pharmacopeia (USP)." Today, the USP is a non-profit organization consisting of 800 volunteer scientists, eleven elected officials, and 400 representatives of state associations and colleges of medicine and pharmacy. The USP is located in Rockville, Maryland, and its home page is located at **www.usp.org**. The USP currently provides standards for over 3,700 medications. The resulting USP DI® Advice for the Patient® can be accessed through the National Library of Medicine of the National Institutes of Health. The database is partially derived from lists of federally approved medications in the Food and Drug Administration's (FDA) Drug Approvals database.[38]

While the FDA database is rather large and difficult to navigate, the Phamacopeia is both user-friendly and free to use. It covers more than 9,000 prescription and over-the-counter medications. To access this database, simply type the following hyperlink into your Web browser: **http://www.nlm.nih.gov/medlineplus/druginformation.html**. To view examples of a given medication (brand names, category, description, preparation, proper use, precautions, side effects, etc.), simply follow the hyperlinks indicated within the United States Pharmacopeia (USP).

Commercial Databases

In addition to the medications listed in the USP above, a number of commercial sites are available by subscription to physicians and their institutions. You may be able to access these sources from your local medical library or your child's doctor's office.

Reuters Health Drug Database

The Reuters Health Drug Database can be searched by keyword at the hyperlink: **http://www.reutershealth.com/frame2/drug.html**.

Mosby's GenRx

Mosby's GenRx database (also available on CD-Rom and book format) covers 45,000 drug products including generics and international brands. It provides information on prescribing and drug interactions. Information can be obtained at the following hyperlink: **http://www.genrx.com/Mosby/PhyGenRx/group.html**.

PDR*health*

The PDR*health* database is a free-to-use, drug information search engine that has been written for the public in layman's terms. It contains FDA-approved drug information adapted from the Physicians' Desk Reference (PDR)

---

[38] Though cumbersome, the FDA database can be freely browsed at the following site: **www.fda.gov/cder/da/da.htm**.

database. PDR*health* can be searched by brand name, generic name, or indication. It features multiple drug interactions reports. Search PDR*health* at **http://www.pdrhealth.com/drug_info/index.html**.

Other Web Sites

A number of additional Web sites discuss drug information. As an example, you may like to look at **www.drugs.com** which reproduces the information in the Pharmacopeia as well as commercial information. You may also want to consider the Web site of the Medical Letter, Inc. which allows users to download articles on various drugs and therapeutics for a nominal fee: **http://www.medletter.com/**.

Contraindications and Interactions (Hidden Dangers)

Some of the medications mentioned in the previous discussions can be problematic for children with sudden infant death syndrome--not because they are used in the treatment process, but because of contraindications, or side effects. Medications with contraindications are those that could react with drugs used to treat sudden infant death syndrome or potentially create deleterious side effects in patients with sudden infant death syndrome. You should ask the physician about any contraindications, especially as these might apply to other medications that your child may be taking for common ailments.

Drug-drug interactions occur when two or more drugs react with each other. This drug-drug interaction may cause your child to experience an unexpected side effect. Drug interactions may make medications less effective, cause unexpected side effects, or increase the action of a particular drug. Some drug interactions can even be harmful to your child.

Be sure to read the label every time you give your child a nonprescription or prescription drug, and take the time to learn about drug interactions. These precautions may be critical to your child's health. You can reduce the risk of potentially harmful drug interactions and side effects with a little bit of knowledge and common sense.

Drug labels contain important information about ingredients, uses, warnings, and directions which you should take the time to read and understand. Labels also include warnings about possible drug interactions. Further, drug labels may change as new information becomes avaiable. This is why it's especially important to read the label every time you give your child a medication. When the doctor prescribes a new drug, discuss all over-the-counter and prescription medications, dietary supplements, vitamins, botanicals, minerals and herbals your child takes. Ask your pharmacist for the package insert for each drug prescribed. The package insert provides more information about potential drug interactions.

A Final Warning

At some point, you may hear of alternative medications from friends, relatives, or in the news media. Advertisements may suggest that certain alternative drugs can produce positive results for sudden infant death syndrome. Exercise caution--some of these drugs may have fraudulent claims, and others may actually hurt your child. The Food and Drug Administration (FDA) is the official U.S. agency charged with discovering which medications are likely to improve the health of patients with sudden infant death syndrome. The FDA warns to watch out for[39]:

- Secret formulas (real scientists share what they know)

- Amazing breakthroughs or miracle cures (real breakthroughs don't happen very often; when they do, real scientists do not call them amazing or miracles)

- Quick, painless, or guaranteed cures

- If it sounds too good to be true, it probably isn't true.

If you have any questions about any kind of medical treatment, the FDA may have an office near you. Look for their number in the blue pages of the phone book. You can also contact the FDA through its toll-free number, 1-888-INFO-FDA (1-888-463-6332), or on the World Wide Web at **www.fda.gov**.

General References

In addition to the resources provided earlier in this chapter, the following general references describe medications (sorted alphabetically by title; hyperlinks provide rankings, information and reviews at Amazon.com):

- **Complete Guide to Prescription and Nonprescription Drugs 2001 (Complete Guide to Prescription and Nonprescription Drugs, 2001)** by H. Winter Griffith, Paperback 16th edition (2001), Medical Surveillance;

---

[39] This section has been adapted from **http://www.fda.gov/opacom/lowlit/medfraud.html**.

ISBN: 0942447417;
http://www.amazon.com/exec/obidos/ASIN/039952634X/icongroupinter
na

- **The Essential Guide to Prescription Drugs, 2001** by James J. Rybacki, James W. Long; Paperback - 1274 pages (2001), Harper Resource; ISBN: 0060958162;
http://www.amazon.com/exec/obidos/ASIN/0060958162/icongroupinter
na

- **Handbook of Commonly Prescribed Drugs** by G. John Digregorio, Edward J. Barbieri; Paperback 16th edition (2001), Medical Surveillance; ISBN: 0942447417;
http://www.amazon.com/exec/obidos/ASIN/0942447417/icongroupinter
na

- **Johns Hopkins Complete Home Encyclopedia of Drugs 2nd ed.** by Simeon Margolis (Ed.), Johns Hopkins; Hardcover - 835 pages (2000), Rebus; ISBN: 0929661583;
http://www.amazon.com/exec/obidos/ASIN/0929661583/icongroupinter
na

- **Medical Pocket Reference: Drugs 2002** by Springhouse Paperback 1st edition (2001), Lippincott Williams & Wilkins Publishers; ISBN: 1582550964;
http://www.amazon.com/exec/obidos/ASIN/1582550964/icongroupinter
na

- **PDR** by Medical Economics Staff, Medical Economics Staff Hardcover - 3506 pages 55th edition (2000), Medical Economics Company; ISBN: 1563633752;
http://www.amazon.com/exec/obidos/ASIN/1563633752/icongroupinter
na

- **Pharmacy Simplified: A Glossary of Terms** by James Grogan; Paperback - 432 pages, 1st edition (2001), Delmar Publishers; ISBN: 0766828581;
http://www.amazon.com/exec/obidos/ASIN/0766828581/icongroupinter
na

- **Physician Federal Desk Reference** by Christine B. Fraizer; Paperback 2nd edition (2001), Medicode Inc; ISBN: 1563373971;
http://www.amazon.com/exec/obidos/ASIN/1563373971/icongroupinter
na

- **Physician's Desk Reference Supplements** Paperback - 300 pages, 53 edition (1999), ISBN: 1563632950;
http://www.amazon.com/exec/obidos/ASIN/1563632950/icongroupinter
na

Vocabulary Builder

The following vocabulary builder gives definitions of words used in this chapter that have not been defined in previous chapters:

Contraindications: Any factor or sign that it is unwise to pursue a certain kind of action or treatment, e. g. giving a general anesthetic to a person with pneumonia. [NIH]

Appendix B. Researching Nutrition

Overview

Since the time of Hippocrates, doctors have understood the importance of diet and nutrition to health and well-being. Since then, they have accumulated an impressive archive of studies and knowledge dedicated to this subject. Based on their experience, doctors and healthcare providers may recommend particular dietary supplements for sudden infant death syndrome. Any dietary recommendation is based on age, body mass, gender, lifestyle, eating habits, food preferences, and health condition. It is therefore likely that different patients with sudden infant death syndrome may be given different recommendations. Some recommendations may be directly related to sudden infant death syndrome, while others may be more related to general health.

In this chapter we will begin by briefly reviewing the essentials of diet and nutrition that will broadly frame more detailed discussions of sudden infant death syndrome. We will then show you how to find studies dedicated specifically to nutrition and sudden infant death syndrome.

Food and Nutrition: General Principles

What Are Essential Foods?

Food is generally viewed by official sources as consisting of six basic elements: (1) fluids, (2) carbohydrates, (3) protein, (4) fats, (5) vitamins, and (6) minerals. Consuming a combination of these elements is considered to be a healthy diet:

- **Fluids** are essential to human life as 80-percent of the body is composed of water. Water is lost via urination, sweating, diarrhea, vomiting, diuretics (drugs that increase urination), caffeine, and physical exertion.

- **Carbohydrates** are the main source for human energy (thermoregulation) and the bulk of typical diets. They are mostly classified as being either simple or complex. Simple carbohydrates include sugars which are often consumed in the form of cookies, candies, or cakes. Complex carbohydrates consist of starches and dietary fibers. Starches are consumed in the form of pastas, breads, potatoes, rice, and other foods. Soluble fibers can be eaten in the form of certain vegetables, fruits, oats, and legumes. Insoluble fibers include brown rice, whole grains, certain fruits, wheat bran and legumes.

- **Proteins** are eaten to build and repair human tissues. Some foods that are high in protein are also high in fat and calories. Food sources for protein include nuts, meat, fish, cheese, and other dairy products.

- **Fats** are consumed for both energy and the absorption of certain vitamins. There are many types of fats, with many general publications recommending the intake of unsaturated fats or those low in cholesterol.

Vitamins and minerals are fundamental to human health, growth, and, in some cases, disease prevention. Most are consumed in your child's diet (exceptions being vitamins K and D which are produced by intestinal bacteria and sunlight on the skin, respectively). Each vitamin and mineral plays a different role in health. The following outlines essential vitamins:

- **Vitamin A** is important to the health of eyes, hair, bones, and skin; sources of vitamin A include foods such as eggs, carrots, and cantaloupe.

- **Vitamin B[1]**, also known as thiamine, is important for the nervous system and energy production; food sources for thiamine include meat, peas, fortified cereals, bread, and whole grains.

- **Vitamin B[2]**, also known as riboflavin, is important for the nervous system and muscles, but is also involved in the release of proteins from nutrients; food sources for riboflavin include dairy products, leafy vegetables, meat, and eggs.

- **Vitamin B[3]**, also known as niacin, is important for healthy skin and helps the body use energy; food sources for niacin include peas, peanuts, fish, and whole grains

- **Vitamin B[6]**, also known as pyridoxine, is important for the regulation of cells in the nervous system and is vital for blood formation; food sources for pyridoxine include bananas, whole grains, meat, and fish.

- **Vitamin B^{12}** is vital for a healthy nervous system and for the growth of red blood cells in bone marrow; food sources for vitamin B^{12} include yeast, milk, fish, eggs, and meat.

- **Vitamin C** allows the body's immune system to fight various medical conditions, strengthens body tissue, and improves the body's use of iron; food sources for vitamin C include a wide variety of fruits and vegetables.

- **Vitamin D** helps the body absorb calcium which strengthens bones and teeth; food sources for vitamin D include oily fish and dairy products.

- **Vitamin E** can help protect certain organs and tissues from various degenerative diseases; food sources for vitamin E include margarine, vegetables, eggs, and fish.

- **Vitamin K** is essential for bone formation and blood clotting; common food sources for vitamin K include leafy green vegetables.

- **Folic Acid** maintains healthy cells and blood; food sources for folic acid include nuts, fortified breads, leafy green vegetables, and whole grains.

It should be noted that it is possible to overdose on certain vitamins which become toxic if consumed in excess (e.g. vitamin A, D, E and K).

Like vitamins, minerals are chemicals that are required by the body to remain in good health. Because the human body does not manufacture these chemicals internally, we obtain them from food and other dietary sources. The more important minerals include:

- **Calcium** is needed for healthy bones, teeth, and muscles, but also helps the nervous system function; food sources for calcium include dry beans, peas, eggs, and dairy products.

- **Chromium** is helpful in regulating sugar levels in blood; food sources for chromium include egg yolks, raw sugar, cheese, nuts, beets, whole grains, and meat.

- **Fluoride** is used by the body to help prevent tooth decay and to reinforce bone strength; sources of fluoride include drinking water and certain brands of toothpaste.

- **Iodine** helps regulate the body's use of energy by synthesizing into the hormone thyroxine; food sources include leafy green vegetables, nuts, egg yolks, and red meat.

- **Iron** helps maintain muscles and the formation of red blood cells and certain proteins; food sources for iron include meat, dairy products, eggs, and leafy green vegetables.

- **Magnesium** is important for the production of DNA, as well as for healthy teeth, bones, muscles, and nerves; food sources for magnesium include dried fruit, dark green vegetables, nuts, and seafood.

- **Phosphorous** is used by the body to work with calcium to form bones and teeth; food sources for phosphorous include eggs, meat, cereals, and dairy products.

- **Selenium** primarily helps maintain normal heart and liver functions; food sources for selenium include wholegrain cereals, fish, meat, and dairy products.

- **Zinc** helps wounds heal, the formation of sperm, and encourage rapid growth and energy; food sources include dried beans, shellfish, eggs, and nuts.

The United States government periodically publishes recommended diets and consumption levels of the various elements of food. Again, the doctor may encourage deviations from the average official recommendation based on your child's specific condition. To learn more about basic dietary guidelines, visit the Web site: **http://www.health.gov/dietaryguidelines/**. Based on these guidelines, many foods are required to list the nutrition levels on the food's packaging. Labeling Requirements are listed at the following site maintained by the Food and Drug Administration: **http://www.cfsan.fda.gov/~dms/lab-cons.html**. When interpreting these requirements, the government recommends that consumers become familiar with the following abbreviations before reading FDA literature:[40]

- **DVs (Daily Values):** A new dietary reference term that will appear on the food label. It is made up of two sets of references, DRVs and RDIs.

- **DRVs (Daily Reference Values):** A set of dietary references that applies to fat, saturated fat, cholesterol, carbohydrate, protein, fiber, sodium, and potassium.

- **RDIs (Reference Daily Intakes):** A set of dietary references based on the Recommended Dietary Allowances for essential vitamins and minerals and, in selected groups, protein. The name "RDI" replaces the term "U.S. RDA."

- **RDAs (Recommended Dietary Allowances):** A set of estimated nutrient allowances established by the National Academy of Sciences. It is updated periodically to reflect current scientific knowledge.

---

[40] Adapted from the FDA: **http://www.fda.gov/fdac/special/foodlabel/dvs.html**.

What Are Dietary Supplements?[41]

Dietary supplements are widely available through many commercial sources, including health food stores, grocery stores, pharmacies, and by mail. Dietary supplements are provided in many forms including tablets, capsules, powders, gel-tabs, extracts, and liquids. Historically in the United States, the most prevalent type of dietary supplement was a multivitamin/mineral tablet or capsule that was available in pharmacies, either by prescription or "over the counter." Supplements containing strictly herbal preparations were less widely available. Currently in the United States, a wide array of supplement products are available, including vitamin, mineral, other nutrients, and botanical supplements as well as ingredients and extracts of animal and plant origin.

The Office of Dietary Supplements (ODS) of the National Institutes of Health is the official agency of the United States which has the expressed goal of acquiring "new knowledge to help prevent, detect, diagnose, and treat disease and disability, from the rarest genetic disorder to the common cold."[42] According to the ODS, dietary supplements can have an important impact on the prevention and management of medical conditions and on the maintenance of health.[43] The ODS notes that considerable research on the effects of dietary supplements has been conducted in Asia and Europe where the use of plant products, in particular, has a long tradition. However, the overwhelming majority of supplements have not been studied scientifically. To explore the role of dietary supplements in the improvement of health care, the ODS plans, organizes, and supports conferences, workshops, and symposia on scientific topics related to dietary supplements. The ODS often works in conjunction with other NIH Institutes and Centers, other government agencies, professional organizations, and public advocacy groups.

---

[41] This discussion has been adapted from the NIH:
http://ods.od.nih.gov/showpage.aspx?pageid=46.
[42] Contact: The Office of Dietary Supplements, National Institutes of Health, Building 31, Room 1B29, 31 Center Drive, MSC 2086, Bethesda, Maryland 20892-2086, Tel: (301) 435-2920, Fax: (301) 480-1845, E-mail: ods@nih.gov.
[43] Adapted from **http://ods.od.nih.gov/showpage.aspx?pageid=2**. The Dietary Supplement Health and Education Act defines dietary supplements as "a product (other than tobacco) intended to supplement the diet that bears or contains one or more of the following dietary ingredients: a vitamin, mineral, amino acid, herb or other botanical; or a dietary substance for use to supplement the diet by increasing the total dietary intake; or a concentrate, metabolite, constituent, extract, or combination of any ingredient described above; and intended for ingestion in the form of a capsule, powder, softgel, or gelcap, and not represented as a conventional food or as a sole item of a meal or the diet."

To learn more about official information on dietary supplements, visit the ODS site at **http://dietary-supplements.info.nih.gov/**. Or contact:

> **The Office of Dietary Supplements**
> National Institutes of Health
> Building 31, Room 1B29
> 31 Center Drive, MSC 2086
> Bethesda, Maryland 20892-2086
> Tel: (301) 435-2920
> Fax: (301) 480-1845
> E-mail: ods@nih.gov

Finding Studies on Sudden Infant Death Syndrome

The NIH maintains an office dedicated to nutrition and diet. The National Institutes of Health's Office of Dietary Supplements (ODS) offers a searchable bibliographic database called the IBIDS (International Bibliographic Information on Dietary Supplements). The IBIDS contains over 460,000 scientific citations and summaries about dietary supplements and nutrition as well as references to published international, scientific literature on dietary supplements such as vitamins, minerals, and botanicals.[44] IBIDS is available to the public free of charge through the ODS Internet page: **http://ods.od.nih.gov/databases/ibids.html**.

After entering the search area, you have three choices: (1) IBIDS Consumer Database, (2) Full IBIDS Database, or (3) Peer Reviewed Citations Only. We recommend that you start with the Consumer Database. While you may not find references for the topics that are of most interest to you, check back periodically as this database is frequently updated. More studies can be found by searching the Full IBIDS Database. Healthcare professionals and researchers generally use the third option, which lists peer-reviewed citations. In all cases, we suggest that you take advantage of the "Advanced Search" option that allows you to retrieve up to 100 fully explained references in a comprehensive format. Type "sudden infant death syndrome" (or synonyms) into the search box. To narrow the search, you can also select the "Title" field.

---

[44] Adapted from **http://ods.od.nih.gov**. IBIDS is produced by the Office of Dietary Supplements (ODS) at the National Institutes of Health to assist the public, healthcare providers, educators, and researchers in locating credible, scientific information on dietary supplements. IBIDS was developed and will be maintained through an interagency partnership with the Food and Nutrition Information Center of the National Agricultural Library, U.S. Department of Agriculture.

The following information is typical of that found when using the "Full IBIDS Database" when searching using "sudden infant death syndrome" (or a synonym):

- **Caffeine and alcohol as risk factors for sudden infant death syndrome. Nordic Epidemiological SIDS Study.**
  Author(s): Department of Paediatrics, Sahlgrenska University Hospital/Ostra, S-416 85 Goteborg, Sweden.
  Source: Alm, B Wennergren, G Norvenius, G Skjaerven, R Oyen, N Helweg Larsen, K Lagercrantz, H Irgens, L M Arch-Dis-Child. 1999 August; 81(2): 107-11 0003-9888

- **Control of breathing by endogenous opioid peptides: possible involvement in sudden infant death syndrome.**
  Author(s): Laboratoire de Physiologie Nerveuse, C.N.R.S., Gif-sur-Yvette, France.
  Source: Morin Surun, M P Boudinot, E Fournie Zaluski, M C Champagnat, J Roques, B P Denavit Saubie, M Neurochem-Int. 1992 January; 20(1): 103-7 0197-0186

- **Could exogenous melatonin prevent sudden infant death syndrome?**
  Author(s): Department of Pathology, Houston Medical Center, Warner Robins, GA 31093, USA.
  Source: Maurizi, C P Med-Hypotheses. 1997 November; 49(5): 425-7 0306-9877

- **Effects of hypomagnesemia on reactivity of bovine and ovine platelets: possible relevance to infantile apnea and sudden infant death syndrome.**
  Author(s): Department of Animal Science, University of Tennessee, Knoxville 37901-1071.
  Source: Miller, J K Schneider, M D Ramsey, N White, P K Bell, M C J-Am-Coll-Nutr. 1990 February; 9(1): 58-64 0731-5724

- **Effects of nicotine on bacterial toxins associated with cot death.**
  Author(s): School of Biological Sciences, University of Manchester.
  Source: Sayers, N M Drucker, D B Telford, D R Morris, J A Arch-Dis-Child. 1995 December; 73(6): 549-51 0003-9888

- **Heavy caffeine intake in pregnancy and sudden infant death syndrome.**
  Author(s): Community Paediatric Unit, Community Child and Family Service, PO Box 25-265, Christchurch (New Zealand)
  Source: Ford, R.P.K. Schluter, P.J. Mitchell E.A. Taylor, B.J. Scragg, R. Stewart, A.W. Archives-of-Disease-in-Childhood (United Kingdom).

(1998). volume 78(1) page 9-13. caffeine pregnancy death infants coffee mankind tea

- **Impaired cardiac function during postnatal hypoxia in rats exposed to nicotine prenatally: implications for perinatal morbidity and mortality, and for sudden infant death syndrome.**
  Author(s): Department of Pharmacology, Duke University Medical Center, Durham, North Carolina 27710, USA. slotk001@acpub.duke.edu
  Source: Slotkin, T A Saleh, J L McCook, E C Seidler, F J Teratology. 1997 March; 55(3): 177-84 0040-3709

- **Increased density of somatostatin binding sites in respiratory nuclei of the brainstem in sudden infant death syndrome.**
  Author(s): European Institute for Peptide Research (IFRMP no. 23), INSERM U 413, UA CNRS, University of Rouen, Mont-Saint-Aignan, France.
  Source: Carpentier, V Vaudry, H Mallet, E Laquerriere, A Leroux, P Neuroscience. 1998 September; 86(1): 159-66 0306-4522

- **Inherited metabolic diseases in the sudden infant death syndrome.**
  Author(s): Department of Clinical Chemistry, Southmead Hospital, Westbury-on-Trym, Bristol.
  Source: Holton, J B Allen, J T Green, C A Partington, S Gilbert, R E Berry, P J Arch-Dis-Child. 1991 November; 66(11): 1315-7 0003-9888

- **Liver fatty acids and the sudden infant death syndrome [Dihomo-gama-linolenic acid].**
  Source: Fogerty, A.C. Ford, G.L. Willcox, M.E. Clancy, S.L. Am-J-Clin-Nutr. Bethesda : American Society for Clinical Nutrition. February 1984. volume 39 c (2) page 201-208. 0002-9165

- **Magnesium and thermoregulation. I. Newborn and infant. Is sudden infant death syndrome a magnesium-dependent disease of the transition from chemical to physical thermoregulation?**
  Author(s): SDRM, Hopital St. Vincent-de-Paul, Paris, France.
  Source: Durlach, J Durlach, V Rayssiguier, Y Ricquier, D Goubern, M Bertin, R Bara, M Guiet Bara, A Olive, G Mettey, R Magnes-Res. 1991 Sep-December; 4(3-4): 137-52 0953-1424

- **Medium-chain acyl-CoA dehydrogenase deficiency does not correlate with apparent life-threatening events and the sudden infant death syndrome: results from phenylpropionate loading tests and DNA analysis.**
  Author(s): Department of Paediatrics, University of Berne, Switzerland.
  Source: Penzien, J M Molz, G Wiesmann, U N Colombo, J P Buhlmann, R Wermuth, B Eur-J-Pediatr. 1994 May; 153(5): 352-7 0340-6199

- **Melatonin increases cyclic guanosine monophosphate: biochemical effects mediated by porphyrins, calcium and nitric oxide. Relationships to infant colic and the Sudden Infant Death Syndrome.**
  Source: Weissbluth, M Med-Hypotheses. 1994 June; 42(6): 390-2 0306-9877

- **Methylxanthine treatment in infants at risk for sudden infant death syndrome.**
  Author(s): Department of Pediatrics, Children's Memorial Hospital, Northwestern University Medical School, Chicago, Illinois 60614.
  Source: Hunt, C E Brouillette, R T Ann-N-Y-Acad-Sci. 1988; 533119-26 0077-8923

- **Opioid peptides from milk as a possible cause of sudden infant death syndrome.**
  Author(s): Department of Anesthesiology, New York University Medical Center, NY 10016.
  Source: Ramabadran, K Bansinath, M Med-Hypotheses. 1988 November; 27(3): 181-7 0306-9877

- **Recent advances in sudden infant death syndrome: possible autonomic dysfunction of the airways in infants at risk.**
  Author(s): Pediatric Sleep Unit, University Children's Hospital, Free University of Brussels, Belgium.
  Source: Kahn, A Rebuffat, E Sottiaux, M Muller, M F Lung. 1990; 168 Suppl920-4 0341-2040

- **Selenium and glutathione peroxidase in mothers experiencing sudden infant death syndrome.**
  Source: Valentine, J. Faraji, B. Akashi, K. Trace elements in man and animals 6 / edited by Lucille S. Hurley,... [et al.]. New York : Plenum Press, c1988. page 13-14. ISBN: 0306430045

- **Structural changes in lungs of magnesium-deficient weanling rats dying spontaneously or after spontaneous recovery from the seizure-shock episode. Possible methods for sudden infant death syndromes.**
  Author(s): Section of Disorders of Carbohydrate Metabolism, National Institute of Child Health and Human Development, Bethesda, Md.
  Source: Caddell, J L Blanchette Mackie, E J Magnesium. 1988; 7(4): 195-209 0252-1156

- **Sudden infant death syndrome (SIDS) and disordered blood flow.**
  Source: Reid, G M Tervit, H Med-Hypotheses. 1991 November; 36(3): 295-9 0306-9877

- **The apparent impact of gestational magnesium (Mg) deficiency on the sudden infant death syndrome (SIDS).**
  Author(s): Department of Pediatrics, Thomas Jefferson University, Philadelphia, PA 19107-5083, USA.

Source: Caddell, J L Magnes-Res. 2001 December; 14(4): 291-303 0953-1424

- **The iodine-selenium connection: its possible roles in intelligence, cretinism, sudden infant death syndrome, breast cancer and multiple sclerosis.**
  Author(s): Department of Geography, University of Victoria, British Columbia, Canada.
  Source: Foster, H D Med-Hypotheses. 1993 January; 40(1): 61-5 0306-9877

- **The vitamin E and selenium status of infants and the sudden infant death syndrome.**
  Source: Rhead, W.J. Cary, E.E. Allaway, W.H. Saltzstein, S.L. Schrauzer, G.N. Bioinorganic-Chem. New York, N.Y. : Elsevier Science Publishing. 1972. volume 1 (4) page 289-294. 0162-0134

Federal Resources on Nutrition

In addition to the IBIDS, the United States Department of Health and Human Services (HHS) and the United States Department of Agriculture (USDA) provide many sources of information on general nutrition and health. Recommended resources include:

- healthfinder®, HHS's gateway to health information, including diet and nutrition:
  http://www.healthfinder.gov/scripts/SearchContext.asp?topic=238&page=0

- The United States Department of Agriculture's Web site dedicated to nutrition information: **www.nutrition.gov**

- The Food and Drug Administration's Web site for federal food safety information: **www.foodsafety.gov**

- The National Action Plan on Overweight and Obesity sponsored by the United States Surgeon General: **http://www.surgeongeneral.gov/topics/obesity/**

- The Center for Food Safety and Applied Nutrition has an Internet site sponsored by the Food and Drug Administration and the Department of Health and Human Services: **http://vm.cfsan.fda.gov/**

- Center for Nutrition Policy and Promotion sponsored by the United States Department of Agriculture: **http://www.usda.gov/cnpp/**

- Food and Nutrition Information Center, National Agricultural Library sponsored by the United States Department of Agriculture: **http://www.nal.usda.gov/fnic/**

- Food and Nutrition Service sponsored by the United States Department of Agriculture: **http://www.fns.usda.gov/fns/**

Additional Web Resources

A number of additional Web sites offer encyclopedic information covering food and nutrition. The following is a representative sample:

- AOL: **http://search.aol.com/cat.adp?id=174&layer=&from=subcats**

- Family Village: **http://www.familyvillage.wisc.edu/med_nutrition.html**

- Google: **http://directory.google.com/Top/Health/Nutrition/**

- Open Directory Project: **http://dmoz.org/Health/Nutrition/**

- Yahoo.com: **http://dir.yahoo.com/Health/Nutrition/**

- WebMD®Health: **http://my.webmd.com/nutrition**

- WholeHealthMD.com:
  http://www.wholehealthmd.com/reflib/0,1529,,00.html

The following is a specific Web list relating to sudden infant death syndrome; please note that any particular subject below may indicate either a therapeutic use, or a contraindication (potential danger), and does not reflect an official recommendation:

- **Minerals**

    Selenium
    Source: Integrative Medicine Communications; www.drkoop.com

Vocabulary Builder

The following vocabulary builder defines words used in the references in this chapter that have not been defined in previous chapters:

Monophosphate: So called second messenger for neurotransmitters and hormones. [NIH]

Sperm: The fecundating fluid of the male. [NIH]

Valentine: The patient supine and the hips flexed by means of a double inclined plane: used in irrigating the urethra. [NIH]

Wound: Any interruption, by violence or by surgery, in the continuity of the external surface of the body or of the surface of any internal organ. [NIH]

Appendix C. Finding Medical Libraries

Overview

At a medical library you can find medical texts and reference books, consumer health publications, specialty newspapers and magazines, as well as medical journals. In this Appendix, we show you how to quickly find a medical library in your area.

Preparation

Before going to the library, highlight the references mentioned in this sourcebook that you find interesting. Focus on those items that are not available via the Internet, and ask the reference librarian for help with your search. He or she may know of additional resources that could be helpful to you. Most importantly, your local public library and medical libraries have Interlibrary Loan programs with the National Library of Medicine (NLM), one of the largest medical collections in the world. According to the NLM, most of the literature in the general and historical collections of the National Library of Medicine is available on interlibrary loan to any library. NLM's interlibrary loan services are only available to libraries. If you would like to access NLM medical literature, then visit a library in your area that can request the publications for you.[45]

---

[45] Adapted from the NLM: **http://www.nlm.nih.gov/psd/cas/interlibrary.html**.

Finding a Local Medical Library

The quickest method to locate medical libraries is to use the Internet-based directory published by the National Network of Libraries of Medicine (NN/LM). This network includes 4626 members and affiliates that provide many services to librarians, health professionals, and the public. To find a library in your area, simply visit **http://nnlm.gov/members/adv.html** or call 1-800-338-7657.

Medical Libraries in the U.S. and Canada

In addition to the NN/LM, the National Library of Medicine (NLM) lists a number of libraries with reference facilities that are open to the public. The following is the NLM's list and includes hyperlinks to each library's Web site. These Web pages can provide information on hours of operation and other restrictions. The list below is a small sample of libraries recommended by the National Library of Medicine (sorted alphabetically by name of the U.S. state or Canadian province where the library is located)[46]:

- **Alabama:** Health InfoNet of Jefferson County (Jefferson County Library Cooperative, Lister Hill Library of the Health Sciences), **http://www.uab.edu/infonet/**

- **Alabama:** Richard M. Scrushy Library (American Sports Medicine Institute)

- **Arizona:** Samaritan Regional Medical Center: The Learning Center (Samaritan Health System, Phoenix, Arizona), **http://www.samaritan.edu/library/bannerlibs.htm**

- **California:** Kris Kelly Health Information Center (St. Joseph Health System, Humboldt), **http://www.humboldt1.com/~kkhic/index.html**

- **California:** Community Health Library of Los Gatos, **http://www.healthlib.org/orgresources.html**

- **California:** Consumer Health Program and Services (CHIPS) (County of Los Angeles Public Library, Los Angeles County Harbor-UCLA Medical Center Library) - Carson, CA, **http://www.colapublib.org/services/chips.html**

- **California:** Gateway Health Library (Sutter Gould Medical Foundation)

- **California:** Health Library (Stanford University Medical Center), **http://www-med.stanford.edu/healthlibrary/**

---

[46] Abstracted from **http://www.nlm.nih.gov/medlineplus/libraries.html**.

- **California:** Patient Education Resource Center - Health Information and Resources (University of California, San Francisco), http://sfghdean.ucsf.edu/barnett/PERC/default.asp

- **California:** Redwood Health Library (Petaluma Health Care District), http://www.phcd.org/rdwdlib.html

- **California:** Los Gatos PlaneTree Health Library, http://planetreesanjose.org/

- **California:** Sutter Resource Library (Sutter Hospitals Foundation, Sacramento), http://suttermedicalcenter.org/library/

- **California:** Health Sciences Libraries (University of California, Davis), http://www.lib.ucdavis.edu/healthsci/

- **California:** ValleyCare Health Library & Ryan Comer Cancer Resource Center (ValleyCare Health System, Pleasanton), http://gaelnet.stmarys-ca.edu/other.libs/gbal/east/vchl.html

- **California:** Washington Community Health Resource Library (Fremont), http://www.healthlibrary.org/

- **Colorado:** William V. Gervasini Memorial Library (Exempla Healthcare), http://www.saintjosephdenver.org/yourhealth/libraries/

- **Connecticut:** Hartford Hospital Health Science Libraries (Hartford Hospital), http://www.harthosp.org/library/

- **Connecticut:** Healthnet: Connecticut Consumer Health Information Center (University of Connecticut Health Center, Lyman Maynard Stowe Library), http://library.uchc.edu/departm/hnet/

- **Connecticut:** Waterbury Hospital Health Center Library (Waterbury Hospital, Waterbury), http://www.waterburyhospital.com/library/consumer.shtml

- **Delaware:** Consumer Health Library (Christiana Care Health System, Eugene du Pont Preventive Medicine & Rehabilitation Institute, Wilmington), http://www.christianacare.org/health_guide/health_guide_pmri_health_info.cfm

- **Delaware:** Lewis B. Flinn Library (Delaware Academy of Medicine, Wilmington), http://www.delamed.org/chls.html

- **Georgia:** Family Resource Library (Medical College of Georgia, Augusta), http://cmc.mcg.edu/kids_families/fam_resources/fam_res_lib/frl.htm

- **Georgia:** Health Resource Center (Medical Center of Central Georgia, Macon), http://www.mccg.org/hrc/hrchome.asp

- **Hawaii:** Hawaii Medical Library: Consumer Health Information Service (Hawaii Medical Library, Honolulu), **http://hml.org/CHIS/**

- **Idaho:** DeArmond Consumer Health Library (Kootenai Medical Center, Coeur d'Alene), **http://www.nicon.org/DeArmond/index.htm**

- **Illinois:** Health Learning Center of Northwestern Memorial Hospital (Chicago), **http://www.nmh.org/health_info/hlc.html**

- **Illinois:** Medical Library (OSF Saint Francis Medical Center, Peoria), **http://www.osfsaintfrancis.org/general/library/**

- **Kentucky:** Medical Library - Services for Patients, Families, Students & the Public (Central Baptist Hospital, Lexington), **http://www.centralbap.com/education/community/library.cfm**

- **Kentucky:** University of Kentucky - Health Information Library (Chandler Medical Center, Lexington), **http://www.mc.uky.edu/PatientEd/**

- **Louisiana:** Alton Ochsner Medical Foundation Library (Alton Ochsner Medical Foundation, New Orleans), **http://www.ochsner.org/library/**

- **Louisiana:** Louisiana State University Health Sciences Center Medical Library-Shreveport, **http://lib-sh.lsuhsc.edu/**

- **Maine:** Franklin Memorial Hospital Medical Library (Franklin Memorial Hospital, Farmington), **http://www.fchn.org/fmh/lib.htm**

- **Maine:** Gerrish-True Health Sciences Library (Central Maine Medical Center, Lewiston), **http://www.cmmc.org/library/library.html**

- **Maine:** Hadley Parrot Health Science Library (Eastern Maine Healthcare, Bangor), **http://www.emh.org/hll/hpl/guide.htm**

- **Maine:** Maine Medical Center Library (Maine Medical Center, Portland), **http://www.mmc.org/library/**

- **Maine:** Parkview Hospital (Brunswick), **http://www.parkviewhospital.org/**

- **Maine:** Southern Maine Medical Center Health Sciences Library (Southern Maine Medical Center, Biddeford), **http://www.smmc.org/services/service.php3?choice=10**

- **Maine:** Stephens Memorial Hospital's Health Information Library (Western Maine Health, Norway), **http://www.wmhcc.org/Library/**

- **Manitoba, Canada:** Consumer & Patient Health Information Service (University of Manitoba Libraries), **http://www.umanitoba.ca/libraries/units/health/reference/chis.html**

- **Manitoba, Canada:** J.W. Crane Memorial Library (Deer Lodge Centre, Winnipeg), **http://www.deerlodge.mb.ca/crane_library/about.asp**

- **Maryland:** Health Information Center at the Wheaton Regional Library (Montgomery County, Dept. of Public Libraries, Wheaton Regional Library), **http://www.mont.lib.md.us/healthinfo/hic.asp**

- **Massachusetts:** Baystate Medical Center Library (Baystate Health System), **http://www.baystatehealth.com/1024/**

- **Massachusetts:** Boston University Medical Center Alumni Medical Library (Boston University Medical Center), **http://med-libwww.bu.edu/library/lib.html**

- **Massachusetts:** Lowell General Hospital Health Sciences Library (Lowell General Hospital, Lowell), **http://www.lowellgeneral.org/library/HomePageLinks/WWW.htm**

- **Massachusetts:** Paul E. Woodard Health Sciences Library (New England Baptist Hospital, Boston), **http://www.nebh.org/health_lib.asp**

- **Massachusetts:** St. Luke's Hospital Health Sciences Library (St. Luke's Hospital, Southcoast Health System, New Bedford), **http://www.southcoast.org/library/**

- **Massachusetts:** Treadwell Library Consumer Health Reference Center (Massachusetts General Hospital), **http://www.mgh.harvard.edu/library/chrcindex.html**

- **Massachusetts:** UMass HealthNet (University of Massachusetts Medical School, Worcester), **http://healthnet.umassmed.edu/**

- **Michigan:** Botsford General Hospital Library - Consumer Health (Botsford General Hospital, Library & Internet Services), **http://www.botsfordlibrary.org/consumer.htm**

- **Michigan:** Helen DeRoy Medical Library (Providence Hospital and Medical Centers), **http://www.providence-hospital.org/library/**

- **Michigan:** Marquette General Hospital - Consumer Health Library (Marquette General Hospital, Health Information Center), **http://www.mgh.org/center.html**

- **Michigan:** Patient Education Resouce Center - University of Michigan Cancer Center (University of Michigan Comprehensive Cancer Center, Ann Arbor), **http://www.cancer.med.umich.edu/learn/leares.htm**

- **Michigan:** Sladen Library & Center for Health Information Resources - Consumer Health Information (Detroit), **http://www.henryford.com/body.cfm?id=39330**

- **Montana:** Center for Health Information (St. Patrick Hospital and Health Sciences Center, Missoula)

- **National:** Consumer Health Library Directory (Medical Library Association, Consumer and Patient Health Information Section), **http://caphis.mlanet.org/directory/index.html**

- **National:** National Network of Libraries of Medicine (National Library of Medicine) - provides library services for health professionals in the United States who do not have access to a medical library, **http://nnlm.gov/**

- **National:** NN/LM List of Libraries Serving the Public (National Network of Libraries of Medicine), **http://nnlm.gov/members/**

- **Nevada:** Health Science Library, West Charleston Library (Las Vegas-Clark County Library District, Las Vegas), **http://www.lvccld.org/special_collections/medical/index.htm**

- **New Hampshire:** Dartmouth Biomedical Libraries (Dartmouth College Library, Hanover), **http://www.dartmouth.edu/~biomed/resources.htmld/conshealth.htmld**

- **New Jersey:** Consumer Health Library (Rahway Hospital, Rahway), **http://www.rahwayhospital.com/library.htm**

- **New Jersey:** Dr. Walter Phillips Health Sciences Library (Englewood Hospital and Medical Center, Englewood), **http://www.englewoodhospital.com/links/index.htm**

- **New Jersey:** Meland Foundation (Englewood Hospital and Medical Center, Englewood), **http://www.geocities.com/ResearchTriangle/9360/**

- **New York:** Choices in Health Information (New York Public Library) - NLM Consumer Pilot Project participant, **http://www.nypl.org/branch/health/links.html**

- **New York:** Health Information Center (Upstate Medical University, State University of New York, Syracuse), **http://www.upstate.edu/library/hic/**

- **New York:** Health Sciences Library (Long Island Jewish Medical Center, New Hyde Park), **http://www.lij.edu/library/library.html**

- **New York:** ViaHealth Medical Library (Rochester General Hospital), **http://www.nyam.org/library/**

- **Ohio:** Consumer Health Library (Akron General Medical Center, Medical & Consumer Health Library), **http://www.akrongeneral.org/hwlibrary.htm**

- **Oklahoma:** The Health Information Center at Saint Francis Hospital (Saint Francis Health System, Tulsa), **http://www.sfh-tulsa.com/services/healthinfo.asp**

- **Oregon:** Planetree Health Resource Center (Mid-Columbia Medical Center, The Dalles), **http://www.mcmc.net/phrc/**

- **Pennsylvania:** Community Health Information Library (Milton S. Hershey Medical Center, Hershey), **http://www.hmc.psu.edu/commhealth/**

- **Pennsylvania:** Community Health Resource Library (Geisinger Medical Center, Danville), **http://www.geisinger.edu/education/commlib.shtml**

- **Pennsylvania:** HealthInfo Library (Moses Taylor Hospital, Scranton), **http://www.mth.org/healthwellness.html**

- **Pennsylvania:** Hopwood Library (University of Pittsburgh, Health Sciences Library System, Pittsburgh), **http://www.hsls.pitt.edu/guides/chi/hopwood/index_html**

- **Pennsylvania:** Koop Community Health Information Center (College of Physicians of Philadelphia), **http://www.collphyphil.org/kooppg1.shtml**

- **Pennsylvania:** Learning Resources Center - Medical Library (Susquehanna Health System, Williamsport), **http://www.shscares.org/services/lrc/index.asp**

- **Pennsylvania:** Medical Library (UPMC Health System, Pittsburgh), **http://www.upmc.edu/passavant/library.htm**

- **Quebec, Canada:** Medical Library (Montreal General Hospital), **http://www.mghlib.mcgill.ca/**

- **South Dakota:** Rapid City Regional Hospital Medical Library (Rapid City Regional Hospital), **http://www.rcrh.org/Services/Library/Default.asp**

- **Texas:** Houston HealthWays (Houston Academy of Medicine-Texas Medical Center Library), **http://hhw.library.tmc.edu/**

- **Washington:** Community Health Library (Kittitas Valley Community Hospital), **http://www.kvch.com/**

- **Washington:** Southwest Washington Medical Center Library (Southwest Washington Medical Center, Vancouver), **http://www.swmedicalcenter.com/body.cfm?id=72**

APPENDIX D. MORE ON INFANT SLEEPING POSITION AND SIDS[47]

Overview

In 1992, the American Academy of Pediatrics released a statement recommending that all healthy infants be placed down for sleep on their backs (Pediatrics, 1992;89: 1120-1126). This recommendation was based on numerous reports that babies who sleep prone have a significantly increased likelihood of dying of sudden infant death syndrome (SIDS). The recommendation was reaffirmed in 1994 (Pediatrics, 1994;93:820). Health care professionals are encouraged to read both publications for a review of the evidence that led to the recommendation.

A national campaign (the "Back to Sleep" campaign) was launched in 1994 to promote supine positioning during sleep. Periodic surveys have confirmed that the prevalence of prone sleeping among infants in the United States has decreased from approximately 75% in 1992 to less than 25% in 1995. Provisional mortality statistics suggest that the death rate from SIDS has simultaneously decreased by over 25% -- by far the largest decrease in SIDS rates since such statistics have been compiled.

Questions and Answers about Infant Sleep Position and SIDS

Although the recommendation appears simple (most babies should be put to sleep on their backs), a variety of questions have arisen about the practicalities of implementation. The AAP Task Force on Infant Sleep

---

[47] Adapted from the National Institute of Child Health and Human Development (NICHD): http://www.nichd.nih.gov/sids/sids_qa.htm.

Position and SIDS has considered these questions and prepared the following responses. It should be emphasized, however, that for most of these questions there are not sufficient data to provide definitive answers.

Is the Side Position as Effective as the Back?

The vast majority of studies which showed a relationship between sleep position and SIDS examined whether babies were placed "prone" versus "non-prone" (i.e., side or back). However, a few recent reports indicate that the risk of SIDS is greater for babies placed on their sides versus those placed truly supine. There is some evidence that the reason for this difference is that babies placed on their sides have a higher likelihood of spontaneously turning to prone. However, both non-prone positions (side or back) are associated with a much lower risk of SIDS than is prone. If the side position is used, caretakers should be advised to bring the dependent arm forward, to lessen the likelihood of the baby rolling prone.

Are There Any Babies Who Should Be Placed Prone for Sleep?

In published studies, the vast majority of babies examined were born at term and had no known medical problems. Babies with certain disorders have been shown to have fewer problems when lying prone. These babies include:

- Infants with symptomatic gastro-esophageal reflux (reflux is usually less in the prone position).

- Babies with certain upper airway malformations such as Robin syndrome (there are fewer episodes of airway obstruction in the prone position).

There may also be other specific infants in whom the risk/benefit balance favors prone sleeping. The risk of SIDS increases from approximately 0.86 SIDS deaths per 1,000 live births to 1.62 when babies sleep prone* (that is, 998 of every 1,000 prone-sleeping babies will not die of SIDS). This relatively small increased risk may be reasonable to accept, when balanced against the benefit of prone sleeping for certain babies. Health professionals need to consider the potential benefit when taking into account each baby's circumstances.

If it is decided to allow a baby to sleep prone, special care should be taken to avoid overheating or use of soft bedding since these factors are particularly hazardous for prone-sleeping infants.

Should Healthy Babies Ever Be Placed Prone?

Since the initiation of the national campaign, some parents have misinterpreted the recommendation to say that babies should never be placed prone. This is incorrect. Developmental experts advise that prone positioning during the awake state is important for shoulder girdle motor development. Therefore, parents should be advised that a certain amount of "tummy time," when the baby is awake and observed, is good.

Which Sleeping Position Is Best for a Preterm Baby Who Is Ready for Discharge?

There have been studies showing that preterm babies who have active respiratory disease have improved oxygenation if they are prone. However, these babies have not been specifically examined as a group once they are recovered from respiratory problems and are ready for hospital discharge. There is no reason to believe that they should be treated any differently than a baby who was born at term. Unless there are specific indications to do otherwise (see exceptions above), the Task Force believes that such babies should be placed for sleep on their backs.

In What Position Should Babies Be for Sleep in Hospital Full-Term Nurseries?

Nearly all of the studies have been performed on babies who were beyond the neonatal period, mostly babies who were 2 to 6 months of age. However, experience in other countries has shown that mothers generally position their babies at home similar to the way they were placed in the hospital. Therefore, the Task Force recommends that personnel in hospital nurseries place babies in a supine position or on their sides. If there are concerns about possible aspiration in the immediate neonatal period, the baby may be placed on the side and propped against the side of the bassinet for stability.

If a Baby Doesn't Sleep Well in the Supine Position, Is It Okay to Turn Him or Her to a Prone Position?

Positional preference appears to be a learned behavior among infants from birth to 4 to 6 months of age. The infant, being placed in a back or side position in the newborn nursery, will become accustomed to this position.

If the parent finds that the infant has great difficulty going to sleep in the supine position, consider placing the infant prone and moving the infant to a back position when he or she is sleeping. Again, be sure to avoid overheating or use of soft bedding with such an infant.

At What Age Can You Stop Using the Back Position for Sleep?

We are unsure of the level of risk associated with prone positioning at specific ages during the first year of life, although there are some data that suggest that the greatest decrease in SIDS incidence in those countries that have changed to mostly non-prone sleeping has been seen in the younger aged infants (2 to 6 months). Therefore, the first 6 months, when babies are forming sleeping habits, are probably the most important time to focus on. Nevertheless, until more data suggest otherwise, it seems reasonable to continue to place babies down for sleep supine throughout infancy.

Do I Need to Check on a Baby Sleeping in a Non-Prone Position?

We recommend that parents do not keep checking on their baby after he or she is laid down to sleep. Although the infant's risk of SIDS could be increased slightly if he or she spontaneously assumes the prone position, the risk is not sufficient to outweigh the great disruption to the parents, and possibly to the infant, by frequent checking. Also, studies have shown that it is unusual for a baby who is placed in a supine position to roll into a prone position during early infancy.

How Should Hospitals Place Babies Down for Sleep after They Are Readmitted?

We recommend, as a general guideline, that hospitalized infants sleep in the same position that they have used at home, to minimize additional disruption to the infant. There may, however, be extenuating circumstances that would indicate preference for the prone position (e.g., an infant with significant upper airway obstruction).

Will Babies Aspirate on Their Backs?

While this has been a significant concern to health professionals and parents, there is no evidence that healthy babies are more likely to experience serious or fatal aspiration episodes when they are supine. In fact, in the majority of the very small number of reported cases of death due to aspiration, the infant's position at death, when known, was prone. In addition, indirect reassurance of the safety of the supine position for infants comes from the knowledge that this position has been standard in China, India, and other Asian countries for many years. Finally, in countries such as England, Australia, and New Zealand, where there has been a major change in infant sleeping position from predominantly prone to predominantly supine or side sleeping, there is no evidence of any increased number of serious or fatal episodes of aspiration of gastric contents.

Will Supine Sleeping Cause Flat Heads?

There is some suggestion that the incidence of babies developing a flat spot on their occiputs may have increased since the incidence of prone sleeping has decreased. This is almost always a benign condition, which will disappear within several months after the baby has begun to sit up. Flat spots can be avoided by altering the supine head position. Techniques for accomplishing this include turning the head to one side for a week or so and then changing to the other, reversing the head-to-toe axis in the crib, and changing the orientation of the baby to outside activity (e.g., the door of the room). "Positional plagiocephaly" seldom, if ever, requires surgery and is quite distinguishable from craniosynostosis.

Should Products Be Used to Keep Babies on Their Backs or Sides during Sleep?

Although various devices have been marketed to maintain babies in a non-prone position during sleep, the Task Force does not recommend their use. None of the studies that showed a reduction in risk when the prevalence of prone sleeping was reduced used devices. No studies examining the relative safety of the devices have been published.

Experience from sleep position campaigns overseas suggests that most infants can be stabilized in the side position by bringing the infant's dependent arm forward, at right angles to the body, with the infant's back propped against the side of the crib. There should be no need for additional support. Infants who sleep on their backs need no extra support.

Should Soft Surfaces Be Avoided?

Several studies indicate that soft sleeping surfaces increase the risk of SIDS in infants who sleep prone. How soft a surface must be to pose a threat is unknown. Until more information becomes available, a standard firm infant mattress with no more than a thin covering, such as a sheet or rubberized pad, between the infant and mattress is advised.

The US Consumer Product Safety Commission has also warned against placing any soft, plush, or bulky items, such as pillows, rolls of bedding, or cushions, in the baby's immediate sleeping environment. These items can potentially come into close contact with the infant's face, impeding ventilation or entrapping the infant's head and causing suffocation.

For information on sleep position and SIDS risk reduction, call the "Back to Sleep" campaign line: 1-800-505-CRIB.

ONLINE GLOSSARIES

The Internet provides access to a number of free-to-use medical dictionaries and glossaries. The National Library of Medicine has compiled the following list of online dictionaries:

- ADAM Medical Encyclopedia (A.D.A.M., Inc.), comprehensive medical reference: **http://www.nlm.nih.gov/medlineplus/encyclopedia.html**

- MedicineNet.com Medical Dictionary (MedicineNet, Inc.): **http://www.medterms.com/Script/Main/hp.asp**

- Merriam-Webster Medical Dictionary (Inteli-Health, Inc.): **http://www.intelihealth.com/IH/**

- Multilingual Glossary of Technical and Popular Medical Terms in Eight European Languages (European Commission) - Danish, Dutch, English, French, German, Italian, Portuguese, and Spanish: **http://allserv.rug.ac.be/~rvdstich/eugloss/welcome.html**

- On-line Medical Dictionary (CancerWEB): **http://www.graylab.ac.uk/omd/**

- Technology Glossary (National Library of Medicine) - Health Care Technology: **http://www.nlm.nih.gov/nichsr/ta101/ta10108.htm**

- Terms and Definitions (Office of Rare Diseases): **http://rarediseases.info.nih.gov/ord/glossary_a-e.html**

Beyond these, MEDLINEplus contains a very user-friendly encyclopedia covering every aspect of medicine (licensed from A.D.A.M., Inc.). The ADAM Medical Encyclopedia can be accessed via the following Web site address: **http://www.nlm.nih.gov/medlineplus/encyclopedia.html**. ADAM is also available on commercial Web sites such as Web MD (**http://my.webmd.com/adam/asset/adam_disease_articles/a_to_z/a**) and drkoop.com (**http://www.drkoop.com/**). Topics of interest can be researched by using keywords before continuing elsewhere, as these basic definitions and concepts will be useful in more advanced areas of research. You may choose to print various pages specifically relating to sudden infant death syndrome and keep them on file. The NIH, in particular, suggests that patients with sudden infant death syndrome visit the following Web sites in the ADAM Medical Encyclopedia:

- **Basic Guidelines for Sudden Infant Death Syndrome**

  SIDS
  Web site:
  http://www.nlm.nih.gov/medlineplus/ency/article/001566.htm

  Sudden infant death syndrome
  Web site:
  http://www.nlm.nih.gov/medlineplus/ency/article/001566.htm

- **Signs & Symptoms for Sudden Infant Death Syndrome**

  Apnea
  Web site:
  http://www.nlm.nih.gov/medlineplus/ency/article/003069.htm

- **Background Topics for Sudden Infant Death Syndrome**

  Aggravated by
  Web site:
  http://www.nlm.nih.gov/medlineplus/ency/article/002227.htm

  CPR
  Web site:
  http://www.nlm.nih.gov/medlineplus/ency/article/000010.htm

  Incidence
  Web site:
  http://www.nlm.nih.gov/medlineplus/ency/article/002387.htm

  Safety
  Web site:
  http://www.nlm.nih.gov/medlineplus/ency/article/001931.htm

  SIDS - support group
  Web site:
  http://www.nlm.nih.gov/medlineplus/ency/article/002202.htm

Online Dictionary Directories

The following are additional online directories compiled by the National Library of Medicine, including a number of specialized medical dictionaries and glossaries:

- Medical Dictionaries: Medical & Biological (World Health Organization):
  http://www.who.int/hlt/virtuallibrary/English/diction.htm#Medical

- MEL-Michigan Electronic Library List of Online Health and Medical Dictionaries (Michigan Electronic Library):
  http://mel.lib.mi.us/health/health-dictionaries.html

- Patient Education: Glossaries (DMOZ Open Directory Project):
  http://dmoz.org/Health/Education/Patient_Education/Glossaries/

- Web of Online Dictionaries (Bucknell University):
  http://www.yourdictionary.com/diction5.html#medicine

SUDDEN INFANT DEATH SYNDROME GLOSSARY

The following is a complete glossary of terms used in this sourcebook. The definitions are derived from official public sources including the National Institutes of Health [NIH] and the European Union [EU]. After this glossary, we list a number of additional hardbound and electronic glossaries and dictionaries that you may wish to consult.

Ablation: The removal of an organ by surgery. [NIH]

Airway: A device for securing unobstructed passage of air into and out of the lungs during general anesthesia. [NIH]

Alertness: A state of readiness to detect and respond to certain specified small changes occurring at random intervals in the environment. [NIH]

Alternans: Ipsilateral abducens palsy and facial paralysis and contralateral hemiplegia of the limbs, due to a nuclear or infranuclear lesion in the pons. [NIH]

Anchorage: In dentistry, points of retention of fillings and artificial restorations and appliances. [NIH]

Antagonism: Interference with, or inhibition of, the growth of a living organism by another living organism, due either to creation of unfavorable conditions (e. g. exhaustion of food supplies) or to production of a specific antibiotic substance (e. g. penicillin). [NIH]

Antibiotic: A substance usually produced by vegetal micro-organisms capable of inhibiting the growth of or killing bacteria. [NIH]

Antiserum: The blood serum obtained from an animal after it has been immunized with a particular antigen. It will contain antibodies which are specific for that antigen as well as antibodies specific for any other antigen with which the animal has previously been immunized. [NIH]

Apnea: Cessation of breathing. [NIH]

Applicability: A list of the commodities to which the candidate method can be applied as presented or with minor modifications. [NIH]

Attenuated: Strain with weakened or reduced virulence. [NIH]

Autoradiography: A process in which radioactive material within an object produces an image when it is in close proximity to a radiation sensitive emulsion. [NIH]

Bacterium: Microscopic organism which may have a spherical, rod-like, or spiral unicellular or non-cellular body. Bacteria usually reproduce through asexual processes. [NIH]

Berger: A binocular loupe with the lenses mounted at the anterior end of a light-excluding chamber fitting over the eyes and held in place by an elastic headband. [NIH]

Biophysics: The science of physical phenomena and processes in living organisms. [NIH]

Bowen: Intraepithelial epithelioma affecting the skin and sometimes the mucous membranes. [NIH]

Branch: Most commonly used for branches of nerves, but applied also to other structures. [NIH]

Bridge: A form of dental prosthesis which replaces one or more lost or missing teeth, being supported and held in position by attachments to adjacent teeth. [NIH]

CDNA: Synthetic DNA reverse transcribed from a specific RNA through the action of the enzyme reverse transcriptase. DNA synthesized by reverse transcriptase using RNA as a template. [NIH]

Clamp: A u-shaped steel rod used with a pin or wire for skeletal traction in the treatment of certain fractures. [NIH]

Clone: The term "clone" has acquired a new meaning. It is applied specifically to the bits of inserted foreign DNA in the hybrid molecules of the population. Each inserted segment originally resided in the DNA of a complex genome amid millions of other DNA segment. [NIH]

Compassionate: A process for providing experimental drugs to very sick patients who have no treatment options. [NIH]

Confounder: A factor of confusion which blurs a specific connection between a disease and a probable causal factor which is being studied. [NIH]

Consultation: A deliberation between two or more physicians concerning the diagnosis and the proper method of treatment in a case. [NIH]

Consumption: Pulmonary tuberculosis. [NIH]

Contraindications: Any factor or sign that it is unwise to pursue a certain kind of action or treatment, e. g. giving a general anesthetic to a person with pneumonia. [NIH]

Cyanide: An extremely toxic class of compounds that can be lethal on inhaling of ingesting in minute quantities. [NIH]

Density: The logarithm to the base 10 of the opacity of an exposed and processed film. [NIH]

Diaphragm: Contraceptive intra-uterine device. [NIH]

Discrimination: The act of qualitative and/or quantitative differentiation between two or more stimuli. [NIH]

Disparity: Failure of the two retinal images of an object to fall on corresponding retinal points. [NIH]

Duke: A lamp which produces ultraviolet radiations for certain ophthalmologic therapy. [NIH]

Dysostosis: Defective bone formation. [NIH]

EEG: A graphic recording of the changes in electrical potential associated with the activity of the cerebral cortex made with the electroencephalogram. [NIH]

Effector: It is often an enzyme that converts an inactive precursor molecule into an active second messenger. [NIH]

Efferent: Nerve fibers which conduct impulses from the central nervous system to muscles and glands. [NIH]

Electrode: Component of the pacing system which is at the distal end of the lead. It is the interface with living cardiac tissue across which the stimulus is transmitted. [NIH]

ELISA: A sensitive analytical technique in which an enzyme is complexed to an antigen or antibody. A substrate is then added which generates a color proportional to the amount of binding. This method can be adapted to a solid-phase technique. [NIH]

EMG: Recording of electrical activity or currents in a muscle. [NIH]

Endorphin: Opioid peptides derived from beta-lipotropin. Endorphin is the most potent naturally occurring analgesic agent. It is present in pituitary, brain, and peripheral tissues. [NIH]

Essential Tremor: A rhythmic, involuntary, purposeless, oscillating movement resulting from the alternate contraction and relaxation of opposing groups of muscles. [NIH]

Evoke: The electric response recorded from the cerebral cortex after stimulation of a peripheral sense organ. [NIH]

Excitatory: When cortical neurons are excited, their output increases and each new input they receive while they are still excited raises their output markedly. [NIH]

Fatigue: The feeling of weariness of mind and body. [NIH]

Fluoridation: The addition of fluorine usually as a fluoride to something, as the adding of a fluoride to drinking water or public water supplies for prevention of tooth decay in children. [NIH]

Generator: Any system incorporating a fixed parent radionuclide from which is produced a daughter radionuclide which is to be removed by elution or by any other method and used in a radiopharmaceutical. [NIH]

Genetics: The biological science that deals with the phenomena and mechanisms of heredity. [NIH]

Gestational: Psychosis attributable to or occurring during pregnancy. [NIH]

Glutamate: Excitatory neurotransmitter of the brain. [NIH]

Gould: Turning of the head downward in walking to bring the image of the ground on the functioning position of the retina, in destructive disease of the peripheral retina. [NIH]

Gravis: Eruption of watery blisters on the skin among those handling animals and animal products. [NIH]

Growth: The progressive development of a living being or part of an organism from its earliest stage to maturity. [NIH]

Habitat: An area considered in terms of its environment, particularly as this determines the type and quality of the vegetation the area can carry. [NIH]

Hemosiderin: Molecule which can bind large numbers of iron atoms. [NIH]

Hereditary: Of, relating to, or denoting factors that can be transmitted genetically from one generation to another. [NIH]

Heterogeneity: The property of one or more samples or populations which implies that they are not identical in respect of some or all of their parameters, e. g. heterogeneity of variance. [NIH]

Hospice: Institution dedicated to caring for the terminally ill. [NIH]

Hyperpnea: Increased ventilation in proportion to increased metabolism. [NIH]

Impairment: In the context of health experience, an impairment is any loss or abnormality of psychological, physiological, or anatomical structure or function. [NIH]

Infancy: The period of complete dependency prior to the acquisition of competence in walking, talking, and self-feeding. [NIH]

Infections: The illnesses caused by an organism that usually does not cause disease in a person with a normal immune system. [NIH]

Initiation: Mutation induced by a chemical reactive substance causing cell changes; being a step in a carcinogenic process. [NIH]

Insight: The capacity to understand one's own motives, to be aware of one's own psychodynamics, to appreciate the meaning of symbolic behavior. [NIH]

Involuntary: Reaction occurring without intention or volition. [NIH]

Ionizing: Radiation comprising charged particles, e. g. electrons, protons, alpha-particles, etc., having sufficient kinetic energy to produce ionization by collision. [NIH]

Jefferson: A fracture produced by a compressive downward force that is transmitted evenly through occipital condyles to superior articular surfaces of the lateral masses of C1. [NIH]

Joint: The point of contact between elements of an animal skeleton with the parts that surround and support it. [NIH]

Kainate: Glutamate receptor. [NIH]

Ligands: A RNA simulation method developed by the MIT. [NIH]

Linkage: The tendency of two or more genes in the same chromosome to remain together from one generation to the next more frequently than expected according to the law of independent assortment. [NIH]

Loop: A wire usually of platinum bent at one end into a small loop (usually 4 mm inside diameter) and used in transferring microorganisms. [NIH]

Mesencephalic: Ipsilateral oculomotor paralysis and contralateral tremor, spasm. or choreic movements of the face and limbs. [NIH]

Miscarriage: Spontaneous expulsion of the products of pregnancy before the middle of the second trimester. [NIH]

Modeling: A treatment procedure whereby the therapist presents the target behavior which the learner is to imitate and make part of his repertoire. [NIH]

Monitor: An apparatus which automatically records such physiological signs as respiration, pulse, and blood pressure in an anesthetized patient or one undergoing surgical or other procedures. [NIH]

Monogenic: A human disease caused by a mutation in a single gene. [NIH]

Monophosphate: So called second messenger for neurotransmitters and hormones. [NIH]

MRNA: The RNA molecule that conveys from the DNA the information that is to be translated into the structure of a particular polypeptide molecule. [NIH]

Mycotoxins: Toxins derived from bacteria or fungi. [NIH]

Need: A state of tension or dissatisfaction felt by an individual that impels him to action toward a goal he believes will satisfy the impulse. [NIH]

Nerve: A cordlike structure of nervous tissue that connects parts of the nervous system with other tissues of the body and conveys nervous impulses to, or away from, these tissues. [NIH]

Networks: Pertaining to a nerve or to the nerves, a meshlike structure of interlocking fibers or strands. [NIH]

Neurotrophins: A nerve growth factor. [NIH]

Niche: The ultimate unit of the habitat, i. e. the specific spot occupied by an individual organism; by extension, the more or less specialized relationships existing between an organism, individual or synusia(e), and its environment.

[NIH]

Nuclei: A body of specialized protoplasm found in nearly all cells and containing the chromosomes. [NIH]

Nucleus: A body of specialized protoplasm found in nearly all cells and containing the chromosomes. [NIH]

Otology: The branch of medicine which deals with the diagnosis and treatment of the disorders and diseases of the ear. [NIH]

Pacemakers: A center or a substance that controls the rhythm of a body process; the term usually refers to the cardiac pacemaker. [NIH]

Paralysis: Loss or impairment of muscle function or sensation. [NIH]

Patch: A piece of material used to cover or protect a wound, an injured part, etc.: a patch over the eye. [NIH]

Pathologies: The study of abnormality, especially the study of diseases. [NIH]

Pauling: The breath is passed through a cold trap consisting of a stainless-steel tube chilled by dry ice; the condensate is then assayed by gas chromatography and mass spectroscopy. [NIH]

Phenotypes: An organism as observed, i. e. as judged by its visually perceptible characters resulting from the interaction of its genotype with the environment. [NIH]

Physiology: The science that deals with the life processes and functions of organismus, their cells, tissues, and organs. [NIH]

Plasticity: In an individual or a population, the capacity for adaptation: a) through gene changes (genetic plasticity) or b) through internal physiological modifications in response to changes of environment (physiological plasticity). [NIH]

Polymorphism: The occurrence together of two or more distinct forms in the same population. [NIH]

Pontine: A brain region involved in the detection and processing of taste. [NIH]

Potassium: It is essential to the ability of muscle cells to contract. [NIH]

Potentiating: A degree of synergism which causes the exposure of the organism to a harmful substance to worsen a disease already contracted. [NIH]

Potentiation: An overall effect of two drugs taken together which is greater than the sum of the effects of each drug taken alone. [NIH]

Presumptive: A treatment based on an assumed diagnosis, prior to receiving confirmatory laboratory test results. [NIH]

Prion: Small proteinaceous infectious particles that resist inactivation by procedures modifying nucleic acids and contain an abnormal isoform of a cellular protein which is a major and necessary component. [NIH]

Probe: An instrument used in exploring cavities, or in the detection and dilatation of strictures, or in demonstrating the potency of channels; an elongated instrument for exploring or sounding body cavities. [NIH]

Prone: Having the front portion of the body downwards. [NIH]

Protocol: The detailed plan for a clinical trial that states the trial's rationale, purpose, drug or vaccine dosages, length of study, routes of administration, who may participate, and other aspects of trial design. [NIH]

Reassurance: A procedure in psychotherapy that seeks to give the client confidence in a favorable outcome. It makes use of suggestion, of the prestige of the therapist. [NIH]

Restoration: Broad term applied to any inlay, crown, bridge or complete denture which restores or replaces loss of teeth or oral tissues. [NIH]

Rett Syndrome: A neurological disorder seen almost exclusively in females, and found in a variety of racial and ethnic groups worldwide. [NIH]

Salivary: The duct that convey saliva to the mouth. [NIH]

Secretory: Secreting; relating to or influencing secretion or the secretions. [NIH]

Sensor: A device designed to respond to physical stimuli such as temperature, light, magnetism or movement and transmit resulting impulses for interpretation, recording, movement, or operating control. [NIH]

Serotypes: A cause of haemorrhagic septicaemia (in cattle, sheep and pigs), fowl cholera of birds, pasteurellosis of rabbits, and gangrenous mastitis of ewes. It is also commonly found in atrophic rhinitis of pigs. [NIH]

Specialist: In medicine, one who concentrates on 1 special branch of medical science. [NIH]

Sperm: The fecundating fluid of the male. [NIH]

Spike: The activation of synapses causes changes in the permeability of the dendritic membrane leading to changes in the membrane potential. This difference of the potential travels along the axon of the neuron and is called spike. [NIH]

Stillbirth: The birth of a dead fetus or baby. [NIH]

Stimulants: Any drug or agent which causes stimulation. [NIH]

Stimulus: That which can elicit or evoke action (response) in a muscle, nerve, gland or other excitable issue, or cause an augmenting action upon any function or metabolic process. [NIH]

Supine: Having the front portion of the body upwards. [NIH]

Synapse: The region where the processes of two neurons come into close contiguity, and the nervous impulse passes from one to the other; the fibers of the two are intermeshed, but, according to the general view, there is no direct contiguity. [NIH]

Talc: A native magnesium silicate. [NIH]

Temporal: One of the two irregular bones forming part of the lateral surfaces and base of the skull, and containing the organs of hearing. [NIH]

Therapeutics: The branch of medicine which is concerned with the treatment of diseases, palliative or curative. [NIH]

Thorax: A part of the trunk between the neck and the abdomen; the chest. [NIH]

Tractus: A part of some structure, usually that part along which something passes. [NIH]

Transduction: The transfer of genes from one cell to another by means of a viral (in the case of bacteria, a bacteriophage) vector or a vector which is similar to a virus particle (pseudovirion). [NIH]

Trauma: Any injury, wound, or shock, must frequently physical or structural shock, producing a disturbance. [NIH]

Trigeminal: Cranial nerve V. It is sensory for the eyeball, the conjunctiva, the eyebrow, the skin of face and scalp, the teeth, the mucous membranes in the mouth and nose, and is motor to the muscles of mastication. [NIH]

Tropism: Directed movements and orientations found in plants, such as the turning of the sunflower to face the sun. [NIH]

Tuberous Sclerosis: A rare congenital disease in which the essential pathology is the appearance of multiple tumors in the cerebrum and in other organs, such as the heart or kidneys. [NIH]

Unconscious: Experience which was once conscious, but was subsequently rejected, as the "personal unconscious". [NIH]

Valentine: The patient supine and the hips flexed by means of a double inclined plane: used in irrigating the urethra. [NIH]

Vector: Plasmid or other self-replicating DNA molecule that transfers DNA between cells in nature or in recombinant DNA technology. [NIH]

Venom: That produced by the poison glands of the mouth and injected by the fangs of poisonous snakes. [NIH]

Vertebrae: A bony unit of the segmented spinal column. [NIH]

Vitro: Descriptive of an event or enzyme reaction under experimental investigation occurring outside a living organism. Parts of an organism or microorganism are used together with artificial substrates and/or conditions. [NIH]

Vivo: Outside of or removed from the body of a living organism. [NIH]

Wound: Any interruption, by violence or by surgery, in the continuity of the external surface of the body or of the surface of any internal organ. [NIH]

General Dictionaries and Glossaries

While the above glossary is essentially complete, the dictionaries listed here cover virtually all aspects of medicine, from basic words and phrases to more advanced terms (sorted alphabetically by title; hyperlinks provide rankings, information and reviews at Amazon.com):

- **Dictionary of Medical Acronymns & Abbreviations** by Stanley Jablonski (Editor), Paperback, 4th edition (2001), Lippincott Williams & Wilkins Publishers, ISBN: 1560534605, http://www.amazon.com/exec/obidos/ASIN/1560534605/icongroupinterna

- **Dictionary of Medical Terms : For the Nonmedical Person (Dictionary of Medical Terms for the Nonmedical Person, Ed 4)** by Mikel A. Rothenberg, M.D, et al, Paperback - 544 pages, 4th edition (2000), Barrons Educational Series, ISBN: 0764112015, http://www.amazon.com/exec/obidos/ASIN/0764112015/icongroupinterna

- **A Dictionary of the History of Medicine** by A. Sebastian, CD-Rom edition (2001), CRC Press-Parthenon Publishers, ISBN: 185070368X, http://www.amazon.com/exec/obidos/ASIN/185070368X/icongroupinterna

- **Dorland's Illustrated Medical Dictionary (Standard Version)** by Dorland, et al, Hardcover - 2088 pages, 29th edition (2000), W B Saunders Co, ISBN: 0721662544, http://www.amazon.com/exec/obidos/ASIN/0721662544/icongroupinterna

- **Dorland's Electronic Medical Dictionary** by Dorland, et al, Software, 29th Book & CD-Rom edition (2000), Harcourt Health Sciences, ISBN: 0721694934, http://www.amazon.com/exec/obidos/ASIN/0721694934/icongroupinterna

- **Dorland's Pocket Medical Dictionary (Dorland's Pocket Medical Dictionary, 26th Ed)** Hardcover - 912 pages, 26th edition (2001), W B Saunders Co, ISBN: 0721682812, http://www.amazon.com/exec/obidos/ASIN/0721682812/icongroupinterna/103-4193558-7304618

- **Melloni's Illustrated Medical Dictionary (Melloni's Illustrated Medical Dictionary, 4th Ed)** by Melloni, Hardcover, 4th edition (2001), CRC Press-

Parthenon Publishers, ISBN: 85070094X,
http://www.amazon.com/exec/obidos/ASIN/85070094X/icongroupintern
a

- **Stedman's Electronic Medical Dictionary Version 5.0 (CD-ROM for Windows and Macintosh, Individual)** by Stedmans, CD-ROM edition (2000), Lippincott Williams & Wilkins Publishers, ISBN: 0781726328,
  http://www.amazon.com/exec/obidos/ASIN/0781726328/icongroupinter
  na

- **Stedman's Medical Dictionary** by Thomas Lathrop Stedman, Hardcover - 2098 pages, 27th edition (2000), Lippincott, Williams & Wilkins, ISBN: 068340007X,
  http://www.amazon.com/exec/obidos/ASIN/068340007X/icongroupinter
  na

- **Tabers Cyclopedic Medical Dictionary (Thumb Index)** by Donald Venes (Editor), et al, Hardcover - 2439 pages, 19th edition (2001), F A Davis Co, ISBN: 0803606540,
  http://www.amazon.com/exec/obidos/ASIN/0803606540/icongroupinter
  na

INDEX

LaVergne, TN USA
08 December 2009
166266LV00001B/43/A